Timothy J Watson • Paul JL Ong
James E Tcheng
Editors

Primary Angioplasty

A Practical Guide

Editors
Timothy J Watson
Department of Cardiology
HSC Medical Center
Kuala Lumpur
Malaysia

Faculty of Medicine and Health Sciences
University of Auckland
New Zealand

James E Tcheng
Department of Medicine
Duke University
Durham
North Carolina
USA

Paul JL Ong
Department of Cardiology
Tan Tock Seng Hospital
Singapore

https://doi.org/10.1007/978-981-13-1114-7

To our friends, colleagues, mentors who have worked tirelessly to develop and refine acute cardiac care. This work is dedicated to supporting ongoing growth and development of primary PCI as the most effective treatment for myocardial infarction.

Timothy J Watson, Paul JL Ong

To my wife and forever sweetheart Marianne, for her eternal patience and enduring love.

James E Tcheng

Preface

Management of acute myocardial infarction has dramatically evolved over the last 70 years. Advances in the understanding of the aetiologies of myocardial infarction coupled with development of the defibrillator, the introduction of the coronary care unit and the application of various pharmacological interventions that improved both survival and outcomes all represent significant milestones. Arguably though, the most important gains came from the appreciation that outcome is intimately related to the extent of myocardial injury, and that rapid reperfusion of the infarct-related artery offers striking benefits in terms of myocardial salvage and concomitant reductions in morbidity and mortality.

Early attempts at pharmacological reperfusion were unpredictable and were associated with an increased risk of bleeding—an inherent pitfall of the need for systemic fibrinolysis to achieve a focal effect (reperfusion of the occluded coronary artery). With the introduction of coronary angioplasty in 1977, a new treatment paradigm emerged—targeted therapy direct at the focal culprit lesion. Indeed, seminal trials of coronary angioplasty conducted just 15 years following the first procedure demonstrated superior outcomes with the angioplasty approach compared with systemic fibrinolytic therapy. Consequently, the use of coronary angioplasty to achieve reperfusion for acute myocardial infarction, termed primary percutaneous coronary intervention (primary PCI), has represented a major focus for provision of acute cardiac care over the last 15 years. With vastly improved outcomes and lower complication rates as compared with fibrinolytic therapy, primary PCI has evolved to become the gold standard treatment and is increasingly available not only in tertiary centres but also in smaller district hospitals, allowing rapid treatment upon first medical contact.

Adoption of primary PCI did not occur in isolation, but instead is best considered a component of a larger system of emergent healthcare. Partnerships between healthcare providers in the community, emergency department and cardiologists are required. Patient and community education programmes that emphasise early recognition and triage are also necessary. New funding streams for healthcare delivery must also be leveraged. In parallel, the medical device industry has driven rapid evolution in technology of the procedure itself improving outcomes and reducing risks.

Perhaps though, the most critical contribution to a successful primary PCI programme has been emergence of a shared passion for education and teaching within the cardiology community. Learning through our own successes and failures has provided an opportunity to reflect. Dedicated programmes such as the annual and hugely successful Asia Primary Angioplasty Congress offer important platforms to educate each other, and through such activity we have seen successful primary PCI programmes even in countries where healthcare resources are still limited.

This handbook is the result of our cumulative years of experience in the field of primary PCI. We have brought together some of the leading experts in the world and have aimed to make this handbook both practical and relevant to all those involved in delivering the benefit of primary PCI to our patients.

Kuala Lumpur, Malaysia — Timothy J Watson
Singapore, Singapore — Paul JL Ong
Durham, NC — James E Tcheng
April 2018

Acknowledgments

Publication of this book has been supported through an unrestricted educational grant provided by Medtronic Inc.

The Aesculap Academy (Singapore), the appointed secretariat of the Asia Primary Angioplasty Congress (http://www.apac.sg) provided administrative and legal support to editorial team.

Contents

About the Editors

Timothy J Watson is a board-certified interventional cardiologist with a keen interest in novel technologies and research. He qualified at the University of London and completed his internship and residency in various hospitals in London and across the West Midlands region. After becoming a member of the Royal College of Physicians of London, he joined a clinical research training programme where he led a study investigating mechanisms of blood clot formation in atrial fibrillation, a common irregular heartbeat which can increase the risk of stroke. For this work, he has been awarded a Doctor of Medicine (M.D.) degree from the University of Birmingham. Dr. Watson trained in general and interventional cardiology, primarily at Addenbrooke's and Papworth Hospitals in Cambridge. He has subsequently undertaken a fellowship in interventional and structural cardiology at the renowned Green Lane Cardiovascular Unit in Auckland, New Zealand, where he has been involved in various first-in-human studies using exciting and novel technologies, some of which are now being introduced into clinical mainstream practice. He has worked as a consultant (interventional) cardiologist in New Zealand, Malaysia and in Singapore. In addition to his work as a clinical cardiologist, he continues to undertake various research projects as an investigator and maintains active research collaborations with the University of Auckland.

Paul JL Ong graduated from the University of Cambridge. He has been a member of the Royal College of Physicians since 1996 and has been a fellow of Royal College of Physicians (FRCP) in London and fellow of the European Society of Cardiology (FESC) since 2008. He completed his early medical training in some of the most prestigious London teaching hospitals. Dr. Ong completed his cardiology specialist training in NW Thames, gaining dual accreditation in cardiology and general medicine. He was awarded the Certificate of Completion of Specialist Training (CCST) in both specialties in 2004. He was a NHS consultant interventional cardiologist and cath lab director at the Lister Hospital, Herts, and honorary consultant cardiologist at Royal Brompton and Harefield NHS Trust until 2008. He is currently a senior consultant and Head of the Interventional Cardiology service at the Department of Cardiology at Tan Tock Seng Hospital in Singapore. Dr. Ong has lectured and presented at numerous international meetings and has travelled to various parts of Asia to proctor and support new cardiac units. He is the organising chairman of the Asia Primary Angioplasty Congress and course co-director for Asia PCR and the Asian Champion for the Stent Save a Life initiative.

James E Tcheng, M.D. is a professor of medicine in the Department of Medicine (Cardiology division) and professor of community and family medicine in the Department of Community and Family Medicine at the Duke University School of Medicine, and also the Chief Medical Information Officer for the Duke Heart Network. Dr. Tcheng is a practicing interventional cardiologist and member of the faculty of the Duke Clinical Research Institute (DCRI) and the Duke Center for Health Informatics (DCHI). He is Director of the Duke Cardiovascular Databank and Director of Performance Improvement for the Duke Heart Center. He is faculty of the Medical Device Epidemiology Network (MDEpiNet) Coordinating Center of the DCRI. In addition, he is chair of the Informatics and Health IT Task Force of the American College of Cardiology, a member of the ACC National Cardiovascular Data Registry Management Board and the ACC/AHA Task Force on Clinical Data Standards. His clinical interests focus on the management of coronary artery disease, including percutaneous coronary intervention (angioplasty), stent implantation, laser angioplasty and the treatment of chronic total coronary occlusions. His clinical research has focused on antiplatelet and anticoagulant therapies for cardiovascular disease. Dr. Tcheng received his M.D. degree from the Johns Hopkins University School of Medicine in Baltimore, Maryland, and has completed his residency in medicine at Barnes Hospital/Washington University in St. Louis, Missouri. He completed his fellowship training in cardiology at Duke University and has been a member of the Duke faculty since 1988.

1 Historical Perspectives on Management of Acute Myocardial Infarction

Zhen Vin Lee and Bashir Hanif

1.1 Introduction

In 1977, the first successful coronary angioplasty was performed by Andreas Gruentzig using a double-lumen balloon catheter. This pivotal event spurred major advances in the field of percutaneous coronary intervention (PCI) over the subsequent four decades, including in the setting of myocardial infarction (MI) where primary PCI is now the established gold standard therapy. Nonetheless, although reperfusion is the cornerstone of management of acute MI, the role of various adjunctive therapies also needs to be recognized as these have had a substantial influence in improving both morbidity and mortality. This chapter serves to revisit the key historical milestones that have helped shape the modern management of acute MI.

1.2 Angina Pectoris as a Clinical Entity

In 1772, the eminent English physician, William Heberden, described what would later become known as angina pectoris in the most apt manner [1]:

'But there is a disorder of the breast marked with strong and peculiar symptoms, considerable for the kind of danger belonging to it, and not extremely rare, which deserves to be mentioned more at length. The seat of it, and sense of strangling, and anxiety with which it is attended, may make it not improperly be called angina pectoris. They who are afflicted with it, are seized while they are walking, (more especially if it be up hill, and soon after eating) with a painful and most disagreeable

Z.V. Lee (✉)
University Malaya Medical Centre, Kuala Lumpur, Malaysia
e-mail: zhenvin@ummc.edu.my

B. Hanif
Tabba Heart Institute, Karachi, Pakistan

T. J. Watson et al. (eds.), *Primary Angioplasty*,
https://doi.org/10.1007/978-981-13-1114-7_1

sensation in the breast, which seems as if it would extinguish life, if it were to increase or continue; but the moment they stand still, all this uneasiness vanishes...'

As early as 1850, Richard Quain published a comprehensive review on fatty diseases of the heart, describing an observed association between coronary artery sclerosis and myocardial scars. Subsequently, the theory of 'coagulation necrosis' was coined by Cohnheim, who wrote in 1882, that 'the occlusion of a coronary artery, in case it does not prove fatal, leads to the destruction of the contractile substance of that portion of the heart, which is fed by the affected artery, and afterwards to the formation of so-called myocarditic indurations' [2].

Later, advances in imaging technology would make it possible to objectively identify narrowing (sclerosis) of the coronary arteries and actively demonstrate the presence of myocardial ischaemia allowing correlation between symptoms of the various ischaemic heart disease syndromes and the underlying anatomic and physiologic abnormalities [2]. Thus was born our understanding that at least in simplistic terms, restriction of blood flow in the epicardial coronary arteries led to symptomatic onset of disease.

1.3 Development of the Electrocardiogram

Over the late 1800s to early 1900s, cardiology witnessed a great technological breakthrough that was to have a major effect on the understanding of arrhythmia: the electrocardiograph (ECG). Physiologist Augustus Desiré Waller working in St. Mary's Hospital, London, recorded the first human surface ECG using the Lippmann capillary electrometer to deflect a light beam (Fig. 1.1). Waller had learnt that 'each beat of the heart gives an electric charge, beginning at one end of the organ and ending at the other'. He was convinced that he could measure these electromotive events from the skin surface and proceeded to do so with the electrometer connected between the left and right hands or between the front and back paws of his dog. The clinical significance of the electrocardiogram was not appreciated at the time. Waller himself said: 'I do not imagine that electrocardiography is likely to find any very extensive use in the hospital. It can at most be of rare and occasional use to afford a record of some rare anomaly of cardiac action' [3].

Another physiologist, Willem Einthoven, shares the honour with Waller of having a pivotal role in founding this new diagnostic modality. Einthoven recorded the first human ECG in 1892 using the Lippmann capillary electrometer. He initially indicated the four observed deflections with the characters A, B, C and D but later instead adopted the middle characters of the alphabet: P, Q, R, S and T. In 1902, he made the first direct recording of the true human ECG using a modified string galvanometer (Fig. 1.2) [4]. Although there was wide scepticism by the contemporary scientific community against his methods, Einthoven continued publishing, in 1913 described the Einthoven triangle as the basis for calculations of ECGs and introduced the bipolar electrode system. Classic rhythms were obtained and published. In 1924, he was awarded the Nobel Prize for Physiology and Medicine for his pioneering work in developing the string galvanometer [3].

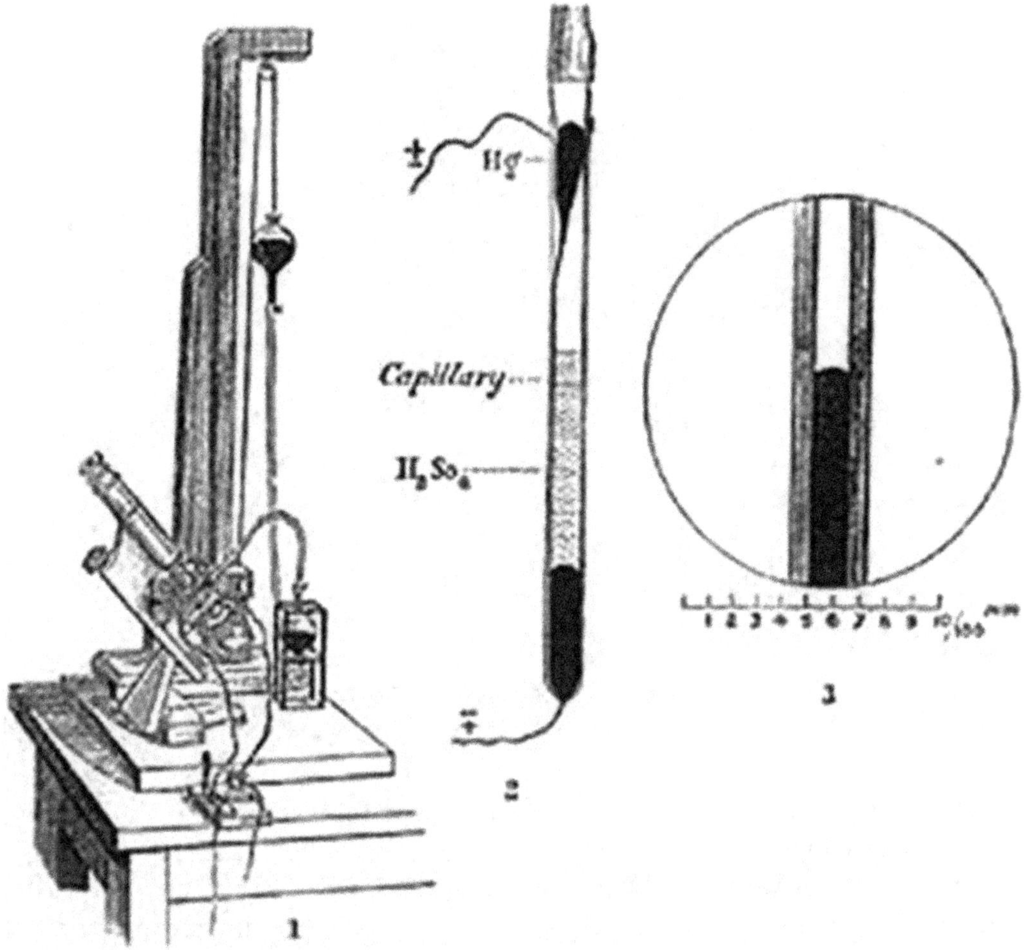

Fig. 1.1 Lippmann capillary electrometer (Source: Aquilina O. A brief history of cardiac pacing. *Images Pardiatr Cardiol.* 2006;8 (2): 17–81)

1.4 Evolving Concepts in Pathophysiology of Myocardial Infarction

Although, even in the nineteenth century, coronary thrombosis was recognized as a cause of death, it was predominantly regarded as a medical curiosity. On the basis of animal experiments involving ligation of a major coronary artery and of limited observations in human beings at necropsy, for many years the condition was considered to be immediately and universally fatal. However, in 1901, Krehl reported that coronary thrombosis did not always result in sudden death and that symptoms were more severe when arterial occlusion was sudden as opposed to progressive. He also recognized that MI may be complicated by ventricular aneurysm formation and myocardial rupture [4].

Once it became clear that survival from acute myocardial infarction (AMI) was possible, attention naturally began to be directed towards management. In his 1912 paper, Herrick stated that after AMI, 'the importance of absolute rest in bed for several days is clear'. This dictum would become the cornerstone of therapy for the

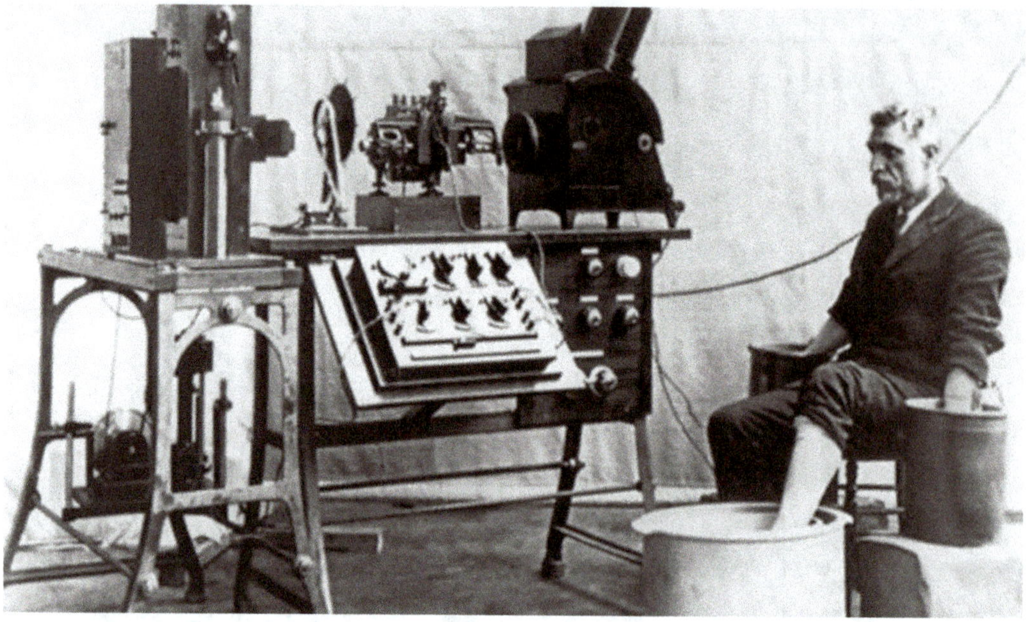

Fig. 1.2 ECG recording using a modified string galvanometer (Source: AlGhatrif M, Lindsay J. A brief review: history to understand fundamentals of electrocardiography. *Journal of Community Hospital Internal Medicine Perspectives*. 2012;2(1). Available from: doi:https://doi.org/10.3402/jchimp.v2i1.14383)

next half-century. Herrick also recognized that hope for restoration of the integrity of the damaged myocardium was possible where collateral blood supply developed. In the course of his work, Herrick also reported ECG findings consistent with acute MI, enabling the ECG to become a powerful diagnostic test in the recognition of this condition [4].

In the early 1920s, Wearn described the first significant series of patients with AMI, in all 19 of whom clinical-pathological correlations had been made. He recommended that 'every effort [be made] to spare the patient any bodily exertion' to prevent sudden death from cardiac rupture. In patients with pulmonary rales, fluid intake was restricted and digitalis given. Caffeine and camphor, two stimulants (vasopressors) then available, were used to prevent hypotension, syncope and heart block. Later that decade, Samuel Levine described a series of his own patients with acute MI. He identified the frequency of, and risk posed by, various cardiac arrhythmias. He recommended quinidine to treat ventricular tachycardia and intramuscular adrenaline to treat heart block and syncope [4].

By the 1930s and 1940s, as outcomes slowly started to improve, there was considerable debate about when in the course of the illness patients could be permitted to sit in a chair, use a commode, ambulate, be discharged from the hospital and ultimately resume their normal activities. In 1952, when Levine and Lown proposed the 'armchair treatment' of AMI, this suggestion, quite radical at the time, provoked heated debate. However, by the mid-twentieth century, it had become clear that although MI was now the most common cause of death in the industrialized world, concepts for post MI care needed to evolve. Cardiac rupture, although almost universally fatal, was relatively uncommon; absolute limitation of physical activity was not truly required; long-term bed rest might itself be associated with serious and occasionally fatal complications such as venous thromboembolism. As a consequence, practice gradually changed. Ambulation was accelerated and convalescence shortened; post-infarction rehabilitation made possible a more rapid return to regular lifestyle [4].

1.5 Cardiopulmonary Resuscitation and External Defibrillation

Coupled with advances in understanding of natural history of CAD and MI, Beck and colleagues in 1947 had resuscitated, by electric shock, a 14-year-old boy in whom ventricular fibrillation developed during surgery. Beck's group was also successful in correcting ventricular fibrillation, using open thoracotomy, in a 65-year-old physician with a myocardial infarction [5]. Soon after, Zoll introduced external defibrillation demonstrating that 'ventricular tachycardia and fibrillation' could be successfully terminated by externally applied electric countershock. This of course was not always successful, but it was recognized that early application of the shock was required to maximize efficacy and that cardiac monitoring provided opportunity for immediate recognition of cardiac arrest and identification of the arrhythmia [6]. A further advance observation was efficacy of mouth-to-mouth breathing, sternal compression and closed-chest electrical defibrillation in restoring normal cardiac function in some victims of ventricular fibrillation. It was this advance that triggered the interest in intensive care for myocardial infarction [7].

1.6 The Coronary Care Unit

The coronary care unit (CCU) is, perhaps, the single most important advancement in the treatment of MI and encompasses clinical application of four separate developments, namely, the appreciation of the importance of arrhythmias as the principal cause of early death in MI; ability to monitor the ECG continuously with the cathode-ray oscilloscope; development of closed-chest cardiac resuscitation; and delegation of the treatment of life-threatening arrhythmias, particularly ventricular fibrillation, to trained nurses in the absence of physicians [4].

Desmond Julian of the Royal Infirmary of Edinburgh is largely credited as the pioneer in the development of the CCU and wrote in his 1961 that 'Many cases of cardiac arrest associated with acute myocardial ischaemia could be treated successfully if all medical, nursing and auxiliary staff were trained in closed chest cardiac massage and if the cardiac rhythm of patients with MI were monitored by an ECG linked to an alarm system… Such units should be staffed by suitably experienced people throughout the 24 hours' [8]. Julian's colleagues in Edinburgh were unenthusiastic about his concept, and subsequently he moved to Australia where he launched a programme of continuous monitoring of patients who presented to Sydney Hospital with MI [9]. The first presentation of coronary care given to the British Cardiovascular Society was at the Autumn Meeting in 1964 when the Sydney experience was described [10].

It was clearly apparent that the new treatment technologies had to be used immediately to save lives. To achieve this goal, doctors had to abandon traditional notions of a nurse's limited role in clinical decision-making and transition to a system where the CCU nurse was able to implement therapeutic measures by herself *without* specific orders, including sometimes the definitive treatment for ventricular fibrillation. The CCU-inspired empowerment of nurses represented a critical first step in the evolution of team-based care that is such a conspicuous part of current-day cardiology practice [9].

With improving survival from MI, Myocardial Infarction Research Units (MIRU) were created in the United States, and a large programme of research was initiated into the investigation of the haemodynamic effects of myocardial infarction. It was quickly shown that the commonly used right atrial and central venous pressures provided an unreliable index of left-sided function. The introduction of the Swan-Ganz flow-guided catheter was a major advancement in the evaluation of cardiac performance in the CCU, allowed more precise delineation of the various haemodynamic subsets of patients with MI and facilitated their more rational treatment [10].

1.7 Concept of Reduction of Infarct Size

Left ventricular function emerged as a critical factor in the outcome in patients who were nursed in the CCU and in whom fatal primary arrhythmias were prevented. Infarct size became recognized as the major determinant of mortality and morbidity, and the concept was put forwards that even after the onset of infarction the quantity of damaged myocardium could be influenced by interventions designed to improve the balance between oxygen supply and demand in the jeopardized zone [4]. Preservation of left ventricular function became the major predictive factor of prognosis. The size of the infarct was then defined as the major determinant of mortality and morbidity. The use of injectable and oral beta blockers not only to treat arrhythmias but also to limit myocardial damage induced by the ischemic area arose as a therapeutic possibility. These drugs reduce oxygen consumption by the myocardium and enhance blood redistribution from the epicardium to the myocardium, diminishing the area of infarct and increasing survival [11].

1.8 Advent of Thrombolysis and Role of Aspirin

In the 1950s and 1960s, Fletcher and Verstraete pioneered the experimental use of streptokinase for thrombolysis. By the 1970s, Chazov and Rentrop were driving what would become a revolution in cardiology, demonstrating that intracoronary infusion of streptokinase could dissolve intracoronary thrombi, thereby limiting the infarct extension and size. This work was corroborated by the studies of De Wood et al. according to which 90% of patients with clinical findings of infarction and alterations in the ST segment had occlusive thrombi in the coronary arteries. The need for a direct intracoronary injection, however, was the major obstacle to its use. Intravenous infusion, which was easier and faster, quickly proved to be equivalent to the intracoronary infusion [11].

The ISIS-2 trial represented a significant milestone in rapid treatment of AMI with streptokinase and aspirin. This trial demonstrated that streptokinase and aspirin alone each produced a significant reduction in 5-week vascular mortality. The combination of streptokinase and aspirin was synergistic and markedly better than either treatment alone. The differences in vascular and in all-cause mortality produced by streptokinase and aspirin remained highly significant, even after a median of 15 months of follow-up [12]. This trial was followed by the GISSI study, which again proved the benefits of streptokinase and indicated that earlier treatment led to greater benefit [13].

Streptokinase though was known to have limitations, including propensity to induce hypotension, high rates of allergy, prolonged anticoagulant effect and development of neutralizing antibodies. It was clear that more efficacious and safer agents were needed. This paved the way for the GUSTO trial series which led to the introduction of differing thrombolytic regimens including the use of accelerated tissue plasminogen activator (t-PA) with intravenous heparin. Although bleeding remained a concern, accelerated t-PA given with intravenous heparin seemed to confer a survival benefit [14, 15]. As agents were further refined, recombinant tissue-type plasminogen activator (rt-PA) was introduced and showed a significantly reduced 1-month mortality in a cohort of patients with suspected AMI who were randomized to receive either rt-PA plus heparin or placebo plus heparin. Whilst there was an excess of bleeding complications in the rt-PA group of patients, the incidence of stroke was similar [16]. The introduction of single-bolus injection of tenecteplase (a genetically engineered variant of alteplase with slower plasma clearance) would facilitate more rapid treatment of AMI both in hospital and in the community setting [17].

These results together with the low incidence of severe adverse effects made the use of thrombolytic agents unquestionable in the first hours of AMI. In addition to significantly reducing mortality, thrombolytic agents protect against associated morbid events, such as cardiogenic shock and heart failure, in a direct relation to the speed with which they are administered. In regard to adverse effects, thrombolytic therapy is related to a small and significant increase in the occurrence of cerebral strokes [11].

1.9 Coronary Angiography and Percutaneous Revascularization

Accurate depictions of the epicardial coronary arteries are present in the historical works of Leonardo da Vinci and Andreas Vesalius; however, smaller intramural branches were difficult to be demonstrated by simple dissection. Later, post-mortem injection techniques facilitated in-depth study of coronary circulation [18].

With the discovery of X-rays in 1895 by Wilhelm Röntgen, a new approach to the study of cardiac anatomy would, with time, become possible. These experiments were made possible by development of a technique for human right heart catheterization by the German physician Werner Forssmann who undertook catheterization of his own heart in 1929. Forssmann soon extended his experiments to include the intracardiac injection of contrast material. Forssmann's contributions together with the development of nontoxic contrast materials and steady advances in X-ray equipment and technique set the stage for the development of cardiac angiography and subsequently coronary arteriography [18].

In the 1950s, Mason Sones developed more selective coronary imaging. Whilst performing aortographic examinations in patients with rheumatic valvular disease, Sones discovered that some injections would preferentially fill one coronary artery and that this caused no apparent harm to the patient. After his studies of semi-selective coronary arteriography, Sones began to perform true selective coronary arteriography in 1958. Sones combined anatomic and physiologic considerations in developing his method of selective coronary arteriography and designed a preformed catheter with a tapered tip permitted selective entry into the coronary ostia but avoided complete obstruction of the coronary artery—an event much feared by earlier physicians who were not using tapered catheters. Furthermore, Sones introduced continual pressure monitoring combined with fluoroscopy to alert the operator to inadvertent complete obstruction of the coronary artery [18].

This has paved the way for the progressive advancement and modernization in the field of coronary angiography and angioplasty. Diagnostic catheters, guiding catheters, coronary guidewires, balloon catheters and coronary stents were invented and upgraded. Techniques of PCI were invented, modified and improved upon, details of which will be further elaborated in subsequent chapters of this handbook.

1.10 Progress of Adjunctive Pharmacotherapy

1.10.1 Beta Blockade

In 1984, the International Collaborative Study Group reported the benefits of timolol. Given as a bolus followed by oral maintenance, this agent was shown to reduce myocardial ischaemia and infarct size as measured by an accelerated reduction of ST-vector magnitude, a significant reduction of maximal cumulative creatine kinase release and significantly smaller changes in QRS-vector variables. Timolol was also associated with significant reductions in pain and was well tolerated overall [19]. Further studies demonstrated efficacy for other beta blockers, notably metoprolol and atenolol, which proved to be even more effective with markedly improved longer-term outcomes through to 1 year [20, 21].

1.10.2 ACE Inhibitors

The role of angiotensin converting enzyme (ACE) inhibitors was established in a number of studies. The AIRE study found that ramipril resulted in a significant reduction in all-cause mortality as well as a significant reduction in the first validated outcome, namely, death, severe or resistant heart failure, MI or stroke in patients with clinical heart failure. These benefits were seen as early as 30 days [22] . Similarly, administration of captopril after AMI was shown to attenuate the process of progressive ventricular enlargement and was able to confer improvement in left ventricular (LV) systolic function in those patients where LV dysfunction was most marked [23, 24]. Later, the HOPE study would report that ramipril significantly reduced the rates of death, myocardial infarction and stroke in a broad range of high-risk patients who were not known to have a low ejection fraction or heart failure [25].

1.10.3 HMG Co-A Reductase Inhibitors

The 4S trial reported that in stable patients with angina or previous MI with elevated serum cholesterol, on a lipid-lowering diet, simvastatin significantly improved survival and reduced the risk of undergoing myocardial revascularization procedures and established the role of statins in management of coronary artery disease (CAD) [26]. Subsequent studies indicated similar advantage from other statins, even where serum cholesterol levels were in the normal or low range [27–29]. Later data would emerge indicating that early administration of statin may offer advantage in the early phase after onset of AMI.

1.10.4 Thienopyridines

Aggregating platelets have long been suspected of having an important role in the development of coronary thrombi, but it remained for the ISIS-2 trial to show unequivocally the enormous effectiveness of aspirin which is a simple, well-tolerated and inexpensive drug in reducing mortality in AMI [4].

The CAPRIE trial randomized 19,185 patients with atherosclerotic vascular disease manifested as either recent ischaemic stroke, recent MI or symptomatic peripheral arterial disease to either clopidogrel at dose of 75 mg once daily or aspirin at dose of 325 mg once daily. The authors reported that clopidogrel is more effective than aspirin in reducing the combined risk of ischaemic stroke, MI or vascular death and the overall safety profile of clopidogrel is at least as good as that of medium-dose aspirin [30].

In the PLATO trial, 18,624 patients who were admitted with an acute coronary syndrome (ACS), with or without ST-segment elevation, were randomized to receive either clopidogrel or ticagrelor, which is an oral, reversible, direct-acting inhibitor of the adenosine diphosphate receptor, P2Y12, that has a more rapid onset and more pronounced platelet inhibition than clopidogrel. Ticagrelor was found in the trial to have significantly reduced the rate of death from vascular causes, MI or stroke without an increase in the rate of overall major bleeding but with an increase in the rate of non-procedure-related bleeding compared to clopidogrel [31] .

In the TRITON-TIMI 38 trial, 13,608 patients with moderate- to high-risk ACS with scheduled PCI were randomized to receive a new thienopyridine and prasugrel or to receive clopidogrel. It was found that prasugrel therapy was associated with significantly reduced rates of ischemic events, including stent thrombosis, but with an increased risk of major bleeding, including fatal bleeding. Overall mortality did not differ significantly between treatment groups [32].

1.10.5 Glycoprotein IIb/IIIa Inhibitors

The EPIC trial randomized 2099 patients who were scheduled to undergo coronary angioplasty or atherectomy in high-risk clinical situations such as severe unstable angina, evolving AMI or high-risk coronary morphologic characteristics to either a bolus and an infusion of placebo, a bolus of a chimeric monoclonal-antibody Fab fragment (c7E3 Fab) directed against the platelet glycoprotein IIb/IIIa receptor and an infusion of placebo or a bolus and an infusion of c7E3 Fab. The investigators concluded that ischemic complications of coronary angioplasty and atherectomy were reduced with the usage of c7E3 Fab, although the bleeding complications were increased [33].

The RAPPORT trial demonstrated that in a cohort of patients suffering from AMI of less than 12 h duration, who underwent primary percutaneous transluminal coronary angioplasty (PTCA), administration of abciximab resulted in a significant reduction in the incidence of death, reinfarction or urgent target vessel revascularization at 30 days compared to placebo albeit at a cost of higher bleeding rates. The 6-month primary end point however was the same for both treatment groups [34].

The EPILOG trial on the contrary was terminated early as abciximab, together with both low-dose and standard-dose heparin, significantly reduced the risk of acute ischemic complications compared to placebo and standard-dose heparin in 2792 patients who underwent either urgent or elective percutaneous coronary revascularization [35].

Conclusion

The last 120 years have witnessed considerable progress in our understanding and management of CAD and MI. Modern treatment algorithms have encompassed and refined techniques to achieve rapid reperfusion and salvage-threatened myocardium and enhance prospects for patient stability and recovery.

References

1. Classics in cardiology: description of angina pectoris by William Heberden. Heart Views 2006;7:118–9.
2. Chopra HK, Nanda NC. Textbook of cardiology (a clinical & historical perspective). New Delhi: Jaypee Brothers Medical Pub; 2013.
3. Aquilina O. A brief history of cardiac pacing. Images Pardiatr Cardiol. 2006;8(2):17–81.
4. Braunwald E. Evolution of the management of acute myocardial infarction: a 20th century saga. Lancet. 1998;352:1771–4. https://doi.org/10.1016/S0140-6736(98)03212-7.
5. Beck CF, Weckesser EC, Barry FM. Fatal heart attack and successful defibrillation: new concepts in coronary artery disease. JAMA. 1956;161:434–6. https://doi.org/10.1001/jama.1956.62970050001008.
6. Zoll PM, Linenthal AJ, Zarsky LRN. Ventricular fibrillation—treatment and prevention by external electric currents. N Engl J Med. 1960;262:105–12. https://doi.org/10.1056/NEJM196001212620301.
7. Julian DG. The evolution of the coronary care unit. Cardiovasc Res. 2001;51(4):621–4. https://doi.org/10.1016/S0008-6363(01)00365-0.
8. Julian DG. Treatment of cardiac arrest in acute myocardial ischaemia and infarction. Lancet. 1961;2:840–4.
9. Fye WB. Resuscitating a circulation abstract to celebrate 50th anniversary of the coronary care unit concept. Circulation. 2011;124:1886–93. https://doi.org/10.1161/CIRCULATIONAHA.111.033597.
10. Julian DG. The history of coronary care units. Br Heart J. 1987;57(6):497–502.
11. Sarmento-Leite R, Krepsky AM, Gottschall CAM. Acute myocardial infarction. One century of history. Arq Bras Cardiol. 2001;77:602–10. https://doi.org/10.1590/S0066-782X2001001200011.
12. ISIS-2 Collaborative Group. Randomized trial of intravenous streptokinase, oral aspirin, both, or neither among 17187 cases of suspected acute myocardial infarction: ISIS-2. Lancet. 1988;2:349–60.
13. Gruppo Italiano per lo Studio Della Streptochinasi Nell' Infarto Miocardico (GISSI). Effectiveness of intravenous thrombolytic treatment in acute myocardial infarction. Lancet. 1986;327:397–402. https://doi.org/10.1016/S0140-6736(86)92368-8.
14. The GUSTO investigators. An international randomized trial comparing four thrombolytic strategies for acute myocardial infarction. The GUSTO trial. N Engl J Med. 1993;329:673–80. https://doi.org/10.1056/NEJM199309023291001.
15. The Global Use of Strategies to Open Occluded Coronary Arteries (GUSTO III) Investigators. A comparison of reteplase with alteplase for acute myocardial infarction. N Engl J Med. 1997;337:1118–23. https://doi.org/10.1056/NEJM199710163371603.
16. Anglo-Scandinavian Study of Early Thrombolysis (ASSET). Trial of tissue plasminogen activator for mortality reduction in acute myocardial infarction. Lancet. 1988;2:525–30.
17. Assessment of the Safety and Efficacy of a New Thrombolytic (ASSENT-2) Investigators. Single-bolus tenecteplase compared with front-loaded alteplase in acute myocardial infarction: the ASSENT-2 double-blind randomised trial. Lancet. 1999;354:716–22.
18. Fye WB. Coronary arteriography-it took a long time! Circulation. 1984;70:781–7. https://doi.org/10.1161/01.CIR.70.5.781.
19. The International Collaborative Study Group. Reduction of infarct size with the early use of timolol in acute myocardial infarction. N Engl J Med. 1984;310:9–15. https://doi.org/10.1056/NEJM198401053100103.
20. The MIAMI Trial Research Group. Metoprolol in acute myocardial infarction (MIAMI). A randomized placebo controlled international trial. Eur Heart J. 1985;6:199–226. https://doi.org/10.1093/oxfordjournals.eurheartj.a061845.

21. ISIS-1 (First International Study of Infarct Survival) Collaborative Group. Randomized trial of intravenous atenolol among 16 027 cases of suspected acute myocardial infarction. Lancet. 1986;2:57–65.
22. The Acute Infarction Ramipril Efficacy (AIRE) Study Investigators. Effect of ramipril on mortality and morbidity of survivors of acute myocardial infarction with clinical evidence of heart failure. Lancet. 1993;342:821–8.
23. Pfeffer MA, Lamas GA, Vaughan DE, et al. Effect of captopril on progressive ventricular dilatation after anterior myocardial infarction. N Engl J Med. 1988;319:80–6. https://doi.org/10.1056/NEJM198807143190204.
24. Sharpe N, Smith H, Murphy J, et al. Early prevention of left ventricular dysfunction after myocardial infarction with angiotensin-converting enzyme inhibition. Lancet. 1991;337:872–6.
25. The Heart Outcomes Prevention Evaluation (HOPE) Study Investigators. Effects of an angiotensin-converting-enzyme inhibitor, ramipril, on cardiovascular events in high-risk patients. N Engl J Med. 2000;342:145–53. https://doi.org/10.1056/NEJM200001203420301.
26. Pedersen TR, Kjekshus J, Berg K, et al. Randomized trial of cholesterol lowering in 4444 patients with coronary heart disease: the Scandinavian simvastatin survival study (4S). Lancet. 1994;344:1383–9.
27. Sacks FM, Pfeffer MA, Moye LA, et al. The effect of pravastatin on coronary events after myocardial infarction in patients with average cholesterol levels. The cholesterol and recurrent events trial (CARE). N Engl J Med. 1996;335:1001–9. https://doi.org/10.1056/NEJM199610033351401.
28. The Long-Term Intervention with Pravastatin in Ischemic Disease (LIPID) Study Group. Prevention of cardiovascular events and death with pravastatin in patients with coronary heart disease and a broad range of initial cholesterol levels. N Engl J Med. 1998;339:1349–57. https://doi.org/10.1056/NEJM199811053391902.
29. Bybee KA, Lee JH, O'Keefe JH. Cumulative clinical trial data on atorvastatin for reducing cardiovascular events: the clinical impact of atorvastatin. Curr Med Res Opin. 2008;24:1217–29. https://doi.org/10.1185/030079908X292001.
30. CAPRIE Investigators. A randomized, blinded trial of clopidogrel versus aspirin in patients at risk of ischaemic events (CAPRIE). Lancet. 1996;348:1329–39.
31. Wallentin L, Becker RC, Budaj A, for the PLATO Investigators, et al. Ticagrelor versus clopidogrel in patients with acute coronary syndromes. N Engl J Med. 2009;361:1045–57. https://doi.org/10.1056/NEJMoa0904327.
32. Wiviott SD, Braunwald E, McCabe CH, for the TRITON-TIMI 38 Investigators, et al. Prasugrel versus clopidogrel in patients with acute coronary syndromes. N Engl J Med. 2007;357:2001–15. https://doi.org/10.1056/NEJMoa0706482.
33. The EPIC Investigators. Use of a monoclonal antibody directed against the platelet glycoprotein IIb/IIIa receptor in high-risk coronary angioplasty. N Engl J Med. 1994;330:956–61. https://doi.org/10.1056/NEJM199404073301402.
34. Brener SJ, Barr LA. Burchenal JEB, et al. on behalf of the ReoPro and primary PTCA organization and randomized trial (RAPPORT) investigators. Randomized, placebo-controlled trial of platelet glycoprotein IIb/IIIa blockade with primary angioplasty for acute myocardial infarction. Circulation. 1998;98:734–41.
35. The EPILOG Investigators. Platelet glycoprotein IIb/IIIa receptor blockade and low-dose heparin during percutaneous coronary revascularization. N Engl J Med. 1997;336:1689–96. https://doi.org/10.1056/NEJM199706123362401.

Prehospital Diagnosis and Management of Acute Myocardial Infarction

2

Adam J. Brown, Francis J. Ha, Michael Michail, and Nick E. J. West

2.1 Introduction

The outcomes of patients suffering from acute myocardial infarction are contingent on the time taken to deliver definitive treatment. Evidence has shown that the extent of myocardial salvage is greatest if patients are reperfused in the first 3 h from the onset of symptoms [1]. For every 30-min delay in coronary reperfusion, the relative 1-year mortality rate increases by 7.5% [2]. This has driven physicians and policy-makers to popularize phrases such as ‘time is myocardium’ and concepts such as ‘door-to-balloon’ time—the latter representing the time to reperfusion with an intra-coronary device from the arrival of the patient at hospital (Fig. 2.1). The biggest delays and challenges in reducing the time to reperfusion, however, are in fact mostly seen in the prehospital setting. This consists of the time from the onset of symptoms to first medical contact (FMC) and subsequently the time from FMC to diagnosis and then reperfusion treatment—termed ‘system delay’. Patient delay may be multifactorial and depends on a host of issues including socioeconomic factors and access to healthcare. The rapid patient assessment and field diagnosis of myocardial infarction has become a crucial factor in time to reperfusion as it dictates the decision on the most appropriate form of reperfusion treatment accounting for geographical factors and available facilities. Importantly, the prehospital role in

A. J. Brown (✉) · F. J. Ha · M. Michail
MonashHeart, Monash Health and Monash Cardiovascular Research Centre, Monash University, Clayton, VIC, Australia

Department of Interventional Cardiology, Papworth Hospital, Cambridge, UK
e-mail: ajdbrown@me.com

N. E. J. West
Department of Interventional Cardiology, Papworth Hospital, Cambridge, UK

T. J. Watson et al. (eds.), *Primary Angioplasty*,
https://doi.org/10.1007/978-981-13-1114-7_2

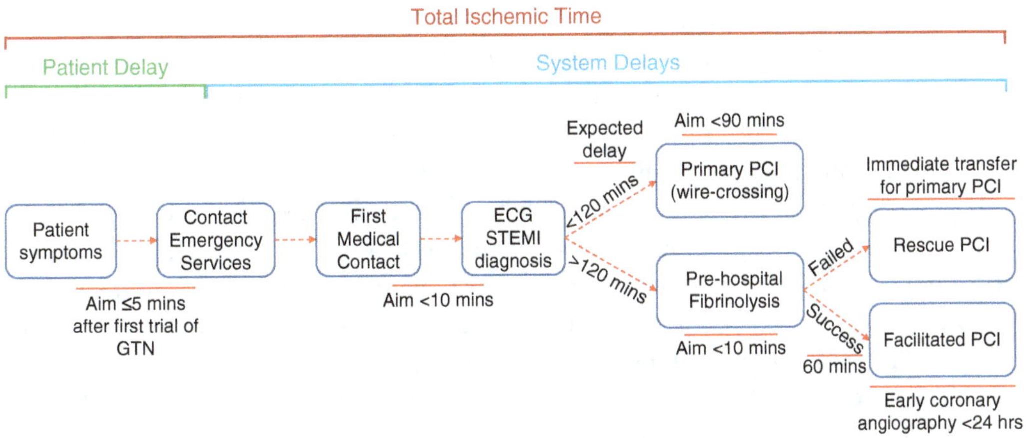

Fig. 2.1 The key components of symptom to revascularization time indicating recommended timing for optimal outcomes. Note that optimization of each component offers an opportunity to minimize total ischaemic time

the management of acute myocardial infarction also involves the initiation of therapy, the upstream of the hospital-delivered treatment. This commonly involves the administration of antiplatelet and anticoagulant therapy in metropolitan areas, while in remote areas where patients cannot be transferred to hospital facilities in a reasonable time, there are policies in place for administration of field thrombolytic agents. Other aspects of the management may involve intravenous access or, indeed in the cases of cardiac arrest, cardiopulmonary resuscitation. In this chapter we will discuss the management of patients presenting with acute myocardial infarction, in the crucial period ahead of their arrival at the heart attack centre.

2.2 Activation of Emergency Services

2.2.1 The Call for Help

The diagnosis and treatment of acute myocardial infarction (MI) in the community is dependent on the recognition of clinical symptoms. Awareness of potential warning signs is largely dependent on the patient, yet it is not uncommon for patients to wait 2 h or more after symptom onset before contacting emergency medical services (EMS) [3]. Reasons for delayed presentation include perception of the 'Hollywood heart attack' (despite up to one-third of patients presenting without angina), differing symptoms compared with previous experiences in patients with known ischaemic heart disease, fear of embarrassment or troubling others and persistent attempts at self-medication. Thus, community awareness and patient education remain a cornerstone of early diagnosis. Public health initiatives encompass identification of key warning signs such as chest discomfort radiating to relevant areas, light headedness or dyspnoea, as well as advocacy of contacting EMS within 5 min of symptom onset. Furthermore, targeted health campaigns towards higher-risk individuals such as those with relevant cardiovascular comorbidities, alongside their families, are a fundamental aspect of primary and secondary prevention. However, systemic factors such as access to EMS, provision of health insurance and socioeconomic background also influence the time to presentation, and policy-makers hold a substantial role in determining patient outcomes.

Following symptom recognition, prompt contact with EMS is necessary. Where previously prescribed, patients may be given a trial of nitroglycerine; however, the worsening or persistence of symptoms (usually beyond 5 min after administration) is indicative of non-response and mandates EMS contact. There is also the risk of systemic hypotension after repeated nitroglycerin administration which may precipitate cardiogenic shock in the context of acute myocardial infarction. Private transportation as opposed to EMS transfer is unsafe given the risk of cardiac arrest in the absence of any trained medical support. Other benefits of prompt EMS contact include the opportunity to perform an ECG leading to earlier diagnosis, subsequent assessment of timely transfer to primary PCI centre and early fibrinolytic therapy by adequately trained healthcare providers.

2.2.2 First Medical Contact

First medical contact (FMC) is the time at which trained EMS providers who can obtain and interpret the ECG arrive at the patient's side. The task faced by EMS providers upon initial patient contact should not be underestimated. An assessment of the patient's need for immediate life support, attainment of key history from the patient and witnessing bystanders and focused clinical examination must be performed efficiently and accurately for appropriate triage. This evaluation may be complicated by atypical but not uncommon presentations such as those in elderly, female, diabetic or cognitively impaired patients. The availability of a defibrillator is a mandatory part of EMS given the initial presentation may be cardiac arrest. Subsequently, a prehospital 12- or 18-lead ECG is crucial in the context of relevant symptoms and can be electronically transmitted to a hospital doctor or interpreted by EMS personnel with adequate training. A prehospital diagnosis of STEMI combined with direct referral to a primary PCI centre reduces time to device intervention and all-cause mortality [4]. In brief, significant ST-segment changes or left bundle branch block with sufficient clinical suspicion warrants exclusion of acute myocardial infarction. At this point and ideally less than 10 min from FMC, EMS providers should activate the 'STEMI pathway' in which patients may be transferred to a centre capable of primary PCI, a non-PCI centre for fibrinolysis, or receive prehospital fibrinolysis during transfer. While immediate transfer to a primary PCI centre is ideal, this is largely dependent on the presence of an established STEMI activation pathway, a coordinated hospital network and regional geography. Moreover, local protocols that facilitate prehospital registration may be in place to transfer patients directly to the catheterization lab, effectively bypassing the emergency department and further reducing unnecessary delays. Current guidelines recommend a FMC to device intervention time of 120 min or less when considering

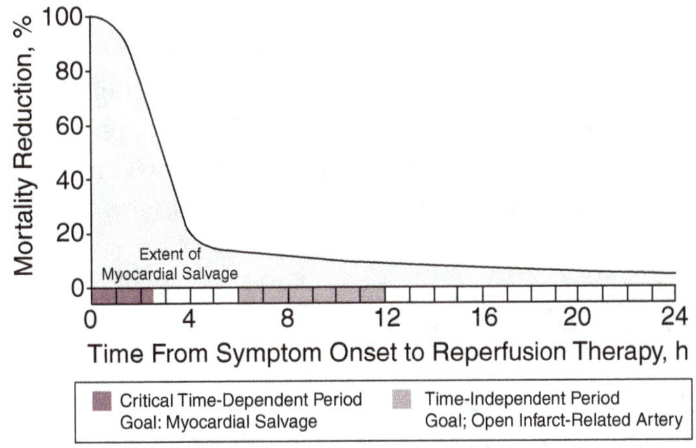

Fig. 2.2 Mortality reduction as a function of total ischaemic time. Note that extent of myocardial salvage dramatically reduces within the first 4 h but that up to 24 h, the salvage of a smaller proportion of myocardium is still possible

primary PCI [5]; however, any system must ultimately focus on reducing total ischaemic time irrespective of the mode of reperfusion therapy (Fig. 2.2). Caution should be exercised concerning overdependence on primary PCI where facilities may not be within reasonable accessibility.

2.3 Diagnosis of Myocardial Infarction

The diagnosis of an acute myocardial infarction is made when a patient has elevated blood serum levels of cardiac enzymes (preferably cardiac troponin) and one or more of the following: (a) symptoms suggestive of myocardial ischaemia, (b) ECG demonstrating new significant ST-T changes or new left bundle branch block (LBBB), (c) new pathological Q waves on ECG, (d) imaging evidence of new loss of viable myocardium or new regional wall motion abnormality or finally (e) identification of intracoronary thrombus on angiography or autopsy [6]. The suspicion of myocardial infarction usually begins from the point at which a call is made to the emergency medical services (EMS). At the point of FMC, a working diagnosis of STEMI must be made as soon as possible, and therefore a focused history and 12-lead electrocardiogram must be performed with a maximum target delay of 10 min. The clinical history is a critical component of the diagnosis of STEMI, with particular emphasis on the nature of the chest pain. While other mimics of STEMI such as myopericarditis or aortic dissection would be important to consider at an early stage as they would affect the subsequent management, acute myocardial infarction should remain at the forefront of the differential diagnoses as it remains common and is time critical in its management.

2.3.1 History and Examination

A focused history and examination must be carried out promptly at FMC. Symptoms suggestive of myocardial ischaemia may include chest pain which can radiate to the left arm, neck and/or jaw. Chest pain may be associated with shortness of breath, diaphoresis, nausea, vomiting, palpitations or even syncope. The early recognition of patients with decompensated heart failure may enable the early administration of diuretics. Pulse rate, blood pressure monitoring and oxygen pulse oximetry should be monitored. It is recommended that as soon as the suspicion of a diagnosis of acute myocardial infarction is made, that ECG monitoring (with defibrillator capacity) is carried out as these patients are at high risk of malignant arrhythmias.

2.3.2 ECG Diagnosis

The 12-lead ECG should be calibrated at 10 mm/mV with a standard paper (or screen) speed of 25 mm/s. The interpretation of the ECG should be made by a trained medical professional; otherwise, field transmission of the ECG should be done for immediate diagnosis. An ECG diagnosis of STEMI is made with new ST-segment elevation at the J point in two contiguous leads at (a) $\geq$0.2 mV in $\geq$40 years, $\geq$0.25 mV in men $<$40 years or $\geq$ 0.15 mV in women in leads V_2–V_3 and/or (b) $\geq$0.1 mV in all other leads (Fig. 2.3). The presence of reciprocal ST depression helps confirm the diagnosis and differentiates myocardial ischaemia from other causes of ST-segment abnormalities, such as left ventricular aneurysm or even non-cardiac causes such as subarachnoid haemorrhage. New LBBB in the context of a highly suggestive history should be treated as acute myocardial infarction. While LBBB is not specific for an MI, one which is related to an infarct is more likely to be inferred a larger infarct size with poorer prognosis. Associated features such as decompensated cardiac failure and cardiogenic shock should raise clinical suspicion [7]. While various algorithms have been proposed to aid the diagnosis in the context of LBBB, they do not offer sufficient diagnostic certainty. Findings in the

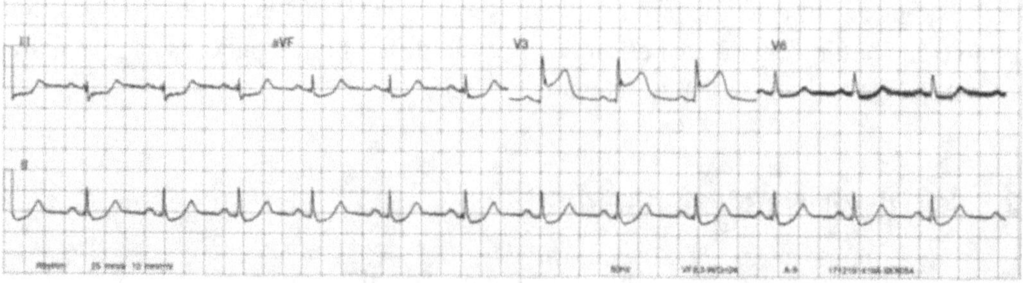

Fig. 2.3 Anterior ST-segment-elevation ECG. More marked ST-segment elevation V_1–V_4 with reciprocal change in other leads

Table 2.1 Localizing of myocardial infarction on ECG

Infarct location	ECG changes	Affected coronary artery
Septal	V_1–V_2	Septal LAD
Anterior	V_3–V_4	LAD
Lateral	I, aVL, V_5, V_6	LCx, diagonals
Inferior	II, III, aVF	LCx (15%), RCA (85%)
Posterior	V_7, V_8, V_9 (posteriorly placed)	RCA

context of LBBB which should raise clinical suspicion include (a) concordant ST-segment elevation ≥1 mm in leads with positive QRS complex, (b) concordant ST-segment depression ≥1 mm in V_1–V_3 and (c) discordant ST-segment elevation ≥5 mm in leads with a negative QRS complex. Given that right bundle branch block (RBBB) in the context of a STEMI often has ambiguous ST segments and has also been associated with a poor prognosis, recent guidelines have advised a change in approach in the management of such patients. In the context of persistent ischaemic symptoms, they should be treated in a similar fashion to LBBB with emergent coronary angiography and PCI if indicated. Likewise, patients with permanent pacemaker devices that are set up for right ventricular pacing will exhibit ECG changes similar to that of left bundle branch block. Of note, a patient with an ECG demonstrating ST-segment elevation in aVR and/or V_1 with otherwise widespread ST-segment depression should raise the suspicion of left main coronary artery obstruction, particularly if coupled with haemodynamic compromise. The localization of myocardial infarction can be also be deduced from the ECG as in table (Table 2.1).

While those with STEMI are at greatest risk from morbidity and mortality, patients presenting with non-ST elevation acute coronary syndromes (NSTEACS) also benefit from angiography and revascularization for prognostic advantage. It has become evident however that patients with NSTEACS and high-risk features benefit from early intervention, and as such, guidelines are now advocating angiography for this group within 24 h of presentation [8, 9]. In order to deliver this high standard of care, select ambulance services have recently adopted a direct access pathway which facilitates patients with certain high-risk clinical and ECG features to be brought directly to a heart attack centre. These protocols frequently include patients with (a) persistent ST depression >1 mm or transient ST elevation, (b) pathological T-wave inversion in V_1–V_4, (c) dynamic T-wave inversion >2 mm in two or more contiguous leads or (d) haemodynamic (e.g. sustained hypotension >15 min, pulmonary oedema, heart failure) or electrical (e.g. sustained ventricular tachycardia or fibrillation) instability thought to be secondary to cardiac ischaemia.

2.3.3 Cardiac Biomarkers

Point-of-care cardiac biomarkers are well established and demonstrate excellent diagnostic performance compared with lab-based assays. Their use in the prehospital setting is still being evaluated, but use of these tests may provide some guidance in the appropriate triaging of patients with suspected acute myocardial infarction, especially in cases where there is diagnostic uncertainty, such as ambiguous chest pain or in the unconscious patient. Some cardiologists have raised concerns that serum levels of cardiac biomarkers may be undetectable or below reference range if they are measured very early in an evolving myocardial infarction, which may in turn provide false reassurance to the practitioner assessing the patient. Their use has therefore been limited to few ambulance services, and their benefit to patient care will continue to be appraised.

2.4 Prehospital Treatment of Myocardial Infarction

2.4.1 Principles of Prehospital Therapy

Prehospital therapy for acute MI focuses on reducing thrombus burden and coagulation cascade hyperactivity prior to coronary reperfusion treatment. Potential therapies include antiplatelets, anticoagulants and glycoprotein (GP) IIb/IIIa inhibitors; the combination in which they are used is often institution or even operator dependent (Table 2.2). The evidence to support each type of therapy and specific drugs within each class varies, although current class 1 guideline recommendations are prompt dual antiplatelet therapy in the form of aspirin and a potent $P2Y_{12}$ inhibitor and an appropriate anticoagulant after assessment of bleeding risk [5]. Total ischaemic time remains the priority, and administration of these adjunct agents should not delay EMS transfer. While the optimal coronary reperfusion is primary PCI, such facilities may not be readily available to all patients. In such cases, prehospital fibrinolytic therapy can be utilized for initial reperfusion.

2.4.2 Antiplatelet Therapy

The benefits of dual antiplatelet therapy (DAPT) in patients undergoing primary PCI are well established. While initially borne out in the context of reducing the ongoing and persistent risk of stent thrombosis, DAPT also reduces the risk of subsequent spontaneous MI in non-stented coronary segments and all-cause mortality [10]. In the prehospital setting, aspirin should be administered as soon as possible. The dissolved or chewed oral form is preferable over swallowing a whole tablet due to more rapid absorption, with a recommended dose of 150–300 mg. There is a paucity of data evaluating intravenous aspirin therapy in the setting of STEMI although given its 50% oral bioavailability, a corresponding dose between 75 and 150 mg is appropriate in patients unable to tolerate the oral route. In contrast, the timing for initiation of adjunct $P2Y_{12}$ inhibition therapy, including ticagrelor, prasugrel or clopidogrel, is uncertain. The ATLANTIC trial aimed to evaluate the safety, ECG changes and pharmacodynamics based on timing of $P2Y_{12}$ inhibition therapy in the form of ticagrelor in early-presenting STEMI patients [11]. In 1862 patients

Table 2.2 Adjuvant pharmacotherapies used in the prehospital setting

Adjunct pharmacologic therapies	Recommendations in primary PCI	Evidence	Notes
Aspirin	+++	ISIS-2, collaborative meta-analysis	– Dissolved or chewed – Loading dose (≥150 mg)
$P2Y_{12}$ inhibitors			
Clopidogrel	++	COMMIT, CURE	– Slower onset vs. prasugrel/ticagrelor
Prasugrel	+++	Triton–TIMI 38, ETAMI	– Avoid in patients with previous stroke/TIA or high risk of bleeding (previous haemorrhagic stroke, oral anticoagulants, liver disease)
Ticagrelor	+++	PLATO	– Avoid in patients at high risk of bleeding
Cangrelor	++	CHAMPION PHOENIX	– IV administration – Rapid onset and offset
Anticoagulants			
UFH	+++	(Operator familiarity)	– Can measure anticoagulation with ACT
Enoxaparin	+++	ATOLL	– Better clinical outcomes than UFH
Bivalirudin	++	MATRIX	– More expensive than heparin – Consider in patients with HIT
Fondaparinux	–	OASIS 6	– No demonstrated benefit in primary PCI
GP IIb/IIIa inhibitors			
Abciximab	+	FINESSE	– Consider as bailout therapy in angiographic evidence of no or slow reflow or large thrombus
Tirofiban	+	On-TIME 2	

Recommendations range from '+++' strongly recommended to '–' not recommended

randomized to prehospital or in-hospital ticagrelor with a median time difference between strategies of 31 min, there was no between-group difference in the co-primary end point of pre-PCI resolution of ST-segment elevation or absence of TIMI flow grade 3 in infarct-related artery on angiography. However, there was a trend favouring prehospital ticagrelor for the resolution of ST-segment elevation after PCI which is consistent with the pharmacokinetic data of drug onset time. As such, the current practice is prompt prehospital DAPT in STEMI patients undergoing primary PCI. Prasugrel and ticagrelor are superior to clopidogrel in patients with acute coronary syndrome (ACS) across a range of cardiovascular outcomes including recurrent MI and stent thrombosis, while also having a faster onset of action [12–14]. An initial loading dose is needed to rapidly attain a therapeutic concentration; however, patients should be assessed for bleeding risk, exclusion of other possible diagnoses and drug-specific contraindications before administration. Cangrelor is another $P2Y_{12}$ inhibitor administered intravenously with benefits including rapid onset and superiority over clopidogrel for the composite end point of death, MI, ischaemic-driven revascularization or stent thrombosis in patients undergoing PCI [15]. It has yet to be compared with prasugrel or ticagrelor and its use limited to patients yet to receive oral $P2Y_{12}$ inhibition therapy.

2.4.3 Anticoagulants

The use of prehospital anticoagulant therapy for primary PCI has been mostly derived from extensive experience and familiarity rather than established clinical evidence. Despite the lack of a placebo-controlled trial for anticoagulants in primary PCI, they are still frequently used in clinical practice. Unfractionated heparin (UFH) is the standard anticoagulant for primary PCI. Enoxaparin is an alternative and has been associated with a reduction in composite risk of death, recurrent ACS or urgent revascularization at 30 days (7% vs. 11%, respectively; $p = 0.02$) compared with UFH in the ATOLL trial [16]. However, the ability to measure UFH anticoagulation through activated clotting time (ACT) has led to UFH remaining the standard of care for PCI. Bivalirudin may be considered with the MATRIX trial reporting lower mortality and bleeding at the expense of increased absolute stent thrombosis events compared with UFH in 7213 ACS patients [17]. Its comparatively higher cost and lack of prehospital data have limited its use, although it may be preferred in patients at greater risk of bleeding, especially when infused for longer durations (>4 h) post-PCI. Conversely, fondaparinux has shown no benefit in primary PCI and is not recommended in this setting. However it may be an attractive alternative in STEMI patients not suitable for primary PCI with reduced death and re-infarction compared with UFH at 3–6 months (hazard ratio 0.77, 95% CI 0.64–0.93, $p = 0.008$) shown in the OASIS-6 trial [18].

2.4.4 GP IIb/IIIa Inhibitors

Prehospital glycoprotein (GP) IIb/IIIa inhibitors are proposed to reduce thrombus burden and improve reperfusion success in primary PCI given its rapid onset in intravenous administration. Examples include abciximab, eptifibatide and tirofiban. While they are generally associated with a greater reduction in ST-segment deviation post-PCI, data are conflicting as to whether this translates to better clinical outcomes. The FINESSE trial is the largest trial to evaluate the use of upstream GP IIb/IIIa inhibition using abciximab or combination of abciximab-tenecteplase compared with PCI alone in STEMI patients intended for primary PCI [19]. In 2452 patients, there was no difference in mortality between any of the patient groups at 90 days follow-up (between 4.5 and 5.5% for all three groups; $p = 0.49$). Conversely, in the On-TIME 2 trial, pre-PCI tirofiban was associated with fewer major adverse cardiovascular events at 30 days compared with placebo (5.8% and 8.6%, respectively; $p = 0.04$) and a trend towards reduced mortality at 1 year (3.7% and 5.8%, respectively; 0.08) [20]. Given mortality is significantly reduced in patients who receive early compared with late GP IIb/IIIa inhibitors [21], it should be noted that time from symptom onset to drug therapy was 165 min in the FINESSE trial which was much longer compared with ~75 min in On-TIME 2. Further to the conflicting evidence for clinical benefit, these agents are highly potent and could unnecessarily increase the risk of bleeding, particularly where the diagnosis of STEMI is not definitive. In view of these limitations, current guidelines do not recommend the use of GP IIb/IIIa inhibitors in the prehospital setting [5].

2.4.5 Fibrinolytic Therapy

Fibrinolytic therapy was previously the mainstay treatment for STEMI patients with early presentation from symptom onset. Its rapidly waning beneficial effects with ongoing myocardial injury highlight the importance of early administration; mortality is more than halved when given less than 2 h from symptom onset compared with later [22]. However, more than two decades ago, primary coronary angioplasty was shown to significantly reduce death, re-infarction and hospital readmission compared with thrombolysis [23]. While subsequent findings from the CAPTIM trial suggest fibrinolysis may be equivalent if administered early in intermediate-risk STEMI patients and where rescue angioplasty is readily available [24], the further development of stent technology has since established primary PCI as the optimal reperfusion strategy for STEMI patients presenting within 12 h of symptom onset. However, the success of any reperfusion strategy is still dependent on total ischaemic time. Patients should not be delayed with treatment where a primary PCI facility is not within reasonable proximity, either by EMS vehicle or air transportation. Where a predefined time threshold according to local protocols cannot be met, the role of fibrinolytic therapy remains a critical aspect of prehospital STEMI management.

Fibrinolytic therapy should be administered prehospital (preferably <10 min of STEMI diagnosis) and within 12 h of symptom onset in the absence of contraindications if a primary PCI facility is logistically unavailable. Fibrin-specific agents are preferred (e.g. tenecteplase) over systemic lytic agents (e.g. streptokinase) and should be co-administered with age-adjusted doses of dual antiplatelet and anticoagulation therapy. In the PCI-CLARITY study, adjunct clopidogrel significantly reduced the rate of major adverse cardiovascular events compared with aspirin alone in STEMI patients receiving fibrinolytic therapy (relative risk reduction, 40%) [25]. At present, no studies have evaluated the adjunct use of ticagrelor or prasugrel with fibrinolytic therapy, and thus clopidogrel is the preferred choice in this setting. For adjunct anticoagulation, enoxaparin is the preferred treatment and is associated with fewer deaths, re-infarction or urgent revascularization compared with UFH for STEMI patients scheduled for fibrinolysis [26]. When considering fibrinolytics in the context of optimal adjunct therapy, the risk of bleeding, particularly intracranial, must be weighed against the expected benefit. Absolute contraindications include previous intracranial haemorrhage, ischaemic stroke within the last 6 months, any central nervous system malformations, gastrointestinal bleed within the last month, known bleeding disorders or possible aortic dissection. Certain patient characteristics such as elderly, female gender or chronic kidney disease also increase bleeding risk, and risk prediction scores are available although should not unnecessarily delay reperfusion therapy [27]. In STEMI patients with cardiogenic shock, fibrinolysis does not improve clinical outcomes possibly due to decreased coronary perfusion, and in this setting, primary PCI is recommended.

2.4.6 Role of PCI After Fibrinolytic Therapy

The necessity and timing of PCI after administered fibrinolytic therapy has been an area of controversy since the advent of angioplasty. Several trials have sought to evaluate the role of immediate coronary angiographic assessment (i.e. facilitated PCI) compared with conservative, ischaemia-driven angiography after fibrinolysis. The GRACIA-1 trial randomized 500 patients with thrombolysed STEMI to either facilitated PCI or conservative, ischaemia-driven management with the primary end point being death, re-infarction or revascularization at 12 months [28]. Patients in the facilitated PCI group had lower frequency of the primary end point (9% vs. 21%; $p < 0.001$): however, the time from symptom onset to fibrinolysis was 3 h. With such delay, the optimal benefit of fibrinolysis may have passed, thus favouring PCI. The ASSENT-4 PCI trial also evaluated facilitated PCI and reported higher rates of adverse cardiovascular events (19% vs. 13%, respectively; $p = 0.005$) and stroke (1.8% vs. 0%, respectively; $p < 0.0001$) compared with PCI alone in patients with an anticipated PCI delay [29]. Routine fibrinolytic therapy with immediate PCI in patients with anticipated PCI delay could heighten the risk of intracranial bleeding in the context of adjunct DAPT and peri-procedural anticoagulants, which may in turn outweigh the benefits of thorough reperfusion.

Focus has since shifted towards a pharmaco-invasive strategy in which early-presenting STEMI patients receive prehospital fibrinolytic therapy and transfer to a PCI-capable facility for timely, but not necessarily immediate, angiographic assessment. This approach carries the benefit of reducing early procedural risk from PCI, while enabling rapid emergency angiography (i.e. rescue PCI) in those with failed reperfusion after fibrinolysis (<50% ST-segment elevation resolution within 90 min) [30]. The STREAM trial confirmed the safety of this strategy, in which 1892 STEMI patients within 3 h of symptom onset and > 1 h of anticipated PCI delay were randomized to either prehospital fibrinolysis and angiographic assessment within 24 h or primary PCI alone [31]. No difference in the primary end point of death, shock, heart failure or re-infarct at 30 days was detected, although fibrinolysis was still associated with increased risk of intracranial haemorrhage (1.6% vs. 0.5%; $p = 0.03$). Of note, the trial protocol mandated direct EMS transfer to a primary PCI facility which was critical to showing equivalence given more than one-third of patients required rescue PCI. Taken together, there remains a distinct role for early fibrinolytic therapy in STEMI patients with anticipated PCI delay and considered risk of bleeding, although it should be followed by transfer to a PCI-capable centre for routine early angiographic assessment.

2.4.7 Safe Transfer to the Heart Attack Centre

Ensuring patient safety while minimizing total ischaemic time underlies optimal transfer of patients being managed for STEMI. Following attainment of 12-lead ECG and transmission where possible, defibrillator pads should be routinely attached with continuous cardiac monitoring throughout transfer. Supplemental oxygen therapy in hypoxaemic patients (haemoglobin-oxygen saturation <90–94%) is part of routine initial management; however, its effect above this saturation level is currently uncertain (see next section). During immediate assessment and transfer, sublingual nitroglycerin can be administered where there is ongoing chest pain although regular non-invasive blood pressure monitoring for hypotension is needed. Intravenous morphine may also be administered where pain persists. An EMS checklist and transfer report regarding patient presentation, clinical assessment findings and received treatments, including dose, time and route of administration, is common and provides clear documentation and handover to the receiving hospital team. The ability to consistently perform these tasks while monitoring the patient's clinical status is dependent on established regional STEMI protocols. The protocol should also incorporate specific key parameters for time thresholds such that EMS personnel can rapidly determine whether primary PCI is logistically achievable and to enable quantitative and regular assessment of local outcomes compared with performance benchmarks.

2.4.8 Oxygen Therapy in Acute Myocardial Infarction

Oxygen therapy has historically been a part of routine initial management of STEMI patients regardless of haemoglobin-oxygen saturation. This was derived from the belief that increased oxygen delivery to an ischaemic myocardium would reduce myocardial injury. However, the AVOID trial which randomized 441 STEMI patients with ≥94% baseline oxygen saturation to either supplemental oxygen at 8 L/min or no oxygen found that supplemental oxygen was associated with a significant increase in peak creatine kinase [32]. Additionally, recurrent MI (5.5% vs. 0.9%, $p = 0.006$) and cardiac arrhythmias (40.4% vs. 31.4%, $p = 0.05$) at 6 months follow-up were higher in patients receiving supplemental oxygen compared with none, although the study was not powered for clinical outcomes. Subsequently, the much larger DETO2X-AMI trial found no difference with or without supplemental oxygen in patients with suspected myocardial infarction for all-cause mortality (5.0% and 5.1%, respectively) and rehospitalization with MI (3.8% and 3.3%, respectively) [33]. Of note, less than one-half of patients in each arm had a final diagnosis of STEMI, and the lower threshold of oxygen saturation for inclusion was 90%. While it remains unclear whether supplemental oxygen is harmful in patients with oxygen saturation in the normal range, the equivalent lack of benefit suggests that it should be reserved for patients with lower saturation (<90–94%) and we await further randomized data to elucidate this controversy.

2.5 Summary

Patient outcomes following myocardial infarction are heavily dependent on the prehospital phase. Prompt recognition and correct triage of patients suffering from chest pain are paramount, with healthcare networks continually evolving to deliver upfront pharmacological treatment and rapid access to therapies that allow for myocardial reperfusion. As we move into the future, our focus as healthcare providers should remain on reducing the overall duration of myocardial ischaemia while also considering expansion of rapid reperfusion to patients with an acute coronary syndrome not currently served by existing pathways.

References

1. Gersh BJ, Stone GW, White HD, Holmes DR Jr. Pharmacological facilitation of primary percutaneous coronary intervention for acute myocardial infarction: is the slope of the curve the shape of the future? JAMA. 2005;293:979–86.
2. De Luca G, Suryapranata H, Ottervanger JP, Antman EM. Time delay to treatment and mortality in primary angioplasty for acute myocardial infarction: every minute of delay counts. Circulation. 2004;109:1223–5.
3. Goldberg RJ, Spencer FA, Fox KA, et al. Prehospital delay in patients with acute coronary syndromes (from the global registry of acute coronary events [GRACE]). Am J Cardiol. 2009;103:598–603.
4. Sorensen JT, Terkelsen CJ, Norgaard BL, et al. Urban and rural implementation of pre-hospital diagnosis and direct referral for primary percutaneous coronary intervention in patients with acute ST-elevation myocardial infarction. Eur Heart J. 2011;32:430–6.
5. Ibanez B, James S, Agewall S, et al. ESC guidelines for the management of acute myocardial infarction in patients presenting with ST-segment elevation: the task force for the management of acute myocardial infarction in patients presenting with ST-segment elevation of the European Society of Cardiology (ESC). Eur Heart J. 2017;33(20):2569–619.
6. Thygesen K, Alpert JS, Jaffe AS, et al. Third universal definition of myocardial infarction. Circulation. 2012;126:2020–35.
7. Brown AJ, Hoole SP, McCormick LM, et al. Left bundle branch block with acute thrombotic occlusion is associated with increased myocardial jeopardy score and poor clinical outcomes in primary percutaneous coronary intervention activations. Heart. 2013;99:774–8.
8. Katritsis DG, Siontis GC, Kastrati A, et al. Optimal timing of coronary angiography and potential intervention in non-ST-elevation acute coronary syndromes. Eur Heart J. 2011;32:32–40.
9. Roffi M, Patrono C, Collet JP, et al. 2015 ESC guidelines for the management of acute coronary syndromes in patients presenting without persistent ST-segment elevation: task force for the Management of Acute Coronary Syndromes in patients presenting without persistent ST-segment elevation of the European Society of Cardiology (ESC). Eur Heart J. 2016;37:267–315.
10. Mauri L, Kereiakes DJ, Yeh RW, et al. Twelve or 30 months of dual antiplatelet therapy after drug-eluting stents. N Engl J Med. 2014;371:2155–66.
11. Montalescot G, van 't Hof AW, Lapostolle F, et al. Prehospital ticagrelor in ST-segment elevation myocardial infarction. N Engl J Med. 2014;371:1016–27.
12. Wiviott SD, Braunwald E, McCabe CH, et al. Prasugrel versus Clopidogrel in patients with acute coronary syndromes. N Engl J Med. 2007;357:2001–15.
13. Wallentin L, Becker RC, Budaj A, et al. Ticagrelor versus Clopidogrel in patients with acute coronary syndromes. N Engl J Med. 2009;361:1045–57.

14. Zeymer U, Mochmann HC, Mark B, et al. Double-blind, randomized, prospective comparison of loading doses of 600 mg clopidogrel versus 60 mg prasugrel in patients with acute ST-segment elevation myocardial infarction scheduled for primary percutaneous intervention: the ETAMI trial (early thienopyridine treatment to improve primary PCI in patients with acute myocardial infarction). JACC Cardiovasc Interv. 2015;8:147–54.
15. Bhatt DL, Stone GW, Mahaffey KW, et al. Effect of platelet inhibition with Cangrelor during PCI on ischemic events. N Engl J Med. 2013;368:1303–13.
16. Montalescot G, Zeymer U, Silvain J, et al. Intravenous enoxaparin or unfractionated heparin in primary percutaneous coronary intervention for ST-elevation myocardial infarction: the international randomised open-label ATOLL trial. Lancet. 2011;378:693–703.
17. Valgimigli M, Frigoli E, Leonardi S, et al. Bivalirudin or unfractionated heparin in acute coronary syndromes. N Engl J Med. 2015;373:997–1009.
18. Yusuf S, Mehta SR, Chrolavicius S, et al. Effects of fondaparinux on mortality and reinfarction in patients with acute ST-segment elevation myocardial infarction: the OASIS-6 randomized trial. JAMA. 2006;295:1519–30.
19. Ellis SG, Tendera M, de Belder MA, et al. Facilitated PCI in patients with ST-elevation myocardial infarction. N Engl J Med. 2008;358:2205–17.
20. ten Berg JM, van 't Hof AW, Dill T, et al. Effect of early, pre-hospital initiation of high bolus dose tirofiban in patients with ST-segment elevation myocardial infarction on short- and long-term clinical outcome. J Am Coll Cardiol. 2010;55:2446–55.
21. DEL G, Bellandi F, Huber K, et al. Early glycoprotein IIb-IIIa inhibitors in primary angioplasty-abciximab long-term results (EGYPT-ALT) cooperation: individual patient's data meta-analysis. J Thromb Haemost. 2011;9:2361–70.
22. Boersma E, Maas AC, Deckers JW, Simoons ML. Early thrombolytic treatment in acute myocardial infarction: reappraisal of the golden hour. Lancet. 1996;348:771–5.
23. Investigators. TGUoStOOCAiACSAS. A clinical trial comparing primary coronary angioplasty with tissue plasminogen activator for acute myocardial infarction. N Engl J Med. 1997;336:1621–8.
24. Bonnefoy E, Lapostolle F, Leizorovicz A, et al. Primary angioplasty versus prehospital fibrinolysis in acute myocardial infarction: a randomised study. Lancet. 2002;360:825–9.
25. Sabatine MS, Cannon CP, Gibson CM, et al. Effect of clopidogrel pretreatment before percutaneous coronary intervention in patients with ST-elevation myocardial infarction treated with fibrinolytics: the PCI-CLARITY study. JAMA. 2005;294:1224–32.
26. Antman EM, Morrow DA, McCabe CH, et al. Enoxaparin versus unfractionated heparin with fibrinolysis for ST-elevation myocardial infarction. N Engl J Med. 2006;354:1477–88.
27. Moscucci M, Fox KA, Cannon CP, et al. Predictors of major bleeding in acute coronary syndromes: the global registry of acute coronary events (GRACE). Eur Heart J. 2003;24:1815–23.
28. Fernandez-Aviles F, Alonso JJ, Castro-Beiras A, et al. Routine invasive strategy within 24 hours of thrombolysis versus ischaemia-guided conservative approach for acute myocardial infarction with ST-segment elevation (GRACIA-1): a randomised controlled trial. Lancet. 2004;364:1045–53.
29. Assessment of the Safety and Efficacy of a New Treatment Strategy with Percutaneous Coronary Intervention (ASSENT-4 PCI) investigators. Primary versus tenecteplase-facilitated percutaneous coronary intervention in patients with ST-segment elevation acute myocardial infarction (ASSENT-4 PCI): randomised trial. Lancet. 2006;367:569–78.
30. Gershlick AH, Stephens-Lloyd A, Hughes S, et al. Rescue angioplasty after failed thrombolytic therapy for acute myocardial infarction. N Engl J Med. 2005;353:2758–68.
31. Armstrong PW, Gershlick AH, Goldstein P, et al. Fibrinolysis or primary PCI in ST-segment elevation myocardial infarction. N Engl J Med. 2013;368:1379–87.
32. Stub D, Smith K, Bernard S, Nehme Z, Stephenson M, Bray JE, Cameron P, Barger B, Ellims AH, Taylor AJ, Meredith IT, Kaye DM, AVOID Investigators. Air vs. oxygen in ST-segment-elevation myocardial infarction. Circulation. 2015;131(24):2143–50.
33. Hofmann R, James SK, Jernberg T, et al. Oxygen therapy in suspected acute myocardial infarction. N Engl J Med. 2017;377:1240–9.

Primary Angioplasty: Efficacy and Outcomes

3

Ian Patrick Kay and Brittany Georgia Kay

3.1 Introduction

Internationally ischaemic heart disease (IHD) is the single most common cause of death, and its frequency is increasing. The relative incidences of ST-elevation myocardial infarction (STEMI) and non-ST-elevation myocardial infarction (NSTEMI) are decreasing and increasing, respectively. In European countries, the incidence rate for STEMI ranges from 43 to 144 per 100,000 population per year. Similarly, the reported adjusted incidence rates from the USA decreased from 133 per 100,000 in 1999 to 50 per 100,000 in 2008, whereas the incidence of NSTEMI remained constant or increased slightly. STEMI is more common in younger than in older people and is more common in men than in women.

Mortality in STEMI is associated with advanced age, Killip class, time delay to treatment, presence of emergency medical system (EMS)-based STEMI networks, treatment strategy, history of MI, diabetes mellitus, renal failure, number of diseased coronary arteries and left ventricular ejection fraction (LVEF). Overall mortality from STEMI remains substantial with the in-hospital mortality of unselected patients with STEMI in the national registries of the European Society of Cardiology (ESC) member countries varying between 4% and 12%. Whilst reported 1-year mortality among STEMI patients in other registries is approximately 10%.

Although IHD develops later in women compared with men, MI remains a leading cause of death in women. Acute coronary syndrome (ACS) occurs three to four times more often in men than in women below the age of 60 years, but after the age of 75, women represent the majority of patients. Women may present with atypical symptoms—seen in up to 30% in some registries. It is therefore important to be

I. P. Kay (✉)
Mercy Angiography, Auckland, New Zealand

B. G. Kay
University of Tasmania, Hobart, TAS, Australia

T. J. Watson et al. (eds.), *Primary Angioplasty*,
https://doi.org/10.1007/978-981-13-1114-7_3

vigilant when encountering a potential ACS presentation in a female. Women also have a higher bleeding risk peri- and post-PCI. Several studies have suggested a poorer outcome in females suffering MI, related to older age and more comorbidities. Some studies have indicated that women may undergo fewer interventions than men and receive reperfusion therapy less frequently. The guidelines stress the fact that women and men receive equal benefit from a reperfusion strategy and STEMI-related therapy and that both genders must be managed in a similar fashion.

3.2 Treatment of STEMI

Patients with chest pain suggestive of an ACS and having ECG evidence of an acute STEMI are candidates for reperfusion therapy with either primary percutaneous coronary intervention (PPCI) or fibrinolytic therapy. Patients with typical symptoms in the presence of a new left or right bundle branch block or a true posterior STEMI are also considered eligible.

Coronary reperfusion with PPCI or fibrinolytic therapy improves outcomes in patients with acute ST-elevation MI. However, PPCI is the reperfusion therapy of choice compared to fibrinolysis because it achieves a higher rate of TIMI 3 flow (more than 90%), does not carry the risk of intracranial haemorrhage and is associated with improved outcomes. The time to onset of reperfusion therapy is a critical determinant of outcome with both PPCI and fibrinolysis.

Definitions—The delay in treatment delivery between the onset of symptoms and primary percutaneous coronary intervention (PPCI) is termed the treatment delay and has the following components:

- Patient delay—This is the time between onset of symptoms and the call to the emergency medical system (EMS).
- Prehospital system delay—This is the time between the EMS call and the arrival at the PCI centre and is equivalent to the time of EMS evaluation, prehospital electrocardiogram obtainment (if any) and transportation to the hospital. For patients transferred from a local hospital to a PCI centre, this is sum of the time between the EMS call and arrival at the local hospital, the time at the local hospital and the time between hospitals (second transfer time).
- Door-to-balloon delay (D2B)—This is the time between arrival at the PCI centre and PPCI. Time of PPCI refers to the time of coronary intervention with a balloon, stent or other intervention, not to be confused with the time of arrival in the catheterization laboratory or the time of vascular access.
- First medical contact (FMC)—This concept is upgraded in the 2017 version of the ESC guidelines. This is the time point when the patient is initially assessed by a physician, paramedic or nurse who can obtain and interpret an ECG. This can be prehospital or in-hospital. Note if FMC is in the community and if the patient is transferred directly to the catheter laboratory, then the concept of door to balloon is dropped.
- System delay—This is the sum of the prehospital system and door-to-balloon delays.

In this schema, patient delay is not easily corrected by the healthcare system, while strategies to shorten other delays are potentially modifiable. Such an effort will be useful if longer time intervals are associated with worse outcomes.

3.3 Fibrinolytic Therapy

Fibrinolytics are most effective when given within the first 2 h after the onset of symptoms. However, many patients with STEMI present late after the development of symptoms. In different registries of patients, the time from symptom onset to hospital presentation was ≥4 h in 50%, more than 6 h in 40% and more than 12 h in 9–31%. Delay is greatest in women, older adults, low socioeconomic and ethnic minority groups and those with symptoms that occur between 6 P.M. and 6 A.M.

3.4 Late Presentation PPCI

In contrast to fibrinolysis, revascularization after 12 h with PCI may still be beneficial in the 9–31% of patients with STEMI who present more than 12 h after the onset of symptoms. The randomized trials that have evaluated late PCI have included patients at different time periods after symptom onset, ranging from 12 h to up to 28 days. Some have demonstrated an improvement in left ventricular function with PCI, but none have demonstrated a significant benefit on death.

The American College of Cardiology/American Heart Association (ACC/AHA) guidelines suggest that it is reasonable to perform PPCI for patients with onset of symptoms within the prior 12–24 h who have one or more of the following:

- Severe heart failure
- Haemodynamic or electrical instability
- Persistent ischaemic symptoms

In contrast, the task force did **not** recommend PPCI in stable, asymptomatic patients presenting more than 12 h after symptom onset.

3.5 Door-To-Balloon Time (D2B)

D2B is well studied and is predictive of in-hospital mortality. Longer D2B times result in poorer outcomes as evidenced by both observational studies and randomized trials:

- The NRMI-3 and NRMI-4 registries (1999–2002) reported 29,222 ST-elevation myocardial infarction (STEMI) patients who were treated with PCI within 6 h of presentation. Longer D2B times were significantly associated with increased in-hospital mortality (3.0%, 4.2%, 5.7% and 7.4% for D2B time of ≤90 min,

91–120 min, 121–150 min and >150 min, respectively). Patients with D2B times >90 min had a significant increase in mortality compared to those with D2B times ≤90 min (odds ratio 1.42).

- The CADILLAC and HORIZONS-AMI trials analysed 4548 patients; short D2B times (≤90 min) were associated with a significantly lower mortality rate at 1 year compared to longer times (3.1% vs. 4.3%; hazard ratio 0.72, 95% CI 0.52–0.99).

Despite the evidence that longer D2B times lead to worse outcomes, improvement in D2B times has not lead to improvement in survival rates. In a study of nearly 100,000 STEMI patients in the US CathPCI Registry of the National Cardiovascular Data Registry who underwent primary PCI between July 2005 and June 2009, median D2B times fell from 83 to 67 min, comparing the first to the last 12 months of the time period. Despite this significant improvement, there was no change in risk-adjusted in-hospital mortality (5.0% vs. 4.7%, respectively; $p = 0.34$).

Although there is a direct relationship between increasing mortality and longer D2B time, it may be difficult to demonstrate further improvements in survival with shorter D2B times, particularly if they are in the order of magnitude of minutes. This is in part related to the impact of total ischaemic time on mortality.

Outcomes in patient subgroups—The issue of whether the improvement in survival with short D2B times is delivered equally to all patients has been studied, and two subgroups of patients appear to benefit the most: those who present early after symptom onset and those at high risk.

Early versus late presentation—With regard to early versus late presentation, it appears that short D2B time is associated with improved outcome in early presenters more than in late presenters:

- In a study of 2322 patients who underwent PPCI comparing short versus long D2B time (<2 vs. >2 h), there was a significant decrease in 7-year mortality in patients presenting ≤3 hours from symptom onset (15.0% vs. 24.7%), but not in patients presenting after 3 h (18.5% vs. 21.1%).
- Similarly in 4548 patients who underwent PPCI win the CADILLAC and HORIZONS-AMI trials, short (≤90 min) compared to long D2B times were associated with a significantly lower 1-year mortality rate in patients with early presentation (≤90 min vs. ≥90 min), but not those with later presentation (1.9% vs. 3.8%, HR = 0.86, 95% CI 0.26–0.93 and 4.0% vs. 4.6%, HR = 0.86, 95% CI 0.58–1.28, respectively).

Patient risk category—High-risk patients (defined as one or more of Killip class 3 or 4, heart failure, age >70 years or anterior MI) appear to benefit more from short D2B time:

- In the study of 2322 patients discussed above, there was a significant decrease in 7-year mortality with shorter D2B times (<2 vs. ≥2 h) in high-risk (21.5% vs. 32.5%) but not low-risk patients (9.2% vs. 10.8%).

- In the CADILLAC and HORIZONS-AMI trials, short compared to long D2B times showed a trend toward lower 1-year mortality in both high- and low-risk groups (5.7% vs. 7.4% and 1.1% vs. 1.6%, respectively). In patients presenting early (≤90 min), the hazard ratios for mortality rate in patients with short versus long D2B times were identical for high- versus low-risk patients, but the absolute mortality rate differences were greater in high-risk patients (3.3% vs. 0.7%). In patients presenting late (>90 min), mortality was similar with short and long D2B times in both high- and low-risk patients.

The findings above suggest that short D2B times are critically important in patients who present early, especially in high-risk patients.

3.6 Time from First Medical Contact with the Healthcare System (System Delay)

System delay is the sum of the prehospital system and door-to-balloon delays. For patients first brought to a hospital without PCI capability, the system delay has multiple components.

The associations between healthcare delays and mortality were evaluated in a study of 6209 patients with STEMI from 2002 to 2006 by Danish researchers. Approximately one-third of these patients were triaged in the field to a PCI centre, and two-thirds were admitted to a local hospital and then transferred to a PCI centre. The median follow-up time was 3.4 years, and the cumulative 1-year mortality was 9.3%. The following findings were noted:

- In the univariate analysis of the components of delay (system, prehospital system, door-to-balloon, treatment and patient), system delay had the strongest association with mortality (hazard ratios [HR] 1.22, 1.19, 1.13, 1.054 and 1.042, respectively). All HR were significant.
- For system delays of 0–60 min, 61–120 min, 121–180 min and 181–360 min, the long-term cumulative mortality was 15.4%, 23.3%, 28.1% and 30.8%, respectively.
- In the multivariate analysis, treatment delay and patient delay were not associated with mortality, but system delay was independently associated with mortality (HR 1.10, 95% CI 1.01–1.16 per 1-hour delay). The main components of system delay, prehospital system delay and door-to-balloon delay were similarly associated with mortality (HR 1.10, 95% CI 1.02–1.18 and 1.14, 95% CI 1.05–1.24, respectively).

This study demonstrates the negative impact of increasing system delay on mortality. It does not allow any firm conclusion regarding the time at which using a fibrinolytic agent would be preferable. Therefore, the earlier a patient presents (and thus a higher baseline risk), the less D2B delay that is acceptable. Thus, fibrinolytic therapy is an important option for patients who present within the first 3 h and who are at a low risk of bleeding.

3.7 Direct Transfer from the Community

Mortality is improved with direct transfer from the community to a PCI hospital compared with evaluation and treatment at a closer hospital without PCI capability. The feasibility and impact of this strategy on D2B delay were evaluated in a nonrandomized comparison of 344 patients with chest pain of less than 12 h duration and ST-segment elevation characteristic of acute MI in 2005 and 2006. In this study, 135 patients were referred directly from the community by paramedics trained in ECG interpretation, and 209 patients were referred directly from regional emergency departments. The median D2B time, defined as the time between arrival at the first hospital to first balloon inflation, was significantly shorter in patients referred from the community (69 vs. 123 min), and the percent of patients with D2B times of less than 90 min was significantly higher (80 vs. 12).

For patients with STEMI diagnosed with a prehospital ECG who are transported to a PCI-capable hospital, one way to shorten the time to reperfusion is to bypass the emergency department (ED) and take the patient directly to the catheterization laboratory. The efficacy of this approach was addressed in a study of 12,158 STEMI patients, 10.5% of whom bypassed the ED. The time from first medical contact (FMC) to device activation was shorter in these individuals compared to those who went to the ED (68 vs. 88 min; $p < 0.0001$). There was a trend toward lower mortality (2.7% vs. 4.1%; adjusted odds ratio 0.69, 95% CI 0.45–1.03).

Therefore, the optimal strategy for STEMI patients diagnosed with a prehospital ECG should be to transfer the patient directly to the catheterization laboratory of a PCI-capable hospital (bypassing the ED) if the following two criteria are met:

1. The patient is haemodynamically stable.
2. The patient is received by personnel (including one physician) qualified to care for critically ill patients.

Transfer from a non-PCI centre—The poor outcomes seen in patients who are initially evaluated at hospitals without on-site PCI capability are of concern. The time spent at the first hospital, the subsequent transfer time and the time spent at the receiving hospital prior to arrival in the catheterization laboratory are sources of longer D2B. The frequency, magnitude and clinical impact of delays occurring at each of these time intervals were examined in a prospective study of 2034 patients referred to a PCI centre for primary PCI. The following findings were noted:

- Delays occurred most frequently in the ED at the referral hospital, with less delay seen at the PCI centre or in transport (64%, 16% and 13%, respectively).
- For the referral hospital, the most frequent reasons for delay were awaiting transport and ED delays (26% and 14%, respectively).

Interestingly, diagnostic difficulties, including non-diagnostic initial ECGs, led to the greatest delay, but these had limited or no impact on mortality.

3.8 The Door-In to Door-Out (DIDO) Time

This is defined as the duration of time from arrival to discharge at the first (non-PCI capable) hospital. The DIDO time is probably modifiable, as opposed to the non-modifiable delay caused by an additional ambulance ride. The optimum DIDO measure is<30 min, (AHA/ACC 2008). The relationship between DIDO time and outcomes was evaluated in in the Acute Coronary Treatment and Intervention Outcomes Network (ACTION) Registry-Get With the Guidelines (GWTG) between 2007 and 2010. The following results were reported:

- The median DIDO time was 68 min, with only 11% of patients having a goal DIDO time of less than 30 min.
- Predictors of longer DIDO times included older age, female sex, off-hours presentation and non-emergency medical services presentation to the first hospital.
- Patients with DIDO times less than 30 min had significantly shorter door-to-balloon times (85 vs. 127 min) and a lower in-hospital mortality rate (2.7% vs. 5.9%).

AHA/ACC and ESC Recommendations—The 2013 American College of Cardiology Foundation/American Heart Association guideline for the management of ST-elevation myocardial infarction (STEMI) recommends the timely performance of primary percutaneous coronary intervention (PCI) and sets the following time goals:

- For patients who initially arrive at or are transported to a non-PCI-capable hospital, the first medical contact to device time should be 120 min or less.
- For patients who initially arrive at or are transported to a PCI-capable hospital, the first medical contact to device time should be 90 min or less.
- The 2012 European Society of Cardiology guideline on STEMI recommended shorter time intervals of 90 and 60 min, respectively.

ESC 2017 Summary of important time targets	Time targets
Maximum time from FMC to ECG and diagnosis	≤10 min
Maximum time delay from STEMI diagnosis to PPCI (wire crossing) to choose PPCI strategy over fibrinolysis (if this target cannot be met consider fibrinolysis)	≤120 min
Maximum time from STEMI diagnosis to wire crossing in patients presenting to PPCI hospitals	≤60 min
Maximum time from STEMI diagnosis to wire crossing in transferred patients	≤90 min
Maximum time from STEMI diagnosis to bolus or infusion of fibrinolysis in patients unable to meet PPCI target times	≤10 min
Time delay from start of fibrinolysis to evaluation of its efficacy	60–90 min
Time delay from start of fibrinolysis to angiography (if fibrinolysis successful)	2–24 h

Ref: academic.oup.com/eurheartj/advance-article/doi/10.1093/eurheartj/ehx393/4095042

3.9 Non-system Factors Leading to Delay

In a study of nearly 83,000 patients with STEMI in the US PCI Registry (2009–2011), non-system delays occurred in 14.7%. Typical reasons cited included delays in gaining consent, difficult vascular access and difficulty in crossing the lesion. As expected, and consistent with an increase in D2B time, the in-hospital mortality was greater in those with compared to those without non-system delay (15.1% vs. 2.5%; $p < 0.01$) even after PCI.

Prognosis after Primary PCI—In a registry study of 2804 patients, 30-day, 1-year and 5-year all-cause (and cardiac) mortality rates were 7.9 (7.3)%, 11.4 (8.4)% and 23.3 (13.8)%, respectively. In this study, the main causes of cardiac death within the first 30 days were cardiogenic shock and anoxic brain injury. After 30 days, causes of death were predominantly noncardiac, with malignancies and pulmonary diseases dominating.

Other risk factors are discussed below:

TIMI flow grade—Patients with normal blood flow in the infarcted artery at the end of the procedure have a better prognosis than those who do not.

Electrocardiographic markers—Electrocardiographic markers can successfully predict outcome in the broad range of patients with ST-elevation myocardial infarction. The prognostic utility of six different methods for evaluating the extent of ST-segment elevation resolution after PCI was assessed in 4866 patients enrolled in the APEX-AMI trial. All six methods were successful in predicting outcomes of death or the composite of death, cardiogenic shock or heart failure at 90 days. One of these, the measurement of the residual, absolute ST elevation in the single, most affected (worst) lead 30 min after PCI, performed as well as the more complex methods.

Infarct size—Larger infarct size after PPCI is associated with worse outcomes. In a patient-level meta-analysis of ten randomized trials of primary PCI in which infarct size was assessed with cardiac magnetic resonance imaging or technetium-99 m sestaMIBI single-photon emission computed tomography within 1 month of STEMI, the following was noted:

- Median infarct size (percent of left ventricular myocardial mass) was 17.9%.
- One-year estimates of all-cause mortality, re-infarction and heart failure hospitalization were 2.2%, 2.5% and 2.6%, respectively.
- There was a strong, graded response between infarct size and mortality and hospitalization for heart failure at 1 year.

Other risk factors—Other risk factors including Killip class, age and the number of diseased vessels are also important. These parameters have been incorporated into three risk models that have been prospectively validated: the Zwolle risk index, the TIMI risk score and the CADILLAC risk score.

3.10 What Is New in the ESC 2017 Guidelines on AMI-STEMI? New/Revised Concepts

Strategy Selection and Time Delays:

- Clear definition of first medical contact (FMC).
- Definition of "time 0" to choose reperfusion strategy (i.e. the strategy clock starts at the time of "STEMI diagnosis").
- Selection of PCI over fibrinolysis: when anticipated delay from "STEMI diagnosis" to wire crossing is ≤120 min.
- Maximum delay time from "STEMI diagnosis" to bolus of fibrinolysis agent is set in 10 min.
- "Door-to-balloon" term eliminated from guidelines.
- **See** www.escardio.org/guidelines **2017 ESC Guidelines for the Management of AMI-STEMI (European Heart Journal 2017—doi:10.1093/eurheartj/ehx095).**

3.11 Summary

The following conclusions can be reached from the clinical trials and observational studies discussed above:

- Primary percutaneous coronary intervention (PPCI) with stenting, if performed in a timely manner, is associated with better outcomes than fibrinolysis.
- The time from symptom onset to PCI has not been shown to be an important determinant of outcome. At the least, the benefit from PPCI is less dependent upon the time from symptom onset than is fibrinolysis.
- The time from hospital arrival to PCI (D2B) is an important determinant of benefit, with the best outcomes occurring when the time to PCI is 90 min or less. This measure is likely to be replaced with the greater use of FMC.
- Increasing system delay is associated with worse outcomes.
- Patients who are transferred to a PCI centre have better outcomes than those treated with fibrinolysis at the presenting hospital if PPCI is delivered according to guideline standards. Destination protocols for emergency medical system that bypass non-PPCI-capable hospitals and thereby shorten system delays to PPCI have been associated with improved outcomes in ST-elevation myocardial infarction.
- Hospitals should adapt strategies to reduce door-to-balloon times and thereby improve outcomes in STEMI patients treated with PPCI.
- Late PCI to open an occluded artery should be considered in patients with severe heart failure, hemodynamic or electrical instability or persistent ischemic symptoms.

- PPCI should not be performed in hospitals without on-site cardiac surgery unless they meet specific criteria, including having a proven plan for rapid transport to a cardiac surgery operating room in a nearby hospital and having appropriate haemodynamic support capability for transfer.

Conclusion

The acute ischaemia caused by SCAD in the left circumflex artery in this case acts as a physical and emotional stressor resulting in TC. Hence postischaemic myocardial stunning from SCAD may induce TC, and SCAD-induced MI may trigger rather than exclude TC.

Further Readings

Lambert L, Brown K, Segal E, et al. Association between timeliness of reperfusion therapy and clinical outcomes in ST-elevation myocardial infarction. JAMA. 2010;303:2148.

Terkelsen CJ, Sørensen JT, Maeng M, et al. System delay and mortality among patients with STEMI treated with primary percutaneous coronary intervention. JAMA. 2010;304:763.

www.escardio.org/guidelines 2017 ESC Guidelines for the Management of AMI-STEMI (European Heart Journal 2017. doi:https://doi.org/10.1093/eurheartj/ehx095)

4 ST-Elevation Myocardial Infarction Networks and Logistics: Rural and Urban

Jithendra B. Somaratne, James T. Stewart, Peter N. Ruygrok, and Mark W. Webster

4.1 Introduction

The facilities and expertise required for primary percutaneous coronary intervention (PPCI) of the infarct-related artery (IRA) in patients with ST-elevation myocardial infarction (STEMI) are only available at a limited number of hospitals. Fibrinolytic therapy, on the other hand, is more widely deliverable. This creates two distinct reperfusion choices: PPCI or a pharmacoinvasive strategy. The first option relies on immediate transfer to the closest PPCI-capable centre even if it means bypassing a closer non-PPCI centre. The second option is the "drip and ship" strategy. It involves delivery of fibrinolytic therapy by a non-PPCI facility with rapid transfer to a PPCI-capable centre.

In patients with ST-elevation myocardial infarction (STEMI), the primary therapeutic goal is the prompt restoration of coronary blood flow and myocardial perfusion. This limits the total ischaemic time and, thereby, the extent of the myocardial injury. In patients presenting within 12 h of symptom onset, PPCI undertaken within 120 min of diagnosis is the preferred reperfusion strategy. It leads to higher rates of IRA patency and thrombolysis in myocardial infarction (TIMI) 3 flow with lower rates of recurrent ischaemia, reinfarction, emergency repeat revascularisation, intracranial haemorrhage and death. This superiority over fibrinolytic therapy was observed when the delay to treatment was short and when patients were treated in high-volume centres by high-volume operators.

The choice of reperfusion strategy depends mainly on the time delays to treatment (Fig. 4.1), which can be categorised into patient- and system-related delays.

J. B. Somaratne (✉) · J. T. Stewart · P. N. Ruygrok · M. W. Webster
Green Lane Cardiovascular Service, Auckland City Hospital, Auckland, New Zealand

Auckland Mail Centre, Auckland, New Zealand

Green Lane Cardiovascular Service, Auckland City Hospital, Auckland, New Zealand
e-mail: jithendra.somaratne@adhb.govt.nz

T. J. Watson et al. (eds.), *Primary Angioplasty*,
https://doi.org/10.1007/978-981-13-1114-7_4

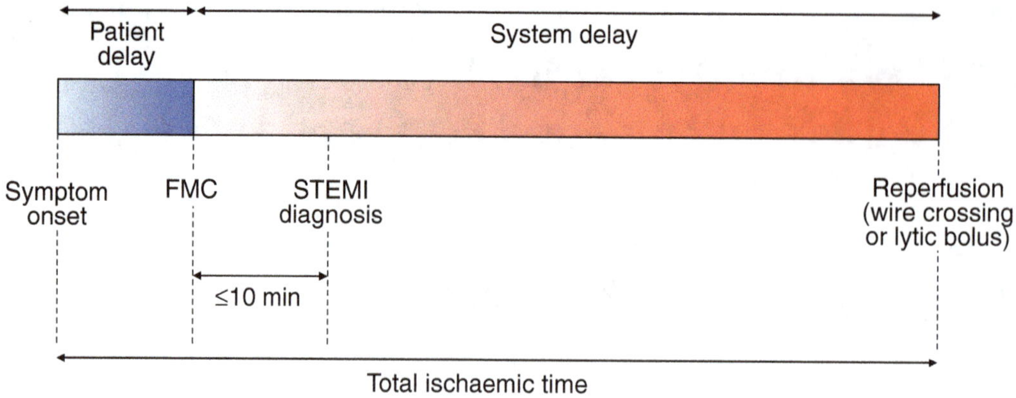

Fig. 4.1 Components of delay in management of patients with STEMI. *FMC* first medical contact, *STEMI* ST-elevation myocardial infarction

Patient delay accounts for the time taken from symptom onset to first medical contact (FMC). The widely accepted definition of FMC is the time of first assessment by a healthcare professional who is able to obtain and interpret a 12-lead electrocardiogram (ECG) and deliver initial interventions. System delay refers to the time from FMC to reperfusion. The time of reperfusion is defined as the commencement of fibrinolytic administration or, in the case of primary PCI, initial wire crossing. The benefit of fibrinolytic therapy has not been established in the context of patient delay >12 h. It could be considered if there is no possibility of PPCI and the patient has ongoing symptoms, particularly when there is a large area of myocardium at risk or there is haemodynamic instability. When the patient delay is between 12 and 48 h, a routine PPCI strategy is recommended. There is no role for PCI to an occluded IRA when the patient delay is >48 h and there are no ongoing symptoms. The task of minimising patient delay rests primarily with public health services. Steps to achieving the goal of reduced delay include increasing public awareness of common symptoms of myocardial ischaemia and the need for early recognition and activation of emergency medical services (EMS). In patients presenting within 12 h of symptom onset, anticipated system delay is the key determinant of reperfusion strategy (Fig. 4.2). If PPCI can be realistically achieved within 120 min of diagnosis, it is clearly preferred to fibrinolytic therapy. On the other hand, a pharmacoinvasive strategy should be adopted if the system delay associated with PPCI is expected to be >120 min.

The well-established relationship between system delay and mortality led to numerous efforts to accelerate the delivery of care. One of the most important advances in addressing system delay is the development of STEMI regional networks or systems of care, which are designed to enhance rapid recognition of STEMI and enable timely reperfusion therapy. Not all hospitals will have the capacity to provide a 24-h PPCI service in any given region. The reasons for this are twofold. Firstly, it is neither practical nor cost-effective to have multiple PPCI services operating within the same region. It leads to duplication of services, a reduction in efficiency and possible confusion of EMS regarding the most appropriate

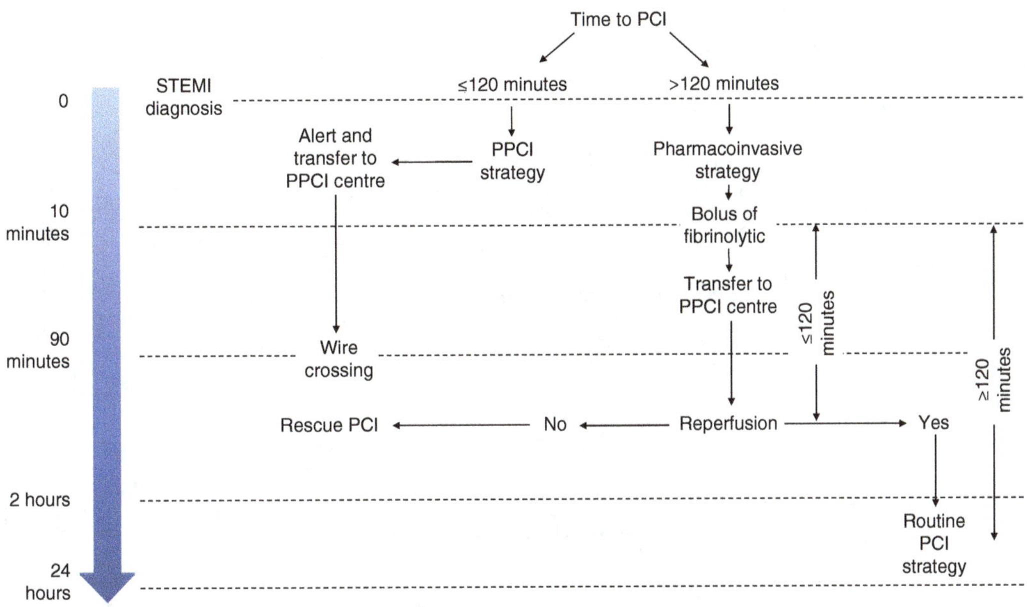

Fig. 4.2 Reperfusion strategy selection and timing. *PCI* percutaneous coronary intervention, *PPCI* primary percutaneous coronary intervention, *STEMI* ST-elevation myocardial infarction

destination. In smaller hospitals, a 24-h PPCI roster may not be possible due to limited staffing. Secondly, there is a need to maintain high operator and institutional case volumes given the link between higher volume and better outcomes. These factors support a hub-and-spoke model of care. The hub is the PPCI-capable centre and the spokes are services that do not have PPCI capability. Each node of the network is linked by technology and by a prioritised and efficient EMS. It relies heavily on active multidisciplinary collaboration between cardiologists, emergency physicians and EMS. A well-organised regional network reduces system delay by using simple management algorithms that are locally developed, practical and acceptable to all stakeholders.

This chapter will describe the organisation and implementation of STEMI networks including the need for ongoing quality control initiatives. A case study is presented to highlight key ideas.

4.2 Organisation of a Regional ST-Elevation Myocardial Infarction Network

A successful STEMI network requires the close interaction of local services. They must be capable of responding to differences in patient presentation and geography (Fig. 4.3). For instance, some patients will self-present to a nearby primary care service or emergency department (ED), while others will call the EMS. The management of these patients will also depend on patient delay and their proximity to a PPCI service at the time they seek medical attention. The essential

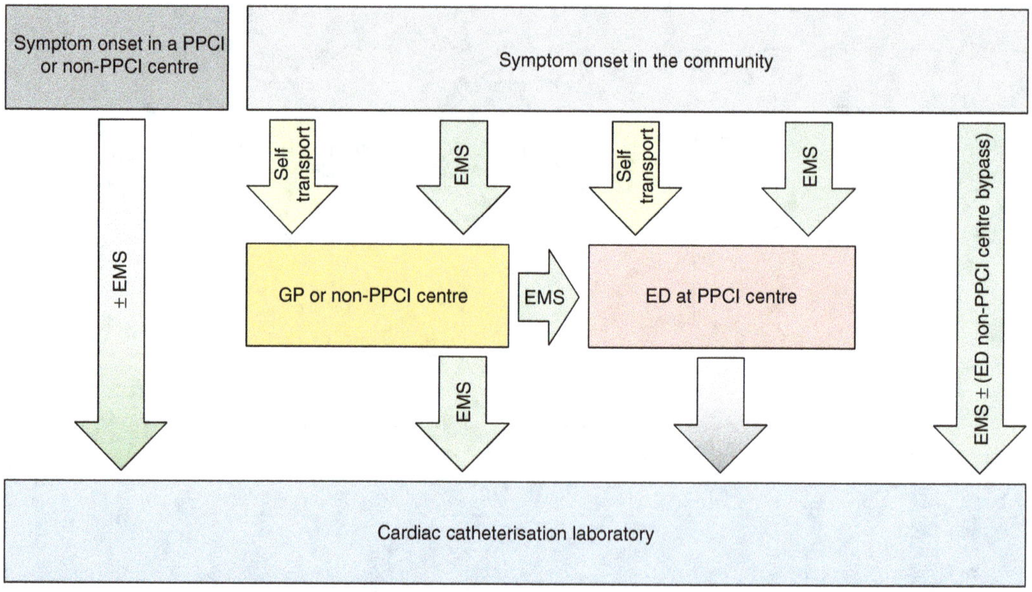

Fig. 4.3 Modes of patient presentation and transfer for primary percutaneous coronary intervention. *ED* emergency department, *EMS* emergency medical service, *GP* general practitioner, *PPCI* primary percutaneous coronary intervention

components of a network are the EMS, primary care facility or non-PPCI-capable centre, ED at a PPCI-capable centre and the cardiac catheterisation laboratory (CCL).

4.3 Emergency Medical Service

The EMS has an important role in early management patients with STEMI, which has evolved from patient transportation to include expedited initial diagnosis, triage and initiation of treatment. Depending upon the geography of the network, transfer of patients to a CCL may require a combination of transport modalities including road ambulances, helicopters and fixed-wing aeroplanes. The EMS may be staffed by suitably trained physicians, nurses or paramedics who are capable of basic and advanced life support.

To facilitate early diagnosis, EMS need to be equipped with a 12-lead ECG recorder and have trained personnel to acquire and interpret a trace correctly. This involves the correct application of leads, operation of the ECG recorder and recognition of different patterns consistent with STEMI or equivalent. Occasionally, paramedic interpretation of the ECG is not possible due to lack of training or experience. In this situation, the diagnosis may be based upon computer algorithm interpretation or physician interpretation of a transmitted ECG. While the computer algorithm output is easy to obtain, it is limited by a higher rate of erroneous interpretations. Wireless transmission and physician interpretation, on the other hand, have the highest level of interpretation accuracy and afford the opportunity for early physician direction of management. Wireless transmission requires transmitting and receiving technology at both ends as well as an available physician for interpretation at the receiving centre. This system is vulnerable to network and technologic failures.

Once the diagnosis has been established, the EMS needs a clear destination protocol to guide transportation to the most appropriate facility. For example, such protocols may authorise EMS units to bypass closer non-PPCI centres and take patients directly to a CCL.

Patients with STEMI are at higher risk of fatal arrhythmias such as ventricular tachycardia (VT) or ventricular fibrillation (VF). Accordingly, EMS providers must have the ability to undertake continuous cardiac rhythm monitoring and administer shocks with an external defibrillator.

Even though PPCI is often the preferred reperfusion strategy, rural paramedics, in particular, should be qualified to administer fibrinolytic therapy. If the delay associated with PPCI is expected to be >120 min, prehospital fibrinolysis is indicated.

4.4 Primary Care Service or Non-primary Percutaneous Coronary Intervention Centre

Sometimes patients with chest pain will transport themselves in a private vehicle to their local primary care service or the ED at a nearby non-PPCI hospital. These facilities are usually capable of recording and interpreting a 12-lead ECG. When a STEMI is diagnosed, the EMS should be activated and initial therapy commenced. This may include opioids and antithrombotic drugs including fibrinolysis. Yet, in comparison to a direct call to the EMS, self-presentation to a non-PPCI-capable facility is usually associated with a greater time delay to reperfusion. As such, patients with symptoms suggestive of a myocardial infarction should be discouraged from transporting themselves to a medical centre, by public health campaigns to raise awareness and understanding.

4.5 Emergency Department at a Primary Percutaneous Coronary Intervention Centre

The major tasks of an ED at a hospital that is PPCI-capable in patients with STEMI relate to diagnosis, initial therapy and immediate transfer to the CCL.

While there may be no doubt about the diagnosis in the majority of patients with STEMI brought into the ED by EMS, some may have an ambiguous clinical presentation. In this scenario, the ED staff assess the patient and clarify the diagnosis, in consultation with the cardiology service. In others, an alternate diagnosis may be found, and the ED physicians redirect patient care accordingly. Infrequently, the ED discover significant comorbidities (e.g. terminal cancer) that warrant de-escalation of care and adoption of a conservative approach. There are patients who present directly to the ED with chest pain. The ED team makes the initial diagnosis of STEMI for such patients.

The two main initial therapies delivered in the ED are symptom relief and antithrombotic therapy. Pain relief is useful to minimise patient discomfort and reduce sympathetic activation. Intravenous opioids such as morphine are used for analgesia. Routine oxygen is no longer indicated although it should be administered in the context of hypoxia ($SpO_2 < 90\%$). Patients are loaded with dual antiplatelet therapy in the form of aspirin and a $P2Y_{12}$ inhibitor (clopidogrel, prasugrel or ticagrelor). Depending on the local protocol, heparin or enoxaparin may also be given in the ED.

In the context of PPCI, the main role of the ED is to facilitate rapid patient transfer to the CCL. If the CCL is available and ready to receive, the patient should bypass ED altogether. However, this approach may not be achievable at all times. For instance, the CCL may be occupied by another patient or the on-call CCL team may not have arrived at the hospital. In this scenario, the ED performs the function of a holding bay until the patient can be transferred to the CCL. While the patient is waiting in ED, possible arterial access sites for coronary angiography should be prepared and initial blood samples sent to the laboratory for assessment. During this time, the patient is carefully observed with continuous cardiac monitoring and defibrillator nearby. The routine insertion of central venous or arterial access should be avoided as it often unnecessary and delays transfer to the CCL.

4.6 Cardiac Catheterisation Laboratory

The CCL is the final common destination for patients with STEMI within a regional network. Each region requires a CCL that is operational at all times even when the hospital is at maximum bed occupancy or the ED is closed due to overcapacity. It is recommended that each network has a single PPCI centre. There are a number of other more complex and less ideal models that may be employed. For instance, in some networks there are multiple PPCI centres or rotation of PPCI centre on a daily or weekly basis. The most recent European Society of Cardiology guidelines for the management of patients with STEMI recommend that any CCL that cannot offer 24-h service should be discouraged from offering PPCI. It is argued that the presence of daytime-only PPCI services may lead to confusion of EMS, affect the quality of intervention and increase system delay. The exception should be for patients admitted to those hospitals for a different reason that develop a STEMI during their hospital stay. However, this model is refuted by those belonging to networks in which alternate arrangements work well. A designated CCL for PPCI within a network should preferably be in a central geographic location within the region. Once the patient arrives on site, easy access to the CCL from the ambulance bay, helipad and ED enhances rapid transfer. Though patients with STEMI rarely require urgent surgical revascularisation, an on-site cardiac surgical facility is an advantage. The support provided by dedicated cardiac intensivists and cardiac anaesthetists at surgical centres is particularly useful when managing critically unwell patients in the CCL. The on-call CCL team usually comprises an interventional cardiologist, scrub nurse, circulating nurse, cardiac technologist and cardiac radiographer.

4.7 Implementation of a Regional ST-elevation Myocardial Infarction Network

Over the last decade, there have been a number of initiatives around the world to develop and implement regional networks with the goal of improving the care of patients with STEMI in accordance with current guidelines. For example, in North America, the American Heart Association promoted Mission: Lifeline® and the American College of Cardiology ran the Door-to-Balloon (D2B): An Alliance for Quality campaign. Similarly, in Europe, the Stent for Life Initiative was a combined joint program by the European Society of Cardiology. To meet the tight guideline-based target times for reperfusion, these initiatives have outlined a number of helpful approaches.

Prior to the designing and implementing a regional network, the Stent for Life Initiative recommends understanding existing local practice with regard to patients with STEMI. This investigation should seek to accurately establish the following statistics:

- Rates of STEMI
- Total number of patients with STEMI per annum
- Number and location of PPCI centres
- Ratio of PPCI centres to overall population
- Time taken patients to arrive at a PPCI centre
- Geographic constraints
- Modes of patient transportation
- Existing transportation protocols
- Equipment available on ambulances
- Level of training EMS personnel
- Proportion of the population served by a PPCI centre within a 90-min travel window
- Variation in the quality of service within the region
- Number of participating interventional cardiologists
- Number of interventional cardiologists per capita
- Reperfusion rates
- Mortality rate

Using the accumulated data, barriers to the delivery of timely reperfusion therapy can be identified. For instance, some of the commonly reported barriers include:

- Insufficient number of 24-h CCLs available for PPCI
- Lack of even geographic distribution of PPCI centres with overconcentration in urban areas
- Variation in the management of patients with STEMI throughout the region
- Delayed or inappropriate EMS response (such as non-adherence to the destination protocol)

- Inadequately equipped or trained EMS
- Lack of EMS motivation to participate in network plans and protocols
- Commercial bias where there are too many CCL offering 24-h PPCI service
- Lack of quality control initiatives
- Poor public awareness of STEMI symptoms leading to delay in seeking medical attention
- Lack of a national registry
- Ineffectual communication and poor collaboration between key stakeholders within network

Once local barriers to timely care have been identified, the next step is to define realistic objectives and prioritise them. For example, the primary objective may be to initially develop a network focussed on a small region. Other possible objectives include setting up a quality control and feedback system or increasing public awareness about the symptoms warranting immediate medical attention. With these objectives in place, a strategic plan should be developed to realise each of them. Such planning has to involve all stakeholders in the networks including medical, transportation, industry and political partners.

Over the last decade, as it has become clear that treatment delays are associated with worse outcome in patients with STEMI, a number of strategies to minimise system delay were examined. Some of the successful approaches that reduce door-to-balloon time and thereby system delay are detailed below.

1. A careful and clear definition of geographic areas of responsibility reduces misunderstanding between each of the stakeholders in a regional network.
2. The use of a prehospital 12-lead ECG to activate the CCL while the patient is in route to the hospital allows time for the team to arrive and prepare to receive the patient in the CCL.
3. Limiting the number of stops on the patient journey from the community to the CCL reduces system delay. At times this will require the EMS to bypass nearby non-PPCI hospitals when a diagnosis of STEMI has been made. Likewise, on arrival at the appropriate hospital, bypassing the ED and heading straight to the CCL saves time. If a prehospital diagnosis was not made, the EMS should await the diagnosis in ED and immediately transfer the patient to a PPCI-capable hospital if the diagnosis is STEMI.
4. A discussion of the case and ECG findings by the ED physician with either a general cardiologist or interventional cardiologist prior to the activation of CCL incurs unnecessary delay. The ideal scenario is that the ED physician diagnoses the STEMI and activates the CCL immediately with consultation only when there is doubt.
5. Current laboratory and radiographic results should not be a prerequisite for activation of the CCL. Waiting for these results to be available leads to a further avoidable delay.
6. Using a single-call system to activate the CCL saves time. Typically, the call is to the hospital switchboard operator who then contacts each member of the

CCL team. A return call can be made by the operator to the activating individual to confirm that the whole team has been notified. An even better option, if available, would be a simultaneous automatic activation system. This bypasses the operator and delivers the activation message simultaneously to each team member.

7. An expectation that the CCL team be available within 20 min of being paged and priority hospital parking during off-hours ensures that CCL staff-related delays are avoided. At some centres, the team is expected to be on site throughout the duration of their on-call period.
8. The initiation of patient transport from ED to CCL after a set time interval following activation rather than awaiting notification that the CCL team are ready was successful at reducing door-to-device time. Another approach is to transport the patient to the CCL when a minimum number of the CCL team arrive. Someone must always available to transport patients from ED to CCL. Whatever the approach adopted, a direct wireless phone line between an ED staff member and a CCL staff member facilitates communication and efficiency of patient transfer.
9. Each regional STEMI network is based on the collaboration of multiple organisations including hospitals, EMS and primary care facilities. The overall success of the network relies on the performance of each organisation. This, in turn, requires the support of senior management and an organisational culture that fosters and sustains change directed at minimising system delays. For those dealing with patients with STEMI directly, having a team-based approach from ambulance to device and a culture of continuous quality improvement is also very useful.
10. A regular multidisciplinary team review of local data with prompt feedback to all involved staff (i.e. EMS, ED and CCL) helps to identify deficiencies in the network and prompts continuous quality improvement initiatives. When significant delays occur in the care of individual patients, the use of a root cause analysis or similar approach helps to prevent recurrences.

4.8 Quality Control

Contemporary guidelines emphasise the importance of robust quality control measures within regional STEMI networks. A useful tool to monitor networks within a country is a national acute coronary syndrome registry. It can be used to ensure that simple quality of care indicators are met and maintained over time. The registry should record demographic data, relevant time points for the calculation of treatment delays, PPCI penetration, morbidity and mortality. Of these parameters, treatment delays are the most straightforward index of quality to audit. A simple comparison of practices and outcomes across different regions and within each region helps to identify outliers. If the continuously recorded quality of care indicators fall short of agreed benchmarks, then specific interventions addressing deficiencies should be devised and implemented to improve the performance of system. The data should be reviewed on a regular basis (e.g. quarterly). All major stakeholders in the network should receive feedback.

4.9 Case Study

The Northern Regional STEMI Network in New Zealand (NZ) includes both the Auckland and Northland regions. The Auckland region has a land area of 4894 km^2 and a population of 1,657,200 in June 2017. This represents the highest population and second smallest land area of any region of NZ. It also has the largest economy in the country. The Northland region has land area of 13,789 km^2 and a population of 175,500 in June 2017. The public hospitals and other health services in NZ are administered by district health boards (DHBs). There are 20 DHBs throughout the country and each is governed by a board of up to 11 members. They plan, manage, provide and purchase health services for the population of their district. The largely urban Auckland region has three DHBs: Auckland DHB (ADHB), Counties Manukau DHB (CMDHB) and Waitemata DHB (WDHB). The population of Northland is largely rural and is serviced by Northland DHB (NDHB). The Northern Regional STEMI Network is comprised of these four DHBs. Each is autonomous and has its own protocols for STEMI. The three urban DHBs (ADHB, CMDHB and WDHB) have CCLs that provide a PPCI service during standard working hours. However, ADHB has the only CCL in the network that offers a 24-h PPCI service. It is also the only one of the four to have on-site cardiac surgery. The NDHB does not have a CCL, and contracts ADHB for all cardiac catheterisation services. Patients with STEMI residing within the Northland region are transported to ADHB via helicopter. Within the Auckland region, PPCI within 120 min of STEMI diagnosis is feasible in the vast majority of patients. As a result, the default reperfusion strategy throughout the region is PPCI. The STEMI protocols for patients residing in the Northland region are necessarily more complex. The much smaller population of Northland is more widely spread out across a larger area. Patients self-presenting to or brought in by EMS to Whangarei Hospital, NDHB's base hospital, receive fibrinolytic therapy unless there is a contraindication. They are then transferred to ADHB for coronary angiography and PCI as indicated. At other smaller hospitals within the NDHB, the anticipated time delay to PPCI is considered and discussed with the on-call interventional cardiologist. If the delay to PPCI is expected to be over 120 min, fibrinolytic therapy is administered, and the patient is transferred to ADHB soon after. Alternately, if the delay is calculated by the EMS to be less than 120 min, the local hospital is bypassed, and the patient is transferred urgently by helicopter to ADHB for PPCI. In the meantime, the on-call CCL team is activated to meet the patient in the CCL on arrival. All out-of-hours (5 p.m. to 8 a.m. and weekends; 73% of the week) PPCI for patients residing within the Auckland and Northland regions are undertaken in the CCL at ADHB. In a unique collaboration, the four interventional cardiologists from WDHB and the three interventional cardiologists from CMDHB join the four interventional cardiologists from ADHB in a network-wide on-call roster. Out-of-hours there is always one interventional cardiologist on call. The on-call CCL team includes a scrub nurse, circulating nurse, cardiac technologist and cardiac radiographer who are all employed by ADHB and work there during standard working hours. The on-call interventional cardiologist can be contacted on a dedicated free call number that is diverted to his/her mobile phone. The on-call interventional cardiologist or ED physician at ADHB is able to activate the CCL by contacting the operator at ADHB. In turn, the operator contacts each individual team member and often confirms with the interventional cardiologist that every team member has been contacted. There is an expectation that every member of the team, including the interventional cardiologist, should arrive within 20 min of the call-out. The individual data for all patients treated within the network are entered electronically into a national registry known as the All NZ Acute Coronary Syndrome Quality Improvement (ANZACS-QI) registry. The data concerning patients with STEMI are analysed and presented to stakeholders on a quarterly basis. In addition, regular network meetings every 6 weeks provide a forum for the discussion of specific concerns as they arise.

4.10 Summary

The management of patients with STEMI is time critical. The choice of reperfusion strategy is contingent upon patient and system delay. Primary PCI is preferred over a pharmacoinvasive approach when the anticipated system delay is short. While public health initiatives help to reduce patient delay, system delay is minimised by well-designed effective regional networks or systems of care. These systems rely on the collaboration of a number of local services such as the EMS, non-PPCI facilities and PPCI hospitals. They lead to better patient outcomes by reducing the time to diagnosis and treatment. Within networks, continuous quality control initiatives with regular feedback to all stakeholders are vital to maintain standards and improve the service.

Further Readings

Bradley EH, Roumanis SA, Radford MJ, Webster TR, McNamara RL, Mattera JA, et al. Achieving door-to-balloon times that meet quality guidelines: how do successful hospitals do It? J Am Coll Cardiol. 2005;46(7):1236–41.

Bradley EH, Herrin J, Wang Y, Barton BA, Webster TR, Mattera JA, et al. Strategies for reducing the door-to-balloon time in acute myocardial infarction. N Engl J Med. 2006;355(22):2308–20.

Bradley EH, Nallamothu BK, Curtis JP, Webster TR, Magid DJ, Granger CB, et al. Summary of evidence regarding hospital strategies to reduce door-to-balloon times for patients with ST-segment elevation myocardial infarction undergoing primary percutaneous coronary intervention. Crit Pathw Cardiol. 2007;6(3):91–7.

Danchin N. Systems of care for ST-segment elevation myocardial infarction: impact of different models on clinical outcomes. JACC Cardiovasc Interv. 2009;2(10):901–8.

Holmes DR, Bell MR, Gersh BJ, Rihal CS, Haro LH, Bjerke CM, et al. Systems of care to improve timeliness of reperfusion therapy for ST-segment elevation myocardial infarction during off hours: the Mayo Clinic STEMI protocol. JACC Cardiovasc Interv. 2008;1(1):88–96.

Ibanez B, James S, Agewall S, Antunes MJ, Bucciarelli-Ducci C, Bueno H, et al. ESC guidelines for the management of acute myocardial infarction in patients presenting with ST-segment elevationThe task force for the management of acute myocardial infarction in patients presenting with ST-segment elevation of the European Society of Cardiology (ESC). Eur Heart J. 2017;33(20):2569–619.

Knot J, Widimsky P, Wijns W, Stenestrand U, Kristensen SD, Van THA, et al. How to set up an effective national primary angioplasty network: lessons learned from five European countries. EuroIntervention. 2009;5(3):299, 301–9.

Nestler DM, Noheria A, Haro LH, Stead LG, Decker WW, Scanlan-Hanson LN, et al. Sustaining improvement in door-to-balloon time over 4 years. Circ Cardiovasc Qual Outcomes. 2009;2(5):508.

O'Gara PT, Kushner FG, Ascheim DD, Casey DE, Chung MK, de Lemos JA, et al. 2013 ACCF/AHA guideline for the management of ST-elevation myocardial infarction. A report of the American College of Cardiology Foundation/American Heart Association task force on practice guidelines. Circulation. 2013;127(4):e362–425.

Utilization of PCI After Fibrinolysis

5

Peter McKavanagh, George Zawadowski, and Warren J. Cantor

5.1 Introduction

It is estimated that there are 1.5 million hospitalizations with acute coronary syndromes (ACS) per year in the United States, with 30–45% being a ST-segment elevation myocardial infarction (STEMI) presentation [1, 2]. STEMI occurs due to an acute occlusion of an infarct-related artery (IRA) that can cause irreversible ischemia-induced myocardial necrosis within 20–60 min of onset. Untreated STEMI patients have higher mortality and poor clinical outcomes compared to those who receive a reperfusion strategy [3–10]. The mainstay of STEMI management is rapid intervention aimed at relieving the IRA thrombotic obstruction and thus reducing infarct size, preserving left ventricular function, and decreasing morbidity and mortality. In the 1980s, fibrinolysis became the standard means to achieve reperfusion. Subsequently, a number of randomized trials and meta-analyses showed that primary PCI (PPCI), when performed rapidly, was associated with improved clinical outcomes compared to fibrinolytic therapy [11–18]. However, the mortality benefit of primary PCI is reduced with treatment delays, with no benefit observed when the difference between time of fibrinolysis and time of PCI exceeds 115 min [19, 20]. Current guidelines recommend the use of fibrinolytic therapy when the time from first medical contact to PCI is anticipated to be greater than 120 min [17, 18]. Despite these recommendations, data from the US National Cardiovascular Data Registry showed that only 51% of STEMI patients transferred for primary PCI

P. McKavanagh
Ulster Hospital, Belfast, UK

G. Zawadowski
Interventional Cardiology, St. Michael's Hospital, University of Toronto, Toronto, ON, Canada

W. J. Cantor (✉)
Southlake Regional Health Centre, University of Toronto, Toronto, ON, Canada
e-mail: cantorw@rogers.com

T. J. Watson et al. (eds.), *Primary Angioplasty*,
https://doi.org/10.1007/978-981-13-1114-7_5

achieved the recommended first door-to-balloon time of <120 min [21]. Similar European data show that 65% of transferred patients had a delay of >120 min, which was associated with increased mortality [22].

Many strategies have been developed to increase the number of patients who can undergo timely primary PCI, including prehospital identification of STEMI and establishment of networks that allow ambulances to bypass the closest hospital and take patients directly to PCI facilities [23–34]. Nevertheless, there will always be a cohort of patients who are too far from PCI centers, and fibrinolytic therapy remains the treatment of choice for these patients [35, 36]. Transporting patients to a PCI center for routine early PCI after fibrinolysis, the so-called pharmacoinvasive strategy, has been shown to reduce the risks of reinfarction and recurrent ischemia with no increase in major bleeding. Within the literature, there exist examples of successful implementation of a combined primary PCI and pharmacoinvasive strategies depending on patient distance from facilities [37], with regional systems proposed [38]. This chapter addresses the evidence for PCI after fibrinolytic therapy, illustrating how and when it should be used.

5.2 Fibrinolytic Therapy

The use of fibrinolytic therapy in STEMI is long established, with pioneering work in 1976 by Chazov et al. showing benefit [39]. Prior to the development of fibrinolytic therapy, treatment of STEMI was limited to analgesia, antiplatelets, anticoagulants, and blood pressure management. The use of fibrinolytic therapy became the standard practice after the pivotal randomized clinical trials Gruppo Italiano per lo Studio della Streptochinasi nell'Infarto Miocardico (GISSI) and Second International Study of Infarct Survival (ISIS-2) [40, 41]. These two studies used intravenous streptokinase (SK) showing a mortality benefit when compared to placebo, especially in combination with aspirin. Based on these studies, SK became standard treatment for STEMI. However there remained concerns about bleeding and limited efficacy, leading to the development of fibrin-specific fibrinolytic agents. These included tissue plasminogen activator (alteplase) [42, 43], recombinant plasminogen activator (reteplase) [44, 45], and tenecteplase [46]. Overall there have been over 40 trials comparing different fibrinolytic regimens. A recent meta-analysis indicated that the lowest mortality and bleeding rates were seen with the use of reteplase, alteplase, and tenecteplase in combination with parenteral anticoagulant therapy [47].

The main advantage of fibrinolytic therapy is the ease of administration, which includes the ability to be given in small rural hospitals and in the prehospital setting. It is most effective when administered early (especially within the first 2 h of symptom onset). To help with appropriate administration, there are time recommendations for each step (Table 5.1). There are however substantial limitations of fibrinolytic therapy, and it is essential that its use is appropriate (Figs. 5.1 and 5.2). Firstly, there is risk of major bleed, including intracranial bleeding, with SK having the highest risk [47]. Secondly, only 40–50% of all patients treated with fibrinolytic

Table 5.1 Time targets for fibrinolytic therapy

Intervals	Time targets
Maximum time from FMC to 1st ECG and STEMI diagnosis	≤10 min
Maximum time from STEMI diagnosis to fibrinolytic therapy	≤10 min
Time from fibrinolytic therapy to assessment of reperfusion efficacy	60–90 min
Time from fibrinolytic therapy to angiography (if fibrinolysis is successful)	2–24 h

FMC first medical contact. Adapted from 2017 ESC STEMI Guidelines [17]

Indications:
- Chest pain or other ischemic symptoms < 12 hours duration
- Persistent ST elevation in ≥ 2 contiguous leads
  - ≥ 2 mm in anterior leads (≥ 1.5mm in women)
  - ≥ 1 mm in inferior leads
  - Absence of LBBB, LVH or other STEMI mimics

Absolute Contraindications:
- Any prior intracranial hemorrhage
- Intracranial vascular or malignant lesion (AVM, tumour)
- Ischemic stroke within 3 months
- Sustained Hypertension: SBP > 180 or DBP > 110 mm Hg
- Active bleeding or bleeding diathesis (not incl menses)
- Significant closed head or facial trauma within 3 months

Relative Contraindications:
- Cardiogenic Shock
- Traumatic or prolonged CPR
- Major surgery within past 3 weeks
- Internal bleeding within past 4 weeks
- Active peptic ulcer disease
- Non-compressible vascular puncture
- Pregnancy
- Current use of anticoagulants

Fig. 5.1 Indications and contraindications for fibrinolytic therapy

1. Use Fibrin-specific Agent (Accelerated tPA, Reteplase, Tenecteplase)
2. Administer ASA 160 mg chewed, Clopidogrel 300 mg (75 mg if patient > 75 years of age)
3. Administer parenteral anticoagulant
   a. UFH 60 U/kg bolus (max 4000 U) then 12 U/kg per hour (max 1000 U/hr)
   b. Enoxaparin 30 mg IV plus 1mg/kg sc (Avoid for elderly patients or renal insufficiency)
   c. Fondaparinux IV bolus followed by 2.5 mg sc dose 24 hours later
4. Transfer patient to PCI center immediately after fibrinolytic therapy for pharmacoinvasive protocol if possible
5. If pharmacoinvasive strategy not possible, transfer to PCI hospital for hemodynamic instability or evidence of failed reperfusion (persistent chest pain or ST elevation) at 60-90 minutes after fibrinolysis

Fig. 5.2 Fibrinolysis checklist

therapy achieve normal TIMI (Thrombolysis in Myocardial Infarction) grade 3 flow, with this figure even lower in elderly patients or those with cardiogenic shock [48–51]. Even patients with TIMI grade 3 flow may have evidence of failed myocardial perfusion [52]. Noninvasive identification of successful reperfusion after fibrinolytic therapy is challenging, with limited positive and negative predictive values for resolution of chest pain and ST-segment elevation. Furthermore, approximately 5% of patients will reinfarct after initial successful reperfusion [53].

5.3 PCI-Based Approaches

Given these limitations of fibrinolytic therapy, and the time dependency of primary PCI, it has been questioned whether combining fibrinolytic therapy and PCI could be the ideal treatment strategy, particularly for patients who cannot undergo timely primary PCI. This combined strategy would minimize treatment delays using rapid administration of fibrinolytic therapy but also achieve complete and sustained reperfusion using PCI. The use of PCI after fibrinolytic therapy can be classified based on the timing and indications for PCI (Table 5.2).

5.3.1 Rescue PCI

Patients who have persistent chest pain and ST elevation after fibrinolytic therapy require urgent cardiac catheterization and rescue PCI to restore flow to the occluded infarct-related artery. Rescue PCI is indicated in the case of suspected failed fibrinolysis (i.e., ST-segment resolution <50% within 60–90 min of fibrinolytic administration) or hemodynamic instability [18]. The landmark rescue PCI trials were Rescue Angioplasty versus Conservative Treatment or Repeat Thrombolysis (REACT) and the Middlesbrough Early Revascularization to Limit Infarction (MERLIN) [54, 55]. REACT compared rescue PCI, medical management, and

Table 5.2 Reperfusion strategies combining fibrinolytic therapy and PCI

Strategy	Definition
Rescue PCI	Emergent PCI performed for failed reperfusion after fibrinolytic therapy
Facilitated PCI	Administration of fibrinolytic therapy (and/or GP IIb/IIIa inhibitors) prior to emergent PCI to bridge PCI-related time delays (PCI within 2 h of fibrinolytic therapy)
Pharmacoinvasive strategy	Administration of fibrinolytic therapy followed by immediate transfer to a PCI center; emergent PCI for patients with evidence of failed reperfusion, hemodynamic instability, or reinfarction; and PCI within 24 h of fibrinolytic therapy for patients who are stable with successful reperfusion

repeat fibrinolytic therapy for patients with clinical evidence of failed reperfusion after fibrinolysis. Rescue PCI was associated with a reduction in reinfarction, with no mortality difference between treatments. The trial was terminated prematurely raising concerns about the true benefit. MERLIN compared rescue PCI and conservative therapy but did not show significant reduction of the primary endpoint, all-cause mortality. In addition, in both trials, patients who underwent rescue PCI had increased bleeding. Meta-analyses have been performed to help guide practice. Patel et al. included five trials and found a 36% decrease in the risk of death with rescue PCI (RR 0.64, 95% confidence interval 0.41–1.00, $p = 0.048$) and a marginally significant 28% decrease in the risk of heart failure (RR 0.72, 95% confidence interval 0.51–1.01, $p = 0.06$) [56]. Wijeysundera et al. analyzed eight trials and found that rescue PCI was not associated with a significant reduction in mortality but was associated with significant reductions in heart failure (RR 0.73, 95% CI 0.54–1.00) and reinfarction (RR 0.58, 95% CI 0.35–0.97) when compared with conservative treatment [57]. Rescue PCI was also associated with an increased risk of stroke (RR 4.98, 95% CI 1.10–22.5) and minor bleeding. Another meta-analysis by Testa et al. had similar findings. Rescue PCI was associated with a 70% reduction in the risk of reinfarction [OR 0.32 (0.14–0.74), $p = 0.008$], with a number needed to treat of 17. On balance rescue PCI is superior to conservative therapy for patients with failed reperfusion after fibrinolytic therapy and has a Class I indication in the guidelines [17, 18].

5.3.2 Facilitated PCI

Initial attempts to routinely combine pharmacological reperfusion therapy and PCI focused on administering fibrinolytic agents and/or glycoprotein IIb/IIIa inhibitors to patients being transferred for immediate PCI to help bridge the treatment delay. This strategy was termed "facilitated PCI" and was assessed in two large randomized trials.

The Assessment of the Safety and Efficacy of a New Treatment Strategy with Percutaneous Coronary Intervention (ASSENT-4 PCI) randomized patients to either PPCI ($n = 838$) or facilitated PCI using full-dose tenecteplase ($n = 829$) [58]. The median time from tenecteplase to first balloon inflation was 104 min. The primary endpoint (death or congestive heart failure or shock within 90 days) was found in 19% of patients assigned to facilitated PCI vs. 13% of those randomized to PPCI (relative risk 1.39, 95% CI 1.11–1.74, $p = 0.0045$). During hospital stay, significantly more strokes (1.8% vs. 0, $p < 0.0001$) were reported in patients assigned to facilitated rather than standard PPCI. There were also more ischemic cardiac complications, such as reinfarction (6% vs. 4%, $p = 0.0279$) or repeat target vessel revascularization (7% vs. 3%, $p = 0.0041$) within 90 days.

The Facilitated Intervention with Enhanced Reperfusion Speed to Stop Events (FINESSE) study randomized 2452 patients to undergo facilitated PCI using a combination of abciximab plus half-dose reteplase, facilitated PCI using abciximab alone, or primary PCI [59]. The primary endpoint was the composite of death from all causes, ventricular fibrillation occurring more than 48 h after randomization, cardiogenic shock, and congestive heart failure during the first 90 days after randomization. The primary endpoint occurred in 9.8, 10.5, and 10.7% of the patients in the combination-facilitated PCI group, abciximab-facilitated PCI group, and primary PCI group, respectively ($p = 0.55$); 90-day mortality rates were 5.2, 5.5, and 4.5%, respectively ($p = 0.49$).

A meta-analysis comparing facilitated and primary percutaneous coronary intervention was published by Keeley et al.[60]. In this they identified 17 trials of patients with STEMI assigned to facilitated ($n = 2237$) or primary ($n = 2267$) PCI. The facilitated PCI group had higher rates of death (5% vs. 3%; 1.38, 1.01–1.87), nonfatal reinfarction rates (3% vs. 2%; 1.71, 1.16–2.51), and urgent target vessel revascularization rates (4% vs. 1%; 2.39, 1.23–4.66). Facilitated PCI was associated with higher rates of major bleeding than PPCI (7% vs. 5%; 1.51, 1.10–2.08). Hemorrhagic stroke was also higher in fibrinolytic therapy facilitated regimens compared with primary PCI (hemorrhagic stroke 0.7% vs. 0.1%, $p = 0.0014$; total stroke 1.1% vs. 0.3%, $p = 0.0008$). The overall conclusion was that facilitated PCI offers no benefit over PPCI and should be avoided.

There are several limitations of the facilitated PCI trials and meta-analysis. Firstly, FINESSE was not included in the meta-analysis, and thus more than half of the patients in the analysis came from the ASSENT-4 trial. Of the 17 trials, 9 used only glycoprotein IIb/IIIa inhibitors and no fibrinolytic, and of the remaining 8 fibrinolytic trials (except ASSENT-4), most of them were small and used balloon angioplasty without coronary stents. Another important limitation to these trials is the absence of up-front clopidogrel loading at the time of fibrinolysis. Fibrinolytic therapy increases platelet activation and aggregation, and without clopidogrel loading, PCI performed early after fibrinolysis may be predisposed toward thrombotic complications [61].

Most patients enrolled in the facilitated PCI studies underwent PCI within 120 min of fibrinolysis. Secondary analyses of the ASSENT-4 and FINESSE study suggested that there may be a subgroup of patients (such as high-risk patients who presented early to non-PCI hospitals) that could benefit from facilitated PCI [62, 63]. However there is no large dataset to support this, and facilitated PCI is not currently recommended in guidelines.

5.3.3 Pharmacoinvasive

The pharmacoinvasive strategy applies to STEMI patients who are treated with fibrinolysis at a non-PCI center. It involves transferring patients to a PCI center right after fibrinolysis (without waiting to see if reperfusion is successful), followed by routine early PCI. For those patients who successfully reperfuse with fibrinolytic therapy, early PCI prevents recurrent ischemia and reinfarction. In the case of failed reperfusion or clinical instability, the patient undergoes emergent PCI on arrival to the PCI center. Figure 5.3 is a checklist for the use of a pharmacoinvasive strategy.

A number of studies have compared routine early PCI after fibrinolysis with an ischemia-driven conservative strategy or delayed PCI [64–68]. The initial studies

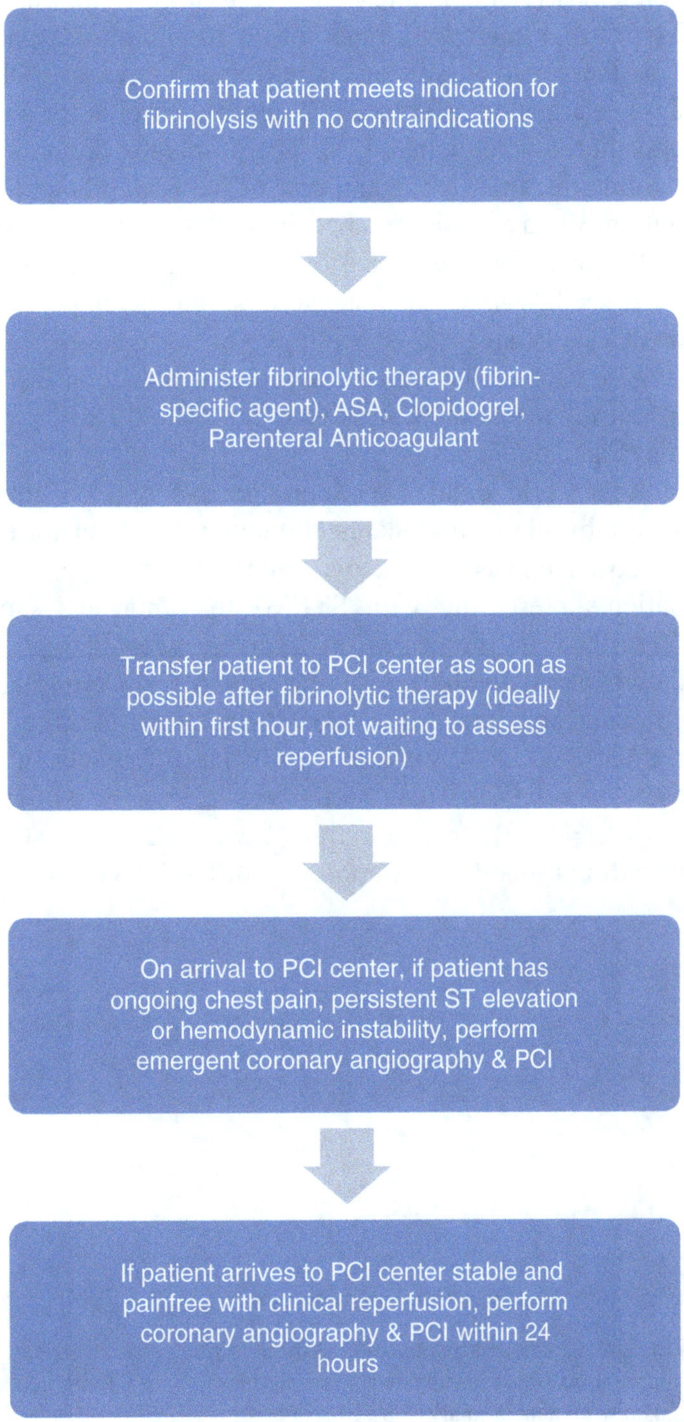

Fig. 5.3 Flow diagram for pharmacoinvasive strategy

were done prior to the use of coronary stents and antiplatelet agents that help maintain infarct artery patency and showed increased rates of emergency bypass surgery and higher mortality when PCI was performed routinely within 24 h of fibrinolysis [69]. Studies that were performed using contemporary PCI techniques (including coronary stenting) and pharmacotherapy have shown improved outcomes with routine early PCI after fibrinolysis [70].

The largest such randomized trial, TRANSFER-AMI (Trial of Routine Angioplasty and Stenting After Fibrinolysis to Enhance Reperfusion in Acute Myocardial Infarction), randomized 1059 high-risk patients who received fibrinolytic therapy to either usual care (including rescue PCI for failed fibrinolytic therapy) or urgent transfer to a PCI-capable hospital for a routine early PCI within 6 h after fibrinolytic therapy [71]. The primary endpoint—a composite of death, reinfarction, recurrent ischemia, new or worsening heart failure, or cardiogenic shock within 30 days—was reached in 17.2% of patients in the usual care group and 11.0% of patients assigned to an early invasive strategy (RR 0.64, 95% CI 0.47–0.87, $p = 0.004$). A meta-analysis of seven contemporary trials comparing a pharmacoinvasive strategy to ischemia-driven (or delayed) PCI after fibrinolytic therapy (Figure 5.1) demonstrated a significant reduction in death or MI at 6 months to 1 year in the pharmacoinvasive group, with no difference in stroke or major bleeding (Fig. 5.4) [72].

Real-world data from a prospective registry involving a rural population served by a large regional health network demonstrated the safety and efficacy of a pharmacoinvasive strategy. Two thousand six hundred twenty-four consecutive patients presenting with STEMI to a non-PCI-capable hospital, more than 60 miles from the nearest PCI center, received aspirin, clopidogrel, unfractionated heparin, and half-dose fibrinolysis and were transferred for PCI. When outcomes were compared to STEMI patients presenting directly to PCI centers for primary PCI, there were no significant differences in 30-day mortality (5.5% vs. 5.6%, $p = 0.94$), stroke (1.1% vs. 1.3%, $P = 0.66$), major bleeding (1.5% vs. 1.8%, $p = 0.65$), or reinfarction (1.2% vs. 2.5%, $p = 0.088$) despite a longer door-to-balloon time [73]. An analysis of the FAST-MI also showed no difference in

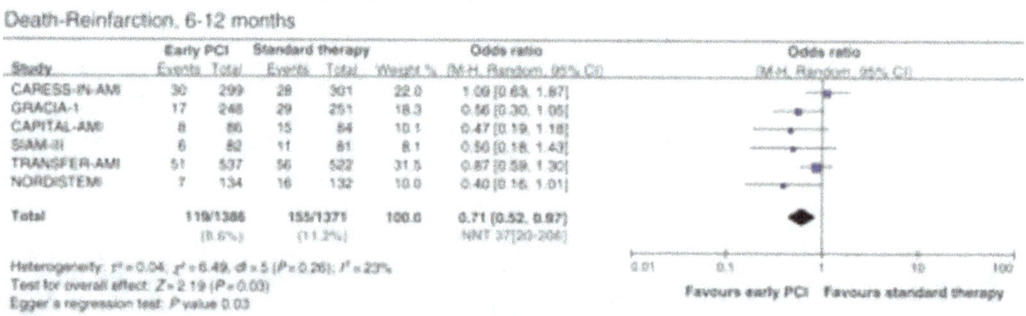

Fig. 5.4 Clinical endpoints at 6–12 months when comparing early routine percutaneous coronary intervention after fibrinolysis vs. standard therapy in ST-segment elevation myocardial infarction. Taken from a meta-analysis by Borgia et al. [72]

risk-adjusted mortality at 1 year with primary PCI compared to a pharmacoinvasive strategy [74].

The STREAM trial was an international, multicenter randomized trial comparing a pharmacoinvasive strategy to primary PCI in 1892 STEMI patients presenting within 3 h from symptom onset but who were unable to undergo PPCI in less than 1 h after first medical contact [75]. The primary outcome was a composite of death, reinfarction, shock, or congestive heart failure. There was no significant difference in the composite primary endpoint between the two groups, 12.4% in the fibrinolysis group versus 14.3% in the primary PCI group ($p = 0.21$, 95% CI 0.68–1.09). There was a higher rate of intracranial hemorrhage in the fibrinolysis group (1.0% vs. 0.2%, $p = 0.004$). However, after a protocol amendment to decrease the fibrinolytic dose by half in patients ≥75 years of age, there was no longer any significant difference in rates of intracranial hemorrhage between groups (0.5% vs. 0.3%, $p = 0.45$). It is important to note that almost one third of patients experienced a PPCI delay of less than 1 h and the average time from first medical contact to balloon inflation was 117 min. As such, the results of the STREAM trial may not be applicable to patients who cannot undergo primary PCI within 120 min of first medical contact.

Based on the results of contemporary pharmacoinvasive trials, current guidelines recommend transfer to a PCI-capable hospital after fibrinolysis "even when hemodynamically stable and with clinical evidence of successful reperfusion," to undergo coronary angiography and revascularization within 24 h after fibrinolysis (Class IIa, Level of Evidence B) [17, 18].

5.4 Antiplatelet Therapy as Adjunct to Fibrinolysis

Current guidelines recommend adjunctive antiplatelet therapy in the setting of fibrinolysis in the form of aspirin 162–325 mg as well as clopidogrel 300 mg (for patients <75 years of age) or 75 mg (for patients >75 years of age) (Class I, Level of Evidence A) [17, 18]. The largest trial studying the use of dual antiplatelet therapy was the CLARITY-TIMI 28 trial [53], published in 2005. In CLARITY, the authors randomized 3491 patients presenting within 12 h of onset of STEMI who were planned for fibrinolysis with adjunctive anticoagulant and aspirin to either clopidogrel (300 mg loading dose followed by 75 mg daily) or placebo. The primary endpoint was a composite of occluded IRA on angiography, death prior to angiography, or recurrent MI prior to angiography. For patients who did not undergo angiography, the primary endpoint was death or recurrent MI by day 8. The primary safety endpoint was TIMI major bleeding. The primary endpoint occurred in 21.7% of the placebo group versus 15.0% in the clopidogrel group (OR 0.64, 95% CI 0.53–0.76, $p < 0.001$), an absolute reduction of 6.7%. There was no difference in the rate of TIMI major bleeding.

In the modern era of primary PCI, two novel oral P2Y12 inhibitors have been studied for use in acute coronary syndrome in conjunction with aspirin as part of a dual antiplatelet strategy, namely, prasugrel and ticagrelor [76, 77]. The safety of combining these more potent P2Y12 inhibitors with fibrinolytic therapy is not known. The TREAT trial randomized 3800 STEMI patients treated with fibrinolytic therapy to ticagrelor or clopidogrel. The primary endpoint is major bleeding. Enrollment was recently completed, and the results of this trial are anticipated in 2018.

More recently, cangrelor, an intravenous, fast-acting, and rapidly reversible P2Y12 inhibitor, has become available for use in the setting of primary PCI, but has not been studied as part of a pharmacoinvasive or fibrinolytic strategy [78].

5.5 Optimal Timing of PCI After Fibrinolytic Therapy

While the current guidelines recommend coronary angiography within 24 h after fibrinolysis as part of a pharmacoinvasive strategy, they discourage performing angiography less than 2–3 h after fibrinolysis, based in part on the adverse outcomes seen in the facilitated PCI trials. However, there remains uncertainty regarding the optimal timing of angiography after fibrinolysis. In TRANSFER-AMI, the median time from randomization to first balloon inflation was 3.2 h, with an interquartile range of 2.5–4.2 h [71]. A meta-analysis evaluating the timing of PCI after fibrinolysis found higher rates of recurrent ischemia and a trend to higher reinfarction when angiography was performed >4 h after fibrinolysis [79].

Conclusions

Fibrinolysis remains a mainstay of STEMI treatment throughout the world and is the initial reperfusion strategy of choice when primary PCI cannot be performed with a first medical contact to balloon time less than 120 min. Fibrin-specific fibrinolytic agents should be used, combined with clopidogrel and parenteral anticoagulant therapy. Patients should be transferred to PCI centers right after receiving fibrinolytic therapy and undergo coronary angiography and revascularization within 24 h. Regional STEMI networks should provide both primary PCI and pharmacoinvasive strategy, based on anticipated first medical contact to balloon times.

References

1. Mozaffarian D, Benjamin EJ, Go AS, et al. Heart disease and stroke statistics-2015 update: a report from the American Heart Association. Circulation. 2015;131:e29–e322.
2. Hong MK. Recent advances in the treatment of ST-segment elevation myocardial infarction. Scientifica. 2012;2012:1–13.
3. Bugiardini R, Badimon L, ISACS-TC Investigators and Coordinators. The International Survey of Acute Coronary Syndromes in Transitional Countries (ISACS-TC): 2010–2015. Int J Cardiol. 2016;217(Suppl:S1–6). https://doi.org/10.1016/j.ijcard.2016.06.219. Epub 2016 Jun 28

4. Roe MT, Messenger JC, Weintraub WS, et al. Treatments, trends, and outcomes of acute myocardial infarction and percutaneous coronary intervention. J Am Coll Cardiol. 2010;56:254–63.
5. Kadakia MB, Desai NR, Alexander KP, et al. Use of anticoagulant agents and risk of bleeding among patients admitted with myocardial infarction: a report from the NCDR ACTION Registry—GWTG (National Cardiovascular Data Registry Acute Coronary Treatment and Intervention Outcomes Network Registry—Get With the Guidelines). J Am Coll Cardiol Intv. 2010;3:1166–77.
6. Farshid A, Brieger D, Hyun K, Hammett C, Ellis C, Rankin J, Lefkovits J, Chew D, French J. Characteristics and clinical course of STEMI patients who received no reperfusion in the Australia and New Zealand SNAPSHOT ACS registry. Heart Lung Circ. 2016;25(2):132–9.
7. Sim DS, Jeong MH, Ahn Y, Kim YJ, Chae SC, Hong TJ, Seong IW, Chae JK, Kim CJ, Cho MC, Rha SW, Bae JH, Seung KB, Park SJ, Korea Acute Myocardial Infarction Registry (KAMIR) Investigators. Pharmacoinvasive strategy versus primary percutaneous coronary intervention in patients with ST-segment-elevation myocardial infarction: a propensity score-matched analysis. Circ Cardiovasc Interv. 2016;9(9). pii: e003508
8. Zubaid M, Rashed W, Alsheikh-Ali AA, Garadah T, Alrawahi N, Ridha M, Akbar M, Alenezi F, Alhamdan R, Almahmeed W, Ouda H, Al-Mulla A, Baslaib F, Shehab A, Alnuaimi A, Amin H. Disparity in ST-segment elevation myocardial infarction practices and outcomes in Arabian gulf countries (Gulf COAST Registry). Heart Views. 2017;18(2):41–6.
9. Xavier D, Pais P, Devereaux PJ, et al. Treatment and outcomes of acute coronary syndromes in India (CREATE): a prospective analysis of registry data. Lancet. 2008;371:1435–42.
10. Mohanan PP, Mathew R, Harikrishnan S, Krishnan MN, Zachariah G, Joseph J, Eapen K, Abraham M, Menon J, Thomas M, Jacob S, Huffman MD, Prabhakaran D, Kerala ACS Registry Investigators. Presentation, management, and outcomes of 25 748 acute coronary syndrome admissions in Kerala, India: results from the Kerala ACS registry. Eur Heart J. 2013;34(2):121–9.
11. Rossellö X, Huo Y, Pocock S, de Werf FV, Chin CT, Danchin N, Lee SW, Medina J, Vega A, Bueno H. Global geographical variations in ST-segment elevation myocardial infarction management and post-discharge mortality. Int J Cardiol. 2017;245:27–34.
12. Zijlstra F, de Boer MJ, Hoorntje JC, Reiffers S, Reiber JH, Suryapranata H. A comparison of immediate coronary angioplasty with intravenous streptokinase in acute myocardial infarction. N Engl J Med. 1993;328:680–4.
13. Grines CL, Browne KF, Marco J, Rothbaum D, Stone GW, O'Keefe J, Overlie P, Donohue B, Chelliah N, Timmis GC. A comparison of immediate angioplasty with fibrinolytic therapy for acute myocardial infarction. The primary angioplasty in myocardial infarction study group. N Engl J Med. 1993;328:673–9.
14. Gibbons RJ, Holmes DR, Reeder GS, Bailey KR, Hopfenspirger MR, Gersh BJ. Immediate angioplasty compared with the administration of a fibrinolytic agent followed by conservative treatment for myocardial infarction. The Mayo Coronary Care Unit and Catheterization Laboratory Groups. N Engl J Med. 1993;328:685–91.
15. Keeley EC, Boura JA, Grines CL. Primary angioplasty versus intravenous fibrinolytic therapy for acute myocardial infarction: a quantitative review of 23 randomised trials. Lancet. 2003;361:13–20.
16. Dalby M, Bouzamondo A, Lechat P, Montalescot G. Transfer for primary angioplasty versus immediate thrombolysis in acute myocardial infarction. A meta-analysis. Circulation. 2003;108:1809–14.
17. Ibanez B, James S, Agewall S, Antunes MJ, Bucciarelli-Ducci C, Bueno H, Caforio ALP, Crea F, Goudevenos JA, Halvorsen S, Hindricks G, Kastrati A, Lenzen MJ, Prescott E, Roffi M, Valgimigli M, Varenhorst C, Vranckx P, Widimský P, ESC Scientific Document Group 2017. ESC guidelines for the management of acute myocardial infarction in patients presenting with ST-segment elevation: the task force for the management of acute myocardial infarction in

patients presenting with ST-segment elevation of the European Society of Cardiology (ESC). Eur Heart J. 2017. https://doi.org/10.1093/eurheartj/ehx393. [Epub ahead of print]
18. O'Gara PT, Kushner FG, Ascheim DD, et al. 2013ACCF/AHA guideline for the management of ST-elevation myocardial infarction: a report of the American College of Cardiology Foundation/American Heart Association Task Force on Practice Guidelines. J Am Coll Cardiol. 2013;61:e78–e140.
19. Pinto DS, Kirtane AJ, Nallamothu BK, et al. Hospital delays in reperfusion for ST-elevation myocardial infarction: implications when selecting a reperfusion strategy. Circulation. 2006;114:2019–25.
20. Chakrabarti AK, Gibson CM, Pinto DS. Optimal selection of STEMI treatment strategies in the current era: benefit of transferring STEMI patients for PCI compared with administration of onsite fibrinolytic therapy. Curr Opin Cardiol. 2012;27(6):651–4.
21. Vora AN, Holmes DN, Rokos I, et al. Fibrinolysis use among patients requiring interhospital transfer for st-segment elevation myocardial infarction care: a report from the us national cardiovascular data registry. JAMA Intern Med. 2015;175:207–15.
22. CJ T, Sørensen JT, Maeng M, Jensen LO, Tilsted HH, Trautner S, Vach W, Johnsen SP, Thuesen L, Lassen JF. System delay and mortality among patients with STEMI treated with primary percutaneous coronary intervention. JAMA. 2010;304(7):763–71.
23. Keeley EC, Grines CL. Primary percutaneous coronary intervention for every patient with ST-segment elevation myocardial infarction: what stands in the way? Ann Intern Med. 2004;141:298–304.
24. Fye WB. Introduction: the origins and implications of a growing shortage of cardiologists. J Am Coll Cardiol. 2004;44:221–32.
25. Person SD, Allison JJ, Kiefe CI, et al. Nurse staffing and mortality for Medicare patients with acute myocardial infarction. Med Care. 2004;42:4–12.
26. Goodacre S, Sampson F, Carter A, et al., Evaluation of the National Infarct Angioplasty Project: National Co-ordinating Centre for NHS Service Delivery and Organisation R&D (NCCSDO), 2008.
27. Selmer R, Halvorsen S, Myhre KI, et al. Cost-effectiveness of primary percutaneous coronary intervention versus fibrinolytic therapy for acute myocardial infarction. Scand Cardiovasc J. 2005;39:276–85.
28. Oh EH, Imanaka Y, Evans E. Determinants of the diffusion of computed tomography and magnetic resonance imaging. Int J Technol Assess Health Care. 2005;21:73–80.
29. Labinaz M, Swabey T, Watson R, et al. Delivery of primary percutaneous coronary intervention for the management of acute ST segment elevation myocardial infarction: summary of the Cardiac Care Network of Ontario consensus report. Can J Cardiol. 2006;22:243–50.
30. Fanaroff AC, Zakroysky P, Dai D, Wojdyla D, Sherwood MC, Roe MT, Wang TY, Peterson ED, Gurm HS, Cohen MG, Messenger JC, Rao SV. Outcomes of PCI in relation to procedural characteristics and operator volumes in the United States. J Am Coll Cardiol. 2017;69(24):2913–24.
31. Boersma E. Does time matter? A pooled analysis of randomized clinical trials comparing primary percutaneous coronary intervention and in-hospital fibrinolysis in acute myocardial infarction patients. Eur Heart J. 2006;27:779–88.
32. Bradley EH, Roumanis SA, Radford MJ, et al. Achieving doorto- balloon times that meet quality guidelines: how do successful hospitals do it? J Am Coll Cardiol. 2005;46:1236–41.
33. Graff LG, Wang Y, Borkowski B, et al. Delay in the diagnosis of acute myocardial infarction: effect on quality of care and its assessment. Acad Emerg Med. 2006;13:931–8.
34. Kalla K, Christ G, Karnik R, et al. Implementation of guidelines improves the standard of care: the Viennese registry on reperfusion strategies in ST-elevation myocardial infarction (Vienna STEMI registry). Circulation. 2006;113:2398–405.
35. Sorensen JT, Terkelsen CJ, Norgaard BL, et al. Urban and rural implementation of pre-hospital diagnosis and direct referral for primary percutaneous coronary intervention in patients with acute ST-elevation myocardial infarction. Eur Heart J. 2011;32:430–6.
36. Le May MR, So DY, Dionne R, Glover CA, Froeschl MP, Wells GA, Davies RF, Sherrard HL, Maloney J, Marquis JF, O'Brien ER, Trickett J, Poirier P, Ryan SC, Ha A, Joseph PG, Labinaz

M. A citywide protocol for primary PCI in ST-segment elevation myocardial infarction. N Engl J Med. 2008;358(3):231–40.

37. Henry TD, Sharkey SW, Burke MN, Chavez IJ, Graham KJ, Henry CR, Lips DL, Madison JD, Menssen KM, Mooney MR, Newell MC, Pedersen WR, Poulose AK, Traverse JH, Unger BT, Wang YL, Larson DM. A regional system to provide timely access to percutaneous coronary intervention for ST-elevation myocardial infarction. Circulation. 2007;116:721–8.
38. Henry TD, Gibson CM, Pinto DS. Moving toward improved care for the patient with ST-elevation myocardial infarction: a mandate for systems of care. Circ Cardiovasc Qual Outcomes. 2010;3:441–3.
39. Chazov EI, Mateeva LS, Mazaev AV. Intracoronary administration of fibrinolysin in acute myocardial infarction. Ter Arkh. 1976;48:8–19.
40. Gruppo Italiano per lo Studio della Streptochinasi nell'Infarto Miocardico (GISSI). Effectiveness of intravenous fibrinolytic treatment in acute myocardial infarction. Lancet. 1986;1:397–402.
41. ISIS-2 (Second International Study of Infarct Survival) Collaborative. Group randomised trial of intravenous streptokinase, oral aspirin, both, or neither among 17,187 cases of suspected acute myocardial infarction:ISIS-2. Lancet. 1988;2:349–60.
42. GUSTO. An international randomized trial comparing four fibrinolytic strategies for acute myocardial infarction. The GUSTO investigators. N Engl J Med. 1993;329:673–82.
43. The GUSTO Angiographic Investigators. The effects of tissue plasminogen activator, streptokinase, or both on coronary-artery patency, ventricular function, and survival after acute myocardial infarction. N Engl J Med. 1993;329:1615–22.
44. Hampton JR, Schroder R, Wilcox RG, Skene AM, Meyer-Sabellek W, Heikkila J, et al. Randomised, double-blind comparison of reteplase double-bolus administration with streptokinase in acute myocardial infarction (INJECT): trial to investigate equivalence. Lancet. 1995;346:329–36.
45. Global Use of Strategies to Open Occluded Coronary Arteries (GUSTO III) Investigators. A comparison of reteplase with alteplase for acute myocardial infarction. N Engl J Med. 1997;337(16):1118–23.
46. Van de Werf F, Adgey J, Ardissino D, Armstrong PW, Aylward P, Barbash G, et al. Single-bolus tenecteplase compared with front-loaded alteplase in acute myocardial infarction: the ASSENT-2 double-blind randomised trial. Lancet. 1999;354:716–22.
47. Jinatongthai P, Kongwatcharapong J, Foo CY, Phrommintikul A, Nathisuwan S, Thakkinstian A, Reid CM, Chaiyakunapruk N. Comparative efficacy and safety of reperfusion therapy with fibrinolytic agents in patients with ST-segment elevation myocardial infarction: a systematic review and network meta-analysis. Lancet. 2017;390(10096):747–59.
48. Bates ER, Topol EJ. Limitations of fibrinolytic therapy for acute myocardial infarction complicated by congestive heart failure and cardiogenic shock. J Am Coll Cardiol. 1991;18:1077–84.
49. Davies CH, Ormerod OJ. Failed coronary thrombolysis. Lancet. 1998;351:1191–6.
50. Simes RJ, Topol EJ, Holmes DR Jr, et al. Link between the angiographic substudy and mortality outcomes in a large randomized trial of myocardial reperfusion. Importance of early and complete infarct artery reperfusion. GUSTO-I Investigators. Circulation. 1995;91:1923–8.
51. Burjonroppa SC, Varosy PD, Rao SV, et al. Survival of patients undergoing rescue percutaneous coronary intervention: development and validation of a predictive tool. J Am Coll Cardiol Intv. 2011;4:42–50.
52. AM L, Topol EJ. Illusion of reperfusion. Does anyone achieve optimal reperfusion during acute myocardial infarction? Circulation. 1993;88(3):1361–74.
53. Sabatine MS, Cannon CP, Gibson CM, López-Sendón JL, Montalescot G, Theroux P, Claeys MJ, Cools F, Hill KA, Skene AM, McCabe CH, Braunwald E, CLARITY-TIMI 28 Investigators. Addition of clopidogrel to aspirin and fibrinolytic therapy for myocardial infarction with ST-segment elevation. N Engl J Med. 2005;352(12):1179–89.
54. Gershlick AH, Stephens-Lloyd A, Hughes S, Abrams KR, Stevens SE, Uren NG, de Belder A, Davis J, Pitt M, Banning A, Baumbach A, Shiu MF, Schofield P, Dawkins KD, Henderson RA,

Oldroyd KG, Wilcox R, REACT Trial Investigators. Rescue angioplasty after failed fibrinolytic therapy for acute myocardial infarction. N Engl J Med. 2005;353(26):2758–68.

55. Sutton AG, Campbell PG, Graham R, Price DJ, Gray JC, Grech ED, Hall JA, Harcombe AA, Wright RA, Smith RH, Murphy JJ, Shyam-Sundar A, Stewart MJ, Davies A, Linker NJ, de Belder MA. A randomized trial of rescue angioplasty versus a conservative approach for failed fibrinolysis in ST-segment elevation myocardial infarction: the Middlesbrough Early Revascularization to Limit INfarction (MERLIN) trial. J Am Coll Cardiol. 2004;44(2):287–96.
56. Patel TN, Bavry AA, Kumbhani DJ, Ellis SG. A meta-analysis of randomized trials of rescue percutaneous coronary intervention after failed fibrinolysis. Am J Cardiol. 2006;97(12):1685–90.
57. Wijeysundera HC, Vijayaraghavan R, Nallamothu BK, Foody JM, Krumholz HM, Phillips CO, Kashani A, You JJ, Tu JV, Ko DT. Rescue angioplasty or repeat fibrinolysis after failed fibrinolytic therapy for ST-segment myocardial infarction: a meta-analysis of randomized trials. J Am Coll Cardiol. 2007;49(4):422–30.
58. Assessment of the Safety and Efficacy of a New Treatment Strategy with Percutaneous Coronary Intervention (ASSENT-4 PCI) investigators. Primary versus tenecteplase-facilitated percutaneous coronary intervention in patients with ST-segment elevation acute myocardial infarction (ASSENT-4 PCI): randomised trial. Lancet. 2006;367:569–78.
59. Ellis SG, Tendera M, de Belder MA, FINESSE Investigators. Facilitated PCI in patients with ST-elevation myocardial infarction. N Engl J Med. 2008;358:2205–17.
60. Keeley EC, Boura JA, Grines CL. Comparison of primary and facilitated percutaneous coronary interventions for ST-elevation myocardial infarction: quantitative review of randomised trials. Lancet. 2006;367(9523):1656.
61. SA C, Cannon CP, Ault KA, Antman EM, Van de Werf F, Adgey AA, Gibson CM, Giugliano RP, Mascelli MA, Scherer J, Barnathan ES, Braunwald E, Kleiman NS. High levels of platelet inhibition with abciximab despite heightened platelet activation and aggregation during thrombolysis for acute myocardial infarction: results from TIMI (thrombolysis in myocardial infarction) 14. Circulation. 2000;101(23):2690–5.
62. Ross AM, Huber K, Zeymer U, et al. The impact of place of enrollment and delay to reperfusion on 90-day post-infarction mortality in the ASSENT-4 PCI trial: assessment of the safety and efficacy of a new treatment strategy with percutaneous coronary intervention. J Am Coll Cardiol Intv. 2009;2:925–30.
63. Herrmann HC, Lu J, Brodie BR, et al. Benefit of facilitated percutaneous coronary intervention in high-risk ST-segment elevation myocardial infarction patients presenting to nonpercutaneous coronary intervention hospitals. J Am Coll Cardiol Intv. 2009;2:917–24.
64. Bøhmer E, Hoffmann P, Abdelnoor M, et al. Efficacy and safety of immediate angioplasty versus ischemia-guided management after thrombolysis in acute myocardial infarction in areas with very long transfer distances results of the NORDISTEMI (NORwegian study on DIstrict treatment of ST-elevation myocardial infarction). J Am Coll Cardiol. 2010;55:102–10.
65. Le May MR, Wells GA, Labinaz M, et al. Combined angioplasty and pharmacological intervention versus thrombolysis alone in acute myocardial infarction (CAPITAL AMI study). J Am Coll Cardiol. 2005;46:417–24.
66. Scheller B, Hennen B, Hammer B, et al. Beneficial effects of immediate stenting after thrombolysis in acute myocardial infarction. J Am Coll Cardiol. 2003;42:634–41.
67. Di Mario C, Dudek D, Piscione F, et al. Immediate angioplasty versus standard therapy with rescue angioplasty after thrombolysis in the combined Abciximab Reteplase stent study in acute myocardial infarction (CARESS-in-AMI): an open, prospective, randomised, multicenter trial. Lancet. 2008;371:559–68.
68. Danchin N, Coste P, Ferrières J, et al. Comparison of thrombolysis followed by broad use of percutaneous coronary intervention with primary percutaneous coronary intervention for ST-segment-elevation acute myocardial infarction: data from the French registry on acute ST-elevation myocardial infarction (FAST-MI). Circulation. 2008;118:268–76.

69. Cantor WJ, Brunet F, Ziegler CP, et al. Immediate angioplasty after thrombolysis: a systematic review. CMAJ. 2005;173(12):1473–81.
70. Armstrong PW. A comparison of pharmacologic therapy with/without timely coronary intervention vs. primary percutaneous intervention early after ST-elevation myocardial infarction: the WEST (which early ST-elevation myocardial infarction therapy) study. Eur Heart J. 2006;27:1530–8.
71. Cantor WJ, Fitchett D, Borgundvaag B, et al. Routine early angioplasty after fibrinolysis for acute myocardial infarction. N Engl J Med. 2009;360:2705–18.
72. Borgia F, Goodman SG, Halvorsen S, et al. Early routine percutaneous coronary intervention after fibrinolysis vs. standard therapy in ST segment elevation myocardial infarction: a meta-analysis. Eur Heart J. 2010;31:2156–69.
73. Larson DM, Duval S, Sharkey SW, et al. Safety and efficacy of a pharmaco-invasive reperfusion strategy in rural ST-elevation myocardial infarction patients with expected delays due to long-distance transfers. Eur Heart J. 2012;33:1232–40.
74. Danchin N, Coste P, Ferrières J, Steg PG, Cottin Y, Blanchard D, Belle L, Ritz B, Kirkorian G, Angioi M, Sans P, Charbonnier B, Eltchaninoff H, Guéret P, Khalife K, Asseman P, Puel J, Goldstein P, Cambou JP, Simon T, FAST-MI Investigators. Comparison of thrombolysis followed by broad use of percutaneous coronary intervention with primary percutaneous coronary intervention for ST-segment-elevation acute myocardial infarction: data from the french registry on acute ST-elevation myocardial infarction (FAST-MI). Circulation. 2008;118(3):268–76.
75. Armstrong PW, Gershlick AH, Goldstein P, et al. Fibrinolysis or primary PCI in ST-segment elevation myocardial infarction. N Engl J Med. 2013;368(15):1379–87.
76. Wallentin L, Becker RC, Budaj A, et al. Ticagrelor versus clopidogrel in patients with acute coronary syndromes. N Engl J Med. 2009;361(11):1045–57.
77. Wiviott SD, Braunwald E, McCabe CH, TRITON-TIMI 38 Investigators, et al. Prasugrel versus clopidogrel in patients with acute coronary syndromes. N Engl J Med. 2007;357(20):2001–15.
78. Bhatt DL, Stone GW, Mahaffey KW, et al. Effect of platelet inhibition with cangrelor during PCI on ischemic events. N Engl J Med. 2013;368(14):1303–13.
79. Madan M, Halvorsen S, Di Mario C, et al. Relationship between time to invasive assessment and clinical outcomes of patients undergoing an early invasive strategy after fibrinolysis for ST-segment elevation myocardial infarction: a patient-level analysis of the randomized early routine invasive clinical trials. J Am Coll Cardiol Interv. 2015;8:166–74.

6 Catheter Laboratory Design, Staffing and Training

Cara Hendry and Rizwan Rashid

6.1 Introduction

Treatment of acute myocardial infarction has improved dramatically in recent years. Primary percutaneous coronary intervention (PPCI) has now become the mainstay of treatment and is available to all but a few geographical catchment areas in the UK. Annually over 24,000 primary PCIs are performed in the UK representing approximately a quarter of the total coronary intervention cases each year [1].

From national registry data in the UK, the reported mortality risk of patients with acute myocardial infarction receiving PPCI is of the order of 6%. Published literature demonstrates that this mortality risk may rise to 40–50% in patients who develop cardiogenic shock.

Patients undergoing primary angioplasty are therefore amongst the highest risk group of patients receiving coronary intervention. It is vital that we should seek to reduce that risk as much as possible by having well-trained teams who work in an optimum environment.

6.2 Personnel: The "Cath Laboratory Team"

The most valuable asset of any catheter laboratory is without doubt the catheter laboratory team. Without a good team, even a catheter laboratory in possession of the most abundant resources will not function as a safe and efficient clinical environment.

C. Hendry (✉) · R. Rashid
Manchester University NHS Foundation Trust, Manchester, UK
e-mail: cara.hendry@cmft.nhs.uk

T. J. Watson et al. (eds.), *Primary Angioplasty*,
https://doi.org/10.1007/978-981-13-1114-7_6

The composition of the catheter laboratory team will vary between centres but, broadly speaking, will consist of the following team members:

- Consultant interventionist
- Interventional trainee (registrar or fellow)
- Nurses (ideally at least two per laboratory)
- Radiographer
- Cardiac physiologist
- Ancillary/domestic staff
- Management/catheter laboratory director

This list is by no means exhaustive. Additional teams may attend the catheter laboratory on a regular basis, for example, the anaesthetic team including anaesthetist and emergency airway practitioner (EAP), who may be required to attend when patients have compromise of their conscious level and/or airway problems or are requiring critical care support. This is a common scenario in most centres, especially when treating patients who have return of spontaneous circulation (ROSC) after suffering an out-of-hospital cardiac arrest. This particular group of patients may deteriorate rapidly and thus require a very high level of clinical suspicion and hence very close supervision.

For procedures requiring conscious sedation (in the UK), the Association of Anaesthetists of Great Britain and Ireland (AAGBI) has issued specific guidance for how these patients should be monitored and managed in the peri-procedural environment, including the need for capnography [2]. The catheter laboratory and recovery area must therefore possess the ability to monitor end-tidal CO_2 to ensure these patients are appropriately monitored and managed.

The time-dependent nature of managing patients with acute STEMI means that catheter laboratory lists must have capacity to be flexible and allow for patients requiring emergency procedures, sometimes with only a few minutes notice. Local arrangements with ambulance services are key aspects in ensuring this is implemented in an efficacious manner. Good working relationships, regular interaction and feedback to and from the ambulance teams are essential to improve and streamline processes. It is useful to have a member of staff allocated on a daily basis to co-ordination of catheter laboratory activity who can act as a contact point for ambulance activation and alter schedules to accommodate emergencies. This can be a complex and stressful role, so ideally this role should be rotated amongst experienced staff to lessen the burden.

The catheter laboratory is an environment where team members may be exposed to situations which are potentially extremely stressful, and it is essential that they are provided with the appropriate training and skills to enable them to deal with this in a way that will protect them from burnout and post-traumatic stress, which are increasingly being recognised as occupational hazards amongst emergency medical teams.

It is important to ensure that the workforce is well supported in terms of education and physical resources (equipment). Of at least equivalent importance is to ensure that emotional support is available. These measures, in turn, will reap rewards in terms of the well-being and retention of staff.

6.2.1 Education

The role of ongoing education in maintaining the highest standards of care in the catheter laboratory cannot be underestimated. In an environment where standards are often updated and evidence rapidly developing, keeping staff up to date must be part of the ongoing catheter laboratory activity.

There are a variety of methods which may be employed in doing so—from teaching during cases (including debrief) to separate educational sessions (which should be considered to be mandatory in maintaining skills and knowledge) with traditional classroom-style teaching and training in practical skills with manikins. Simulation is an extremely useful method of teaching and has obvious advantages in training staff to be familiar with a variety of both routine and emergency scenarios. If using simulation, it is useful to poll the team beforehand to identify any obvious knowledge gaps in order to plan sessions in order of importance. The obvious disadvantage of simulation is that it is resource and personnel-heavy, and therefore it must be planned very carefully. Overall, simulation is felt to be one of the most valuable methods of training and education for the team, and it has the obvious advantage of enhancing communication and relationships between the team members.

There are a variety of simulation courses available for all team members, but there is no substitute for teams being familiar with one another's skills, environment, local arrangements, policies and equipment. The workplace is therefore the ideal environment for simulation.

In addition to the above methods of learning, the role of debrief deserves to be considered separately as it is an important method for team members to discuss their performance (as part of routine clinical practice and after emergencies or simulation) in a safe, noncritical environment. It is important that this is delivered in a supportive environment as participants may feel particularly vulnerable after an event, and early debrief can reduce stress levels and identify individuals requiring extra support early on.

6.2.2 The Workforce

Let us now consider the core (non-medical) members of the team in more detail.

6.2.2.1 Nursing Staff

Nursing staff will be registered with the Nursing and Midwifery Council (in the UK) or equivalent registration body in other countries. They will usually have to work for a minimum of 2 years post-qualification prior to working in the catheter laboratory environment, but this varies widely from centre to centre. Ideally two nurses should be present during primary PCI—one scrubbed or administering drugs and one circulating nurse or "runner" to retrieve necessary drugs and/or equipment. They should be familiar with the administration of drugs required during primary PCI as well as pressors and those required during emergency intubation and resuscitation.

6.2.2.2 Allied Healthcare Professionals

The group of allied health professionals (AHPs) includes radiographers and physiologists and may include operating department practitioners/physician associates. The roles of many of the AHPs and of the nursing team may overlap significantly, and it is very useful for each member of the team to be familiar with the processes which their colleagues must carry out during the procedure to facilitate efficient working. Some centres have also adopted a policy of training AHPs to be proficient in performing the skills of multiple AHP groups in order to improve flexibility and improve patient care. These roles may be named as catheter laboratory practitioners, and training may be nationally by a postgraduate certificate or by local processes.

6.2.2.3 Radiographer

Radiographers in the catheter laboratory will be in possession of a degree in diagnostic radiography which (in the UK) has been approved by HCPC (Health and Care Professions Council) and will have to work post-qualification in imaging radiology for a period of 1–2 years before working in the catheter laboratory environment. After this period, they will usually work in the catheter labs for 3–6 months in order to achieve competency in primary PCI procedures. In the UK, there is usually one radiographer for each catheter laboratory who operates the C-arm and moves the table, but this practice varies in other countries such as North America, where typically the interventionist will operate the C-arm and one radiographer may then be used to cover two labs (where there is a shared control room for two labs).

6.2.2.4 Physiologist

Specialised cardiac physiologists working in the catheter laboratory will possess a degree in physiology (or will have achieved satisfactory competence by local training) or healthcare sciences and will specialise in cardiology. They will be registered with HCPC (UK) and the equivalent body in Europe and beyond. They will usually work under supervision for a period in the catheter laboratory (varies from centre to centre) before being considered sufficiently experienced to participate in catheter laboratory on-call rotas. The role includes monitoring and identifying cardiac rhythm and pressures and in many labs extends to preparing and monitoring adjunctive therapy with devices such as intra-aortic balloon pump or Impella. It is recognised that in some surgical centres, insertion of these devices is supported by the perfusion team.

It is important for the team to work in a cohesive manner and identify as part of a team providing excellent care to patients. All members should remember that although they have been involved in many procedures, for the patient it may be their first and perhaps only one. The impact of this on patients is not to be underestimated, and all should invest their time to ensure patients are dealt with in a sensitive and dignified manner.

6.2.3 Structure and Location of the Catheter Laboratory

The environment of the catheter laboratory and its surroundings should enhance patient care and protect patient and staff from physical harm.

6.2.3.1 Location

Before stepping into the catheter laboratory, it is worth taking into consideration where the catheter laboratory would ideally be housed within a hospital. Ideally, this would be within a short distance from an ambulance entrance which does not require use of an elevator to provide access to the catheter laboratory in order to reduce the transit time for critically unwell patients and minimise delay to reperfusion in ST segment elevation myocardial infarction. For centres receiving patients from helicopter transfers, proximity to the helipad should likewise be given consideration.

For those environments where there is direct access from the community medical services, the ambulance entrance to the cardiac catheter laboratory should be very clearly signposted to enable paramedics unfamiliar with the hospital to easily identify the access route, and additional signposting should make the remainder of the route equally visible. Patients will also frequently be admitted to the catheter laboratory from the emergency department (ED); therefore co-location to the ED would be desirable, as would proximity to the cardiology wards (for inpatient transfers) and the cardiac operating theatres (in tertiary centres) for the rare occasion in which patients are required to be directly transferred from the catheter laboratory for emergency surgery.

As many patients coming to the catheter laboratory are of an acute nature, a waiting area for relatives should be provided. This should be shielded from the public eye and be comfortable with adequate seating provision for larger families. It should be easy for relatives to contact staff if they have any queries. It is advisable that the relatives' room should be close to, but not directly connected to, the catheter laboratory and the catheter laboratory recovery area should not be directly visible to relatives. This will potentially reduce unnecessary anxiety from watching members of staff conducting their duties and relatives overhearing conversations which may or may not apply to their family member.

6.2.3.2 Staff Facilities

Adjacent to the catheter laboratory, there should be adequate facilities for staff to change and securely store personal belongings as well as washing and showering facilities for decontamination purposes. Rest/break facilities should also be provided; again, this would be ideally located in close proximity to the catheter laboratory to avoid time lost by employees in transit and to facilitate contact with teams should there be an emergency requiring support of additional colleagues. Rest facilities should be clean and comfortable and have facilities for preparing and cooking meals.

6.2.4 The Catheter Laboratory

The catheter laboratory area will generally comprise of an access corridor and entrance to the laboratory with a separate entrance to a control room.

6.2.4.1 Entrance

As the catheter laboratory is a designated area where ionising radiation is used, it is mandatory for "X-ray on" illuminated safety warning sign to be placed in a prominent position at each entrance and also at the entrance to the laboratory from the control room. These must be clearly visible and illuminate in red when they are energised. They must state "No Entry" clearly, visible only when illuminated. The lamps are automatically switched on when the X-rays are being utilised and as such are wired into the X-ray activation system. These signs should have power provided in the essential and emergency backup electricity supply.

6.2.4.2 Control Room

In most catheter laboratories, the physiologist will be located along with monitoring equipment and IT equipment. They are separated from the procedure room by lead glass to enable direct visualisation of the patient and equipment while being protected from unnecessary radiation exposure. There should be good vocal contact between the control room and the laboratory—for this reason, it is usual to have a microphone system installed to amplify both operator and physiologist. It is essential that the physiologist has a clear view of the patient table to detect a change in the patient's condition. In some centres, a single control room will be shared between two laboratories. If a shared control room is used, then access to either laboratory should be unobstructed.

6.2.5 The Procedure Room

The recommended minimum dimension for a procedure room is stated to be 50 m^2. This is noted to be sufficient to accommodate the necessary equipment and up to eight members of staff [3]. Sufficient dimensions are required to permit safe passage of staff into and out of the room and for a patient to be transferred in on a trolley or bed with safe access to equipment as necessary.

Basic requirements include piped medicinal gases via adaptors—including pressurised air and oxygen. Traditional wall sources have the potential to get caught in the C-arm operation and must be placed in position to minimise both this and trip hazards. Options exist to pipe these via floor or ceiling. For rooms where implantable devices will be placed (e.g. pacing procedures, trans-catheter valve replacements), air flow and ventilation systems must comply with the standards expected in operating theatres.

6.2.5.1 Safe Practice

An abbreviated form of the World Health Organization safe surgical checklist should be displayed in a prominent position on the wall, and this should be completed as a "team brief" before the patient enters the catheter laboratory. This facilitates safe handover when members of staff may enter or leave the room during a procedure.

Upon the patient entering the laboratory, a safe surgical checklist should be completed to minimise unnecessary risk to the patient and ensure the team are aware of any significant clinical issues which may affect the procedure. In PPCI the paramedics should form part of the check-in as they may have administered drugs or may possess additional information.

6.2.5.2 Clinical Preparation Areas

A scrub trough and gloving-up area, which may be within the procedure room or in an adjacent room, will be required. Ideally this should be placed in a position to minimise the number of staff walking past to avoid de-sterilisation.

6.2.5.3 Radiation

At the time of writing, the legislation regulating the use of ionising radiation (UK) is the Ionising Radiation Regulations, commonly referred to as IRR 99, and these are enforced by the Health and Safety Executive. It is expected that these will be replaced by IRR 17 at the beginning of 2018, subject to parliamentary approval.

The guiding principle of radiation protection remains that of "as low as reasonably practicable" or ALARP as it is commonly described.

The catheter laboratory is defined as a designated area from a radiation protection viewpoint. Its boundaries must be clearly identified. There is a legal obligation to describe the nature of the radiation and the potential risks of exposure. All members of staff working within the designated area must be issued with appropriate training, and this information must be recorded and retained.

Personal protective equipment is also mandatory in this environment to avoid unnecessary radiation exposure to personnel. This may involve traditional lead aprons, which can be issued in a variety of forms, i.e. one or two piece. Additionally, areas particularly sensitive to radiation exposure must be protected by means of lead thyroid collar, lead glasses and leg shields.

In addition to protective clothing, further radiation protection should be available in the form of ceiling-mounted eye shield and a hanging "skirt" which is suspended from the procedural table, and these should be positioned in each case to minimise exposure to operator and assistant.

Should anaesthetic or airway support be required, it is useful to have a mobile screen which can be wheeled into position between the radiation source and assisting team members.

6.3 Protective Equipment

6.3.1 Lead Gowns

Leaded aprons/thyroid/leg shields/leaded glasses should be provided and stored outside of the entrance to the catheter laboratory area. These should be hung on reinforced racks due to their weight. These should be carefully labelled, identifying the level of protection afforded by each.

6.4 Equipment

Each catheter laboratory should contain the necessary equipment in order to safely perform the angioplasty procedure while minimising hazards to staff.

6.4.1 X-Ray Equipment

6.4.1.1 Image Intensifier

The digital angiographic X-ray system may be single or biplane and is usually floor mounted although ceiling-mounted systems are available.

6.4.1.2 Examination Table

This should be fully adjustable capable of multidirectional movement and be placed in a position which allows access to the patient from both sides. When selecting a table, consideration should be given to the treatment of bariatric patients. The C-arm should be able to be moved without restriction. If biplane equipment is installed, the room should be longer along the axis of the table to allow space for movement of the second C-arm. The procedural table should be placed in an area where there is adequate space at the cranial end to allow an area for attending anaesthetist/airway practitioners to perform their duties safely should they be required. At the head end, an anaesthetic machine would be desirable in each catheter laboratory where use of sedation may be required—this allows for additional monitoring, in particular capnography, and the facility to administer anaesthetic gases should they be required (see Fig. 6.1). A power injector system for contrast injections (usually ceiling or table mounted) should also available for use.

6.4.1.3 Monitors

Display equipment for angiographic, ECG and pressure data is commonly ceiling mounted and mobile via an overhead gantry to accommodate for positioning of the C-arm. The number of monitors required will vary from centre to centre—with a minimum of three (pressure and ECG data, current image and stored reference image). Additional screens may be installed for display of intravascular imaging (such as integrated intravascular ultrasound or optical coherence tomography) or pressure wire data. The monitor position should be adjustable to permit the operator to view images comfortably.

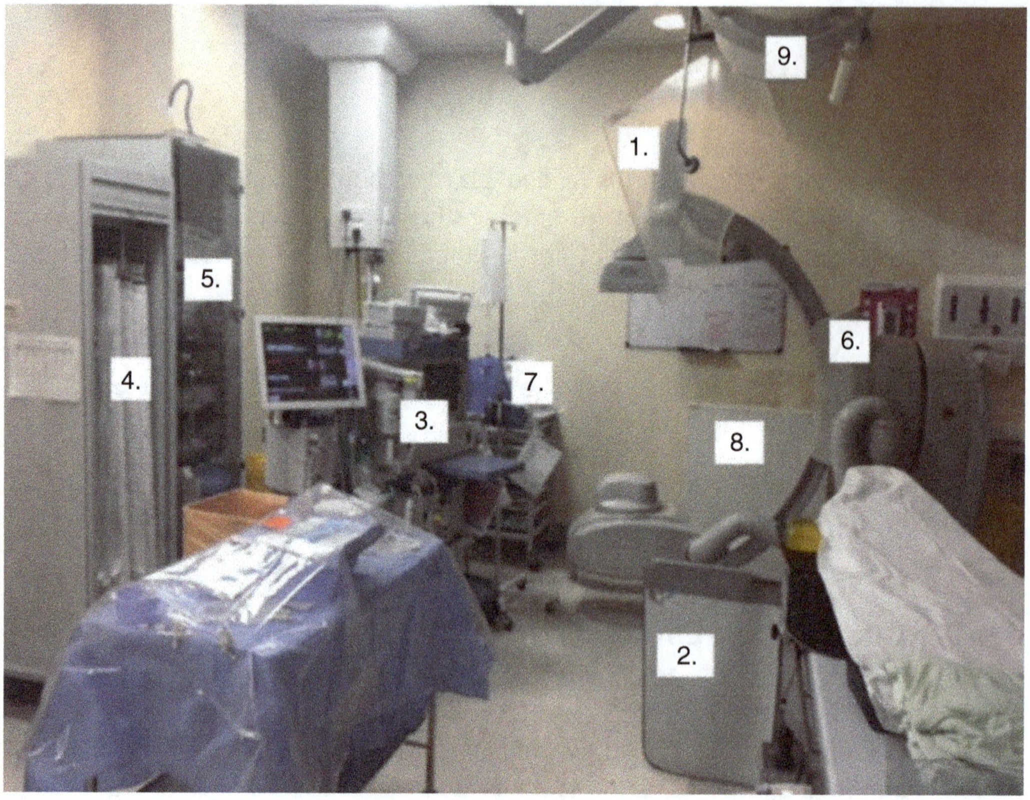

Fig. 6.1 Potential arrangement of catheter laboratory equipment. *1*. Transparent ceiling-mounted protective eye shield. *2*. Leaded radiation—protective skirt mounted on catheter laboratory table. *3*. Anaesthetic machine. *4*. Mobile cabinet containing cardiac catheters. *5*. Mobile cabinet containing stents and balloons. *6*. C-arm in stowed position. *7*. Emergency equipment trolley-containing airway kit, pericardiocentesis set, etc. *8*. Portable adjustable radiation protection screen with leaded glass upper section. *9*. Ceiling-mounted operating light

6.4.1.4 Work Surfaces

A work surface is required for drug preparation and completion of paper documentation.

6.4.2 Storage

6.4.2.1 Drugs

In acute myocardial infarction, opiate analgesia is commonly required; thus the presence of a wall-mounted controlled drug cupboard within the procedure room is desirable to avoid the need for members of nursing staff to leave the operating environment during a procedure to retrieve medications. Similarly, there should be a locked cupboard to store other intravenous fluids and drugs, both injectable and oral, which may be required during the procedure. A heated lotion cabinet should also be available in the procedure room for storage of contrast media.

6.4.2.2 Consumables

Catheters are best stored in hanging racks to enable ease of identification and rapid retrieval for use. These may be housed in mobile units which may be moved to a variety of positions or between labs should this be required. Likewise, miscellaneous equipment, such as for cannulation, vascular access sheaths, balloons and stents, etc. should be available in the procedure room—these may be stored in mobile cabinets or wall-mounted cupboards. Extra storage for additional stock will be required in a separate area (located nearby) to avoid cluttering the procedural room unnecessarily. Items used less frequently may be located in an adjacent storage area.

6.4.2.3 IT Equipment

Computer workstations are required—the number of these will vary—but generally at least two of these will be required. The physiologist will be required to enter contemporaneous data and thus will require a workstation (usually located in the viewing "control" room)—ideally with three screens (one for inputting data, the other for viewing an uninterrupted rhythm and pressure strip and finally a screen for viewing the current fluoroscopic image). The nursing team will also require a computer (ideally a portable workstation on wheels within the procedure room) to enter data and record drug administration, etc. The anaesthetic team may also require a workstation on wheels (ideally this will be incorporated into the anaesthetic machine) to enable data entry and recording of haemodynamic pressures/anaesthetic drug administration, etc. The majority of cables should either run underfloor or overhead to avoid trip hazards.

6.4.2.4 Emergency Equipment

Every laboratory should have an emergency trolley which houses the necessary equipment should there be a life-threatening emergency. This will include (but is not limited to) emergency airway equipment, emergency drug box and pericardiocentesis set. This trolley should be clearly marked and visible. Access should be unimpeded by equipment or personnel. All staff should be familiar with its location and contents. A small stock of covered stents should also be readily available for rapid access in the event of a coronary perforation.

6.4.2.5 Defibrillator

Patients with acute myocardial infarction have a very high risk of arrhythmia, and a defibrillator should be positioned close to the patient to enable rapid defibrillation in the event of a compromising heart rhythm disturbance. All catheter laboratory staff should be familiar with the operation and functionality of the defibrillator. Centres may elect to attach the patient to the defibrillator to prevent delay in defibrillation due to time taken to attach pads to the chest. The capability of the defibrillator should include the ability to externally pace the myocardium should this be required, while more definitive management of bradycardia is arranged (i.e. temporary pacing). Those defibrillators with adhesive pads may be preferable to use of paddles as this facilitates rapid and safe shock delivery while permitting continuation of the PCI procedure. This is particularly relevant for those cases where there are recurrent/frequent bouts of VF/VT.

6.4.2.6 Pacing Equipment

In acute myocardial infarction, particularly those affecting the inferior territory, patients are at high risk of bradycardia and complete heart block. Each laboratory should therefore possess the facility to perform temporary pacing—necessitating pacing box, a stock of temporary wires and batteries for the pacing boxes.

6.4.2.7 Mechanical Chest Compression Device

Provision of effective CPR during a PCI is extremely challenging due to physical factors such as the C-arm placement, table height and the risk of radiation exposure to the person performing CPR. The use of a mechanical device such as LUCAS® or AutoPulse® will enable good-quality CPR to be delivered, while the PCI procedure is continued. This has obvious advantages in any cath laboratory performing PCI. It is suggested that the device would be stored in the catheter laboratory—or if more than one laboratory performing PPCI, in a place which is easily accessible and unobstructed. All staff should be familiar with the device, and it should be checked regularly to ensure all components are present and in good working order.

6.4.2.8 Intra-aortic Balloon Pump (IABP)

Although the IABP is much less commonly used as a result of the SHOCK II trial data, there is still a place for its use in patients with refractory ischaemia/those with post-MI mechanical complications. The pump should be stored near the PPCI catheter laboratory, and its location should be familiar to the catheter laboratory staff. The operator and physiologist (perfusionist in some tertiary centres) ± other team members should be trained in its indications and use and be familiar with the model available.

6.4.2.9 Ventricular Support Devices

The use of ventricular support devices in treatment of patients with cardiogenic shock is increasing worldwide. At the time of writing, there is only one device (Impella®) available for clinical use in the UK, although other devices are in development, both nationally and worldwide. The Impella® device consists of a mobile unit (controller) which is easily transportable via a stand on wheels and the implantable device which is attached by a series of cables. If available, the device and the corresponding consumables should be stored at a location close to the catheter laboratory. This is not considered to be a mandatory device in management of cardiogenic shock; nonetheless in selected cases, it may be extremely valuable and merits consideration.

6.4.3 Adjunctive Devices

6.4.3.1 Rotational Atherectomy

This is less commonly required during primary PCI but is occasionally useful in this setting. Most tertiary centres perform rotational atherectomy, but there are some lower-volume interventional labs where rotablation is not available, and these patients would commonly be referred to the tertiary centre for the procedure. The consumable components to the equipment are usually stored in a shared store room for the catheter labs as they are large, and the console should be housed in a dry storage space which is known to all laboratory staff. If using portable cylinders of pressurised air, they should be housed in a safe location and should be checked regularly to ensure there is an adequate air supply.

6.4.3.2 Intravascular Imaging: Optical Coherence Tomography (OCT) and Intravascular Ultrasound (IVUS)

These widely used systems are both available as mobile console units, and with both technologies, it is possible now to purchase integrated units where the operational equipment is integrated into the catheter laboratory table and monitoring display equipment. There are obvious advantages and disadvantages of integrating the equipment—these being that it limits use of the device to a single procedure room and there is additional cost involved in installation. The advantage is that in doing so, it permits use of co-registration (which although not essential is clearly a desirable property in assessing the nature and extent of complex disease). Additionally, integration allows for more free space in the laboratory, and fewer trip hazards created by free cables, which may be accidentally disconnected. If using mobile consoles, a dedicated storage space in close proximity to the coronary labs which is known to all labs is most useful. If only one of these pieces of equipment is to be purchased, then arguably the most useful device would be intravascular ultrasound, as there are no specific cases in which it cannot be used. OCT and IVUS are extremely useful in detection of malapposition, which is particularly useful as it is one of the main risk factors for stent thrombosis after PPCI. Notably though, neither modality has been definitively proven to alter acute outcomes following primary PCI.

References

1. BCIS database 2013 data
2. Checketts MR, Alladi R, Ferguson K, Gemmell L, Handy JM, Klein AA, Love NJ, Misra U, Morris C, Nathanson MH, Rodney GE, Verma R, Pandit JJ. Recommendations for standards of monitoring during anaesthesia and recovery 2015: Association of Anaesthetists of Great Britain and Ireland. Anaesthesia. 2016;71(1):85–93.
3. Department of Health Publications. Health Building Note 01-01: Cardiac Facilities.

7 Patient Preparation, Vascular Access, and Guiding Catheter Selection

Fuminobu Yoshimachi and Yuji Ikari

7.1 Patient Preparation

Before cardiac catheterization, patient preparation and checking of general condition and appropriateness for procedure should be done. This may not always be possible in emergency cases however.

7.1.1 Changing Clothes

For elective procedure, nurses or assistants help a patient change clothes into hospital gown. However, for emergency cases, patients will usually be taken directly to the catheter laboratory in their usual attire.

7.1.2 Medication

Ideally, it should be confirmed that daily oral medicine is taken by the patient correctly with particular attention to allergies.

7.1.2.1 Dual Antiplatelet Therapy

The use of dual antiplatelet therapy (DAPT) including aspirin and P2Y12 inhibitor must be checked. In case of emergency PCI, aspirin and prasugrel or ticagrelor should be given immediately.

F. Yoshimachi · Y. Ikari (✉)
Department of Cardiology, Tokai University School of Medicine, Isehara, Japan
e-mail: ikari@is.icc.u-tokai.ac.jp

T. J. Watson et al. (eds.), *Primary Angioplasty*,
https://doi.org/10.1007/978-981-13-1114-7_7

7.1.2.2 Metformin

When daily oral medication includes metformin, this should be stopped 48 h after catheterization since it may cause lactic acidosis together with contrast medium. It is a well-known serious complication of contrast medium.

7.1.3 Contrast Medium Allergy

Although an idiosyncratic reaction, prior contrast allergy is important to note, and pre-procedural use of corticosteroids or antihistamine drugs should be considered if this has occurred previously. The presence of asthma does not predict risk of bronchospasm with contrast and does not need routine prophylaxis.

7.1.4 Chronic Kidney Disease

The association of contrast to contrast-induced nephropathy (CIN) and risk factors for this phenomenon are well documented; however, in the emergency setting, knowledge of background renal function is not always available. Intravenous fluids are an important strategy to reduce risk of CIN, but this may be contraindicated in some patients with STEMI or severe cardiac dysfunction. The maximal advisable dose of contrast medium is considered according to kidney function. Traditionally, body weight (kg) × 5/serum creatinine (mg/dL) is a maximum dose of contrast medium. Lower volumes of contrast reduce the likelihood of CIN.

7.1.5 Anemia

Anemia may be a sign of concealed gastrointestinal carcinoma. Since DAPT is required following PCI, gastrointestinal disease should be checked before elective PCI. This is not feasible in the emergency setting, although should blood results be available, the operator may wish to consider a stent where abbreviated DAPT is permissible or use a balloon angioplasty strategy.

7.1.6 Blood Pressure/Oxygen Saturation Monitor/Venous Route

Venous route is necessary for cardiac catheterization, but it should be selected not to disturb the approach site of PCI. Although one route is enough for most of the cases, two or three routes may be necessary for separate administration of continuous catecholamine and others. Saline or Ringer's solution is given as drip infusion. Be careful of volume overload in case of heart failure as less than 100 mL/h is recommended for these cases.

Although arterial pressure monitoring is possible, it is suggested to put manchette on arms or legs. In continuous monitoring of oxygen saturation, 12-lead electronic cardiogram should be put on.

7.1.7 Emergency Cases

Requisite minimum dose of oxygen should be given according to oxygen saturation and/or blood gas analysis [1]. For marked respiratory dysfunction, usually due to acute pulmonary edema which is refractory to immediate intravenous diuretics, intubation and ventilation may be required to facilitate the PCI procedure. Pressor support is sometimes required – usually where the patients have established or early cardiogenic shock. These patients require early comanagement with a cardiac intensivist to ensure that hemodynamic stability is maintained and optimized.

Emergency cases should be connected to a defibrillator – preferably using adhesive pads to allow rapid defibrillation during the PPCI procedure should VT or VF occur. This is particularly common at the reperfusion phase.

7.2 Vascular Access

7.2.1 Access site

Choice of access site is radial, femoral, or brachial arteries. Radial access is favorable because lower access site bleeding complications result in lower mortality rate in patients with acute coronary syndrome [2, 3]. The second choice is femoral artery when radial access is not possible. Brachial access should be avoided because median nerve injury is a critical complication.

7.2.2 Sheath Size

A larger catheter caliber accepts bigger size devices or facilitates complex procedure such as simultaneous two-stent inflation. This has to be counterbalanced with increased chance of vascular complications – particularly bleeding. Recent studies have shown that bleeding complications have predict mortality rates; therefore slender size sheath is suggested for optimal safety. We generally recommend 6F sheath and guide catheter which permit almost all types of complex PCI to be undertaken.

7.2.3 Femoral Artery Puncture

Puncture level proximal to the femoral bifurcation is suggested. However, the level of femoral bifurcation is widely varied in each patient. Femoral puncture point should be carefully determined. One technique is angio-guide positioning using the caput femoris. The other is ultrasound-guided positioning. Front wall puncture must be performed. Penetration to the back wall induces serious bleeding complication and is difficult to manage. It is important to ensure the guidewire correctly passes through the iliac artery and descending aorta under fluoroscopy because the external iliac artery takes a retroperitoneal course. Rarely the guidewire may cause branch perforation and serious bleeding complications, and therefore resistance to wire advancement needs careful and methodical evaluation.

Where there is femoral/iliac calcification, it is desirable to use a long sheath rather than a short sheath to facilitate catheter insertion and exchange and removal. Sometimes a very long sheath or a metallic coil or spring-type long sheath is required. However, we advise these be aspirated and flushed frequently as in situ thrombosis can occur, and this may be transported to the coronary circulation during catheter exchange.

7.2.4 Radial Artery Puncture

Radial artery puncture is often erroneously perceived to be difficult because it is smaller than femoral artery. Radial artery spasm and occlusion are not uncommon complications but can be managed effectively with meticulous attention to care. Notably though, radial artery access is safe because of straight anatomy, no significant branches, or very rare vascular complications such as bleeding – the vessel is easy to tamponade due to its superficial course and bony support posteriorly. Due to the lower complication rate, radial artery is considered as favorable approach site, particularly for primary PCI.

The puncture level is suggested as 1 cm above the radial process, but it is no problem to puncture above or below this point. Extremely low puncture may make application of hemostasis devices such as TR Band more challenging.

The use of sufficient local anesthetic (usually 1% lidocaine) may prevent radial artery spasm, by allowing arterial cannulation without pain. However, large bolus of anesthetic may make palpation of the artery more challenging. We generally use 1–1.5 mL of sc 1% lidocaine. Once the Seldinger wire is passed into the artery, additional sc lidocaine is delivered.

To overcome difficulty due to small caliber, the following techniques are considered to improve puncture efficiency:

7.2.4.1 Ultrasound-Guided Radial Puncture

Due to small caliber, radial artery spasm, or small size, radial puncture is sometimes challenging. Ultrasound-guided radial artery puncture is suggested with high probability of successful puncture [4] (Fig. 7.1). Checking the axis view of radial artery, the needle is advanced in the direction to push and crush the vessel. Even when spasm occurs or where radial palpation is not possible, the radial artery can almost always be detected and successfully punctured by ultrasound.

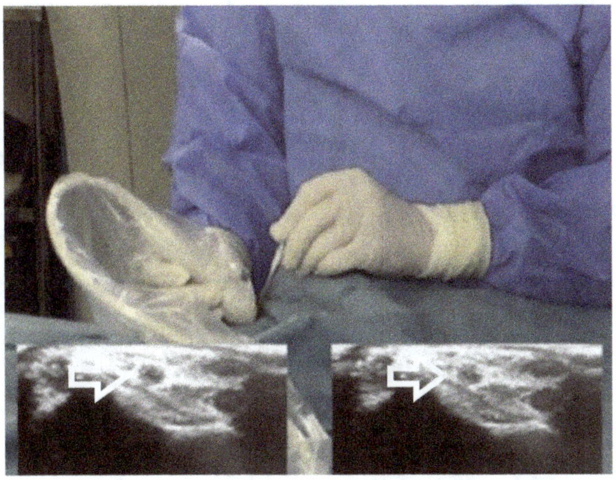

Fig. 7.1 Echo-guided radial artery puncture

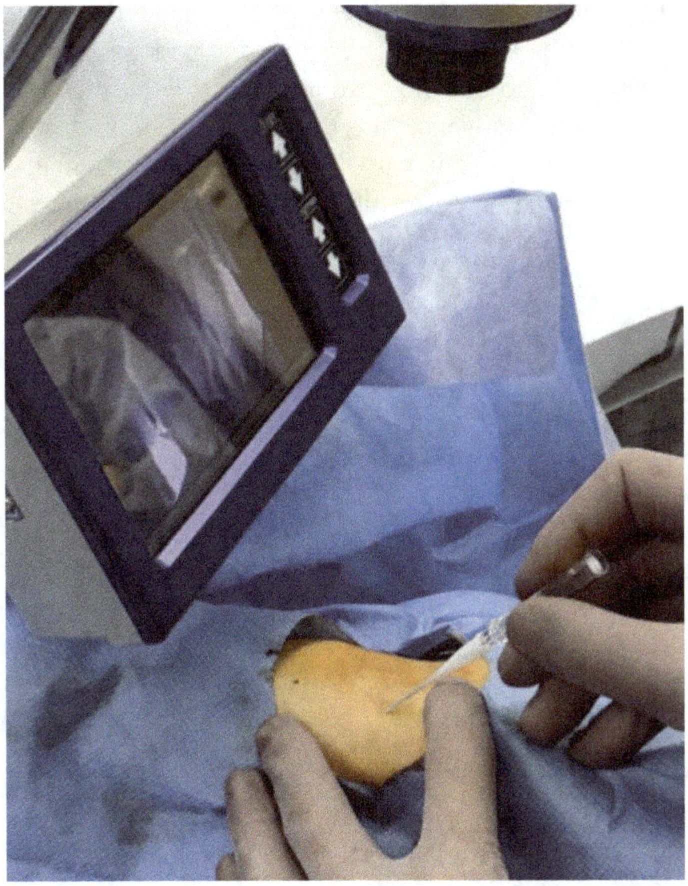

Fig. 7.2 Infrared light-assisted device called Mill Sus

7.2.4.2 Infrared Light-guided Puncture

A recent technology has been developed to visualize radial artery using infrared light, named Mill Sus (Fig. 7.2). A purpose-designed camera detects transmitted near-infrared rays from the back of the wrist. The cardiologist can then puncture the visualized radial artery on the monitor.

7.2.5 Radial Artery Puncture in Cardiopulmonary Arrest

It is very difficult to perform successful radial puncture in pulseless radial arteries due to shock or cardiopulmonary arrest.

7.2.5.1 Angiography-guided Radial Artery Puncture

In case of cardiopulmonary arrest (CPA), femoral artery puncture is also required for intra-aortic balloon pump (IABP) or extracorporeal membrane oxygenation (ECMO) insertion. After femoral access has been achieved and before inserting the IABP, a diagnostic catheter is inserted from the femoral into the subclavian artery to perform angiography of the upper limb. Because of CPA, contrast stasis in the arm allows fluoroscopic puncture of the radial artery.

7.2.5.2 Kenzan Technique

"Kenzan" is a classical, effective, and simple technique (Fig. 7.3).

Because of pulseless artery, the first puncture is made blindly. If first puncture is failed, with no backflow from needle, the needle should be left in situ. A second needle is then advanced next to the first needle. If no backflow is observed, a third needle is advanced next to the second needle. As many needles are used until backflow is observed. A mountain of needles appear like the Kenzan tool designed for Japanese flower arrangements to stand flowers. Quite aptly we call this technique "Kenzan."

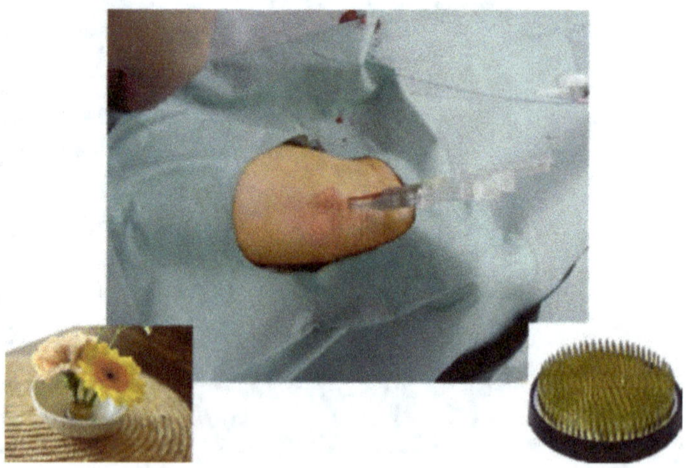

Fig. 7.3 Kenzan radial puncture technique. It is difficult to puncture pulseless radial artery in patients with cardiopulmonary arrest. In that case, puncture using several needles to the area of radial artery. One of the needles may be inside the radial artery. A kenzan, also called spiky frog, is a specific device used in the Japanese art of flower arrangement ikebana for fixing the flowers in the container. It consists of a heavy lead plate with erected brass needles where the stipes are fixed

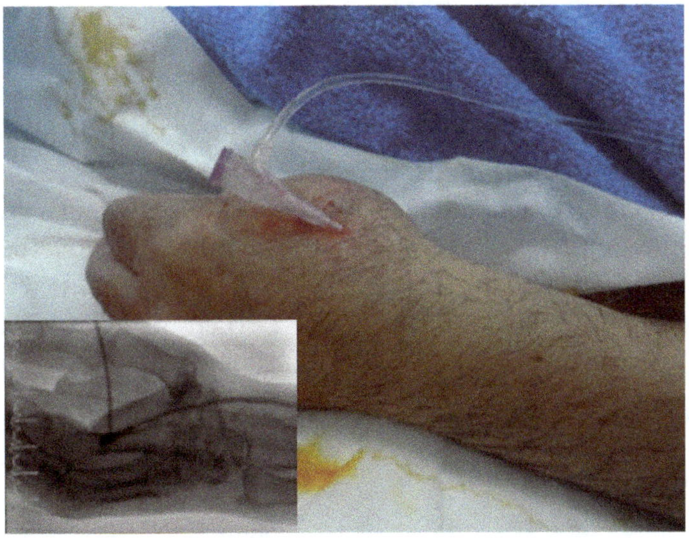

Fig. 7.4 Left distal transradial artery puncture. This is also called as proximal palmar arch puncture (PPAP)

7.2.6 Distal Radial Artery Puncture/Proximal Palm Artery Puncture

This new method of approach has been introduced since 2016. Interchangeable terms of distal radial approach "d-TRI" or proximal palm artery puncture "PPAPp" are used [5] (Fig. 7.4). Hemostasis may be easy, and patient seems to have no discomfort after PCI. Long-term safety, feasibility, complication, and contraindications are unknown.

7.3 Guiding Catheter Selection

An appropriately selected guiding catheter is important for successful PCI either in transfemoral intervention (TFI) or transradial intervention (TRI). The radial approach presents a new set of challenges for the guiding catheter. It is important to understand the basic principles behind guiding catheter selection and the requirements for backup support, coaxial engagement, and the resulting procedural success that can be achieved when using a catheter specifically designed for access from the radial approach.

7.4 Left Coronary Artery

Performance of a guiding catheter can be assessed based on three factors: (1) easy and rapid engagement without specific manipulation, (2) strong backup force, and (3) safety not causing complications such as coronary or aortic dissection. An ideal guiding catheter should be easy to manipulate, supportive, and safe.

7.4.1 Judkins Left

The Judkins left (JL) catheter is an excellent catheter because of its easy engagement and high safety margin. However, the backup force of JL in TRI is poor, although it fairs moderately better in TFI. Why is backup force of the JL in TRI so weak? One study on the physics of backup force in a guide catheter can answer this question (Fig. 7.5) [6]. This showed that the angle between the catheter and the reverse side of the aorta is a key factor to determine the backup force. The JL loses its angle-generating backup force when utilized in TRI. Thus, aside from simple interventions, this catheter is far from ideal in most TRI.

7.4.2 Ikari Left

The Ikari left (IL) guiding catheter was invented in 1995, first applied to PCI in 1996, and commercially available in 2002 [7]. The IL has three modifications from

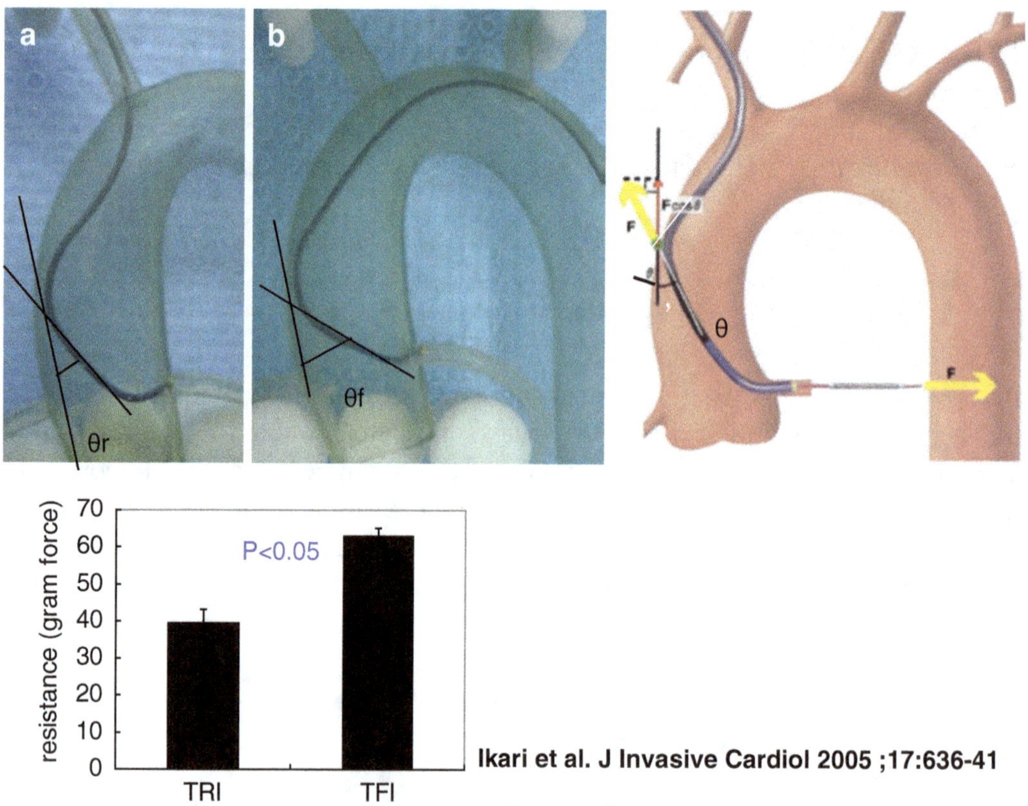

Fig. 7.5 (**a**) Judkins left from right transradial approach. (**b**) Judkins left from femoral approach. (**c**) Force (F) is necessary to pass a stent through a tight lesion. The force comes on the contralateral side of the aorta from where the catheter engages. The vertical segment of F is F cosθ Τηε ϖερτιχαλ σεγμεντ οφ Φ ισ Φ χοσντ τηρουγη α τιγητ λεσιον. Τηε φορχε χομεσ ον τηε ραλ αππροαχη. (X) εβανα φορ φιξινγ τηε φλοωερσ ιν τηε χονταινερ. Ιτ χονσιστσ οφ α ηεαϖψ λεαδ πλατε ωιτη ερεχτεδ βρ (**d**). In vitro measurement of backup force of TRI and TFI using Judkins L

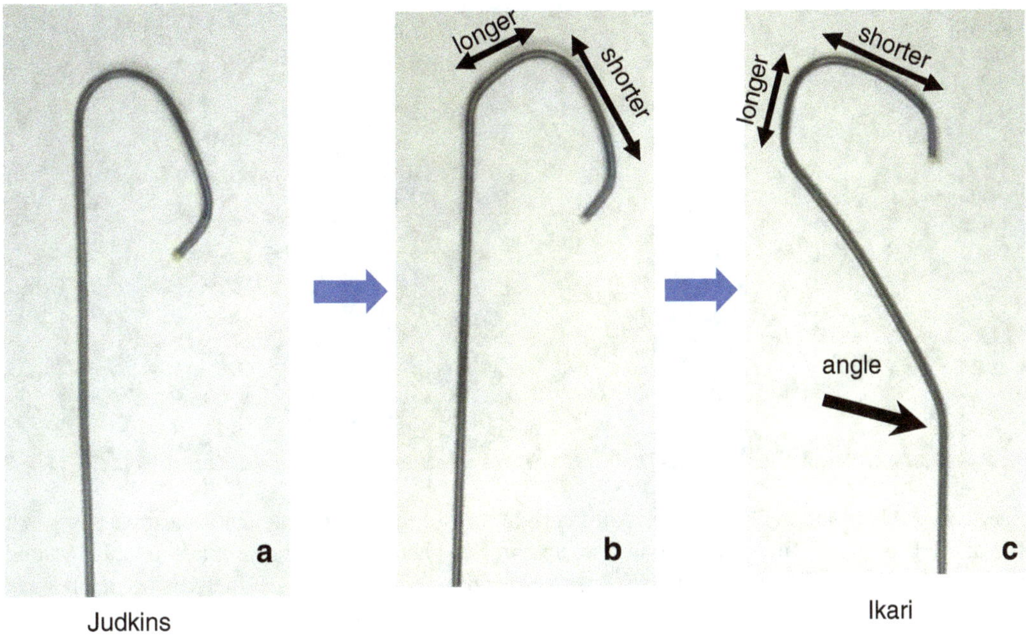

Fig. 7.6 Ikari left has three modifications compared with Judkins left

the JL: (1) shorter length between the third and the forth angles, (2) longer length between the second and the first angles, and (3) a new primary curve that was added to fit the brachiocephalic artery (Fig. 7.6). This means IL is a modified JR catheter designed specifically for TRI. Backup force of the IL is greater than the JL in TRI because the angle between the catheter and the reverse side of the aorta is increased. Furthermore, IL in TRI is shown to be more supportive than a JL in TFI.

7.4.2.1 Engagement Maneuver of Ikari Left

The maneuver is basically the same as JL. Advance the catheter slowly into the left coronary cusp; almost always it can engage the left coronary artery without any other manipulation. There is only a small difference in the gradual angle at the reverse side of the aorta compared with JL. However, this difference enhances safety because of the motion of the engagement. Professor Ikari has trained many people how to use IL; however, for operators familiar with JL, handling the IL will come naturally.

7.4.2.2 Tips to Increase Backup Force in Ikari L (Power Position)

Occasionally, stronger backup force is necessary for an extremely complex lesion. There is an easy manipulation to increase backup force in IL. This technique is as easy as pushing the guiding catheter up to the reverse side angle of 90° (black arrow; Fig. 7.7). At this point the backup force becomes much more significant because the backup force has strong relation with the angle between the guiding catheter and reverse side of the aorta. The power position with IL is safe because the distal tip is never inserted deeply due to its differentiated design since the distance is the same

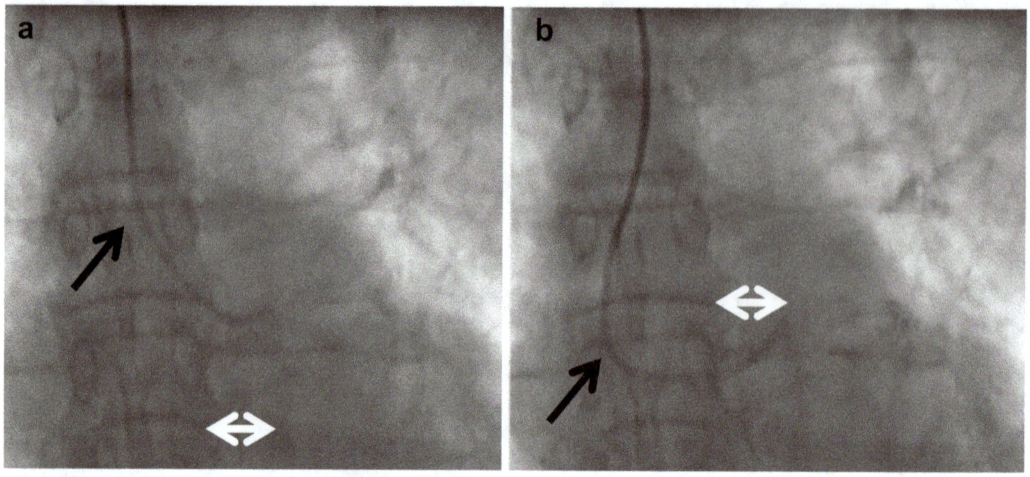

Fig. 7.7 (**a**) Normal position of Ikari left via right transradial approach. A black arrow shows that the angle θ is small. (**b**) When strong backup force is necessary, push the guiding catheter, and make the angle 90° (black arrow). Note that the distal tip of the guiding catheter is not deep since the white arrows show the same distance from the vertebrate both in normal and in power positions

between normal position and power position (white arrow; Fig. 7.7). To date, no left main dissections with IL have been reported in our database (>1000 cases) and in the reports from Youssef et al. (>600 cases) [8] or other studies.

7.4.2.3 Size of Ikari L

The IL 3.5 is a regular size catheter. Most cases can be done successfully with the IL 3.5. If the aorta is elongated, IL 4.0 fits this type of aorta. The elongated aorta is found in severe atherosclerotic patients such as old hypertensive patients or patients with diffuse and complex coronary disease. In the power position, the IL 4.0 will offer even more support than the 3.5. However, we suggest IL 3.5 for your first experience.

7.4.3 Long-tip Catheters as Voda/EBU/XB Type

Guiding catheters can be divided into active or passive manipulation types. The EBU/XB-type guide catheters are passive type, and this may explain why they are utilized so extensively, whereas the IL or JL is an active-type catheter.

What is the benefit of the passive guide catheter? It is not necessary to continually manipulate the guide catheter during the procedure, allowing the operator to concentrate on manipulating other devices such as guidewires, balloon catheters, etc. What is the disadvantage of the passive-type guiding catheter? Common passive guide catheters are the EBU/XB type for the left coronary artery and the Amplatz L for the right coronary artery. Note that these catheters are long-tip catheters. Engagement of long-tip catheters is more difficult than a short-tip catheter. Deep insertion is inevitable with the long-tip catheters, which have higher risk for coronary dissection. Careful engagement is necessary. However, after safe engagement of the guide catheter, the long-tip catheter can safely advance deeper over the guidewire or during balloon catheter removal without any operator manipulation. Operators cannot perfectly control advancement of the catheter, especially during counteraction of pulling devices out from the coronary artery. That being the case, if there is significant plaque at the proximal coronary artery, there is no way to avoid coronary dissection except to avoid using long-tip catheters. The choice of catheter needs to be carefully balanced with regard to the amount of support required and the dangers of potential for pressure damping and dissection.

7.4.4 Right Coronary Artery

The Judkins R (JR) is a standard catheter for the right coronary artery in the transfemoral approach. Easy engagement and safety are benefits of JR. However, in TRI, the JR behaves differently because of different angles and sometimes difficult engagement. This catheter also has weak backup force when used for TRI. Thus, we need a catheter like the JR but more suitable for TRI.

7.4.4.1 Ikari L for Right Coronary Artery

The Ikari L (IL) was originally designed for the left coronary artery, but it is also good for the right coronary artery [9]. The shape of the catheter looks like the JR if a 0.035 inch guidewire is inserted (Fig. 7.8). Thus, catheter manipulation for engagement is similar to the JR. Once the guidewire is removed, the catheter will engage the right coronary artery in a very stable position. When strong backup force is necessary, you can facilitate a power position using the Ikari L catheter with marked deep engagement. Thus, the Ikari L is a strong-type Judkins R for TRI. In vitro experiments showed that the IL in the power position can generate a stronger backup force than JR, Amplatz L, and Ikari R (Fig. 7.9).

Note that Ikari L in the right coronary artery may naturally engage deeply in the power position. This does not happen in the left coronary artery, but you should take care for the right coronary artery. Importantly, you can still control the catheter position and engagement depth. This is markedly different from long-tip catheters.

7.4.4.2 Amplatz L for Right Coronary Artery

The Amplatz L is a passive-type catheter good for the right coronary artery. It is a long-tip catheter and can therefore be inserted deeply into the coronary artery. This can mean a higher risk for coronary dissection. The Ikari L has a similar shape to the JR (Fig. 7.10). When used in a passive way, engagement manipulation of the Ikari L is like JR, but backup force is stronger. If greater backup force is necessary for severe lesions, it is easy to make the power position by pushing the catheter along the guidewire. An in vitro study showed that backup force of the Ikari L at power position was stronger than any other catheters including Amplatz L.

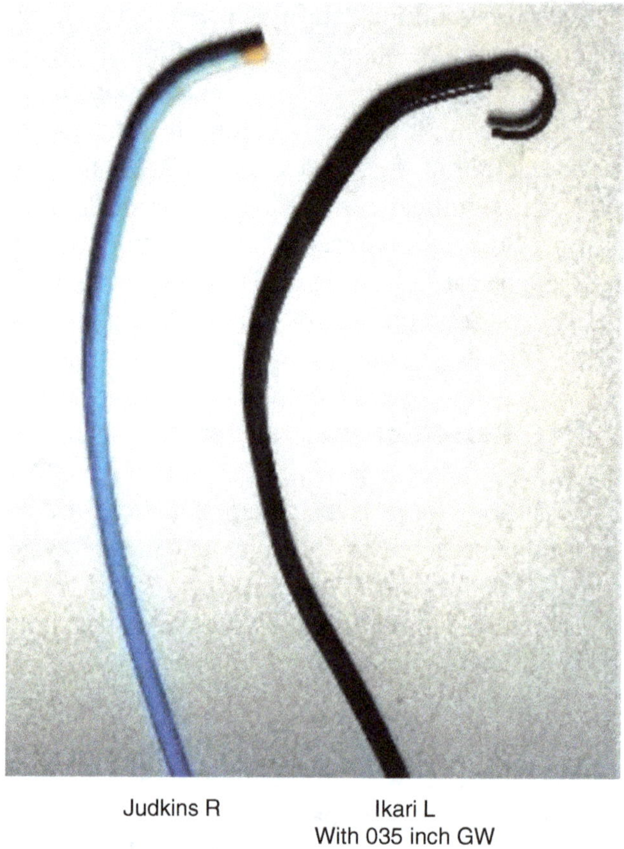

Fig. 7.8 When a 0.035 inch guidewire is inserted, the Ikari L looks like Judkins R

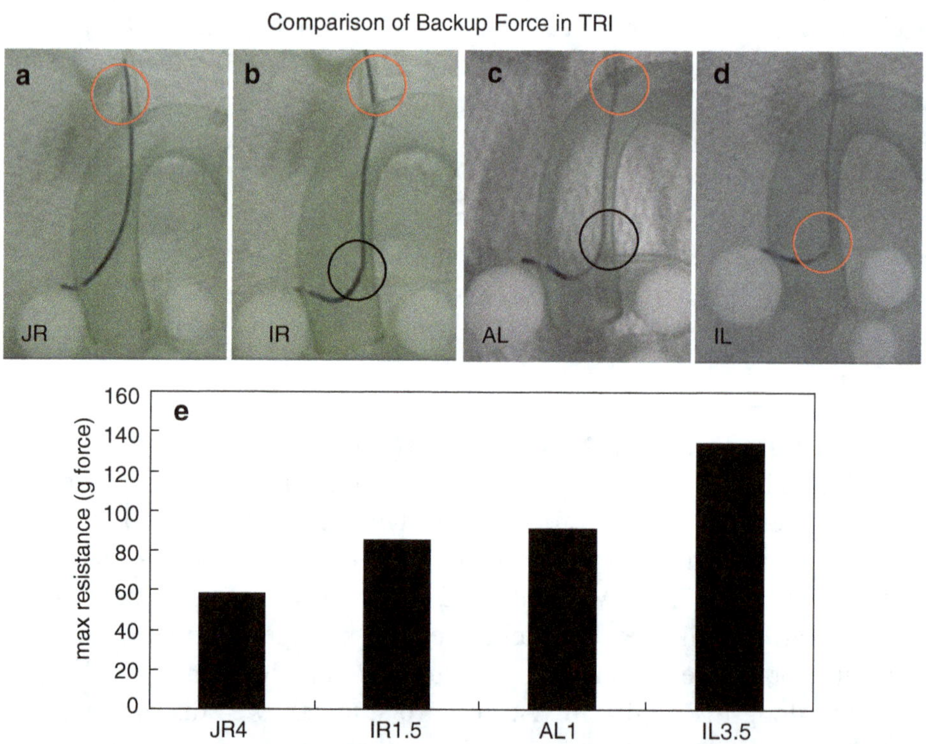

Fig. 7.9 Backup force for the right coronary artery showed Ikari L has the greatest backup force

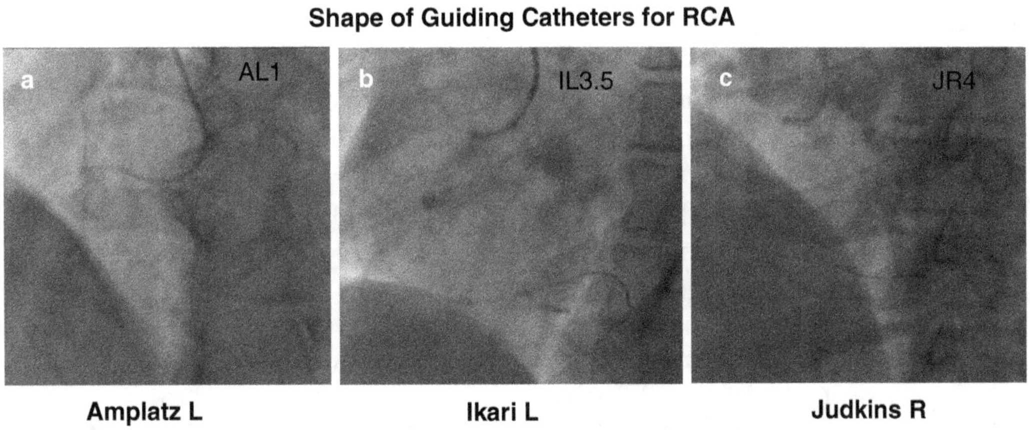

Fig. 7.10 Engagement showed Ikari L looks like Judkins R

7.5 Benefits of Universal Guiding Catheters

Ikari L is a universal catheter both for the left and right coronary arteries. One great benefit is lower cost because of using a single catheter in the procedure. Secondly, a shorter procedure time in TRI may be especially important in patients with ST-segment elevation myocardial infarction. A smart way to reduce door-to-balloon time is to use Ikari L [10]. Only a single catheter is necessary to perform coronary angiography both for the left and right coronary arteries and PCI for the culprit lesion which is found in either the right or left coronary artery. Torii et al. reported puncture-to-reperfusion time was significantly shorter in Ikari L use compared with conventional primary PCI (median 15 min vs. 25 min, $p = 0.001$) [11]. Thus, Ikari L both for the left and right coronary arteries is an ideal catheter for STEMI.

7.6 Case Report: Primary PCI Using an Ikari Guide

Fuminobu Yoshimachi and Yuji Ikari

7.6.1 Introduction

Timely reperfusion is the goal in management of ST elevation myocardial infarction (STEMI). This is best achieved using primary PCI (PPCI) and ideally via a radial approach as this has been shown to reduce procedure-related complications. The Ikari left (IL) guide catheter is a useful adjunctive tool for PPCI and can provide substantial guide support in both the left and right coronary artery positions.

7.6.2 Case Report

A 72-year-old male was admitted to a local hospital with chest pain due to an inferior ST-segment elevation myocardial infarction. An attempt was made to undertake PPCI to the right coronary artery (RCA) in the district hospital from a radial approach. The RCA though was a challenging vessel and due to tortuosity needed an Amplatz 1 guide catheter to gain adequate support. Unfortunately though, the operator was able to engage the RCA, the catheter had weak backup force, and although a wire would cross, a balloon would not track (Fig. 7.11a). The procedure was abandoned, and he was therefore transferred to our center for a second attempt at PPCI.

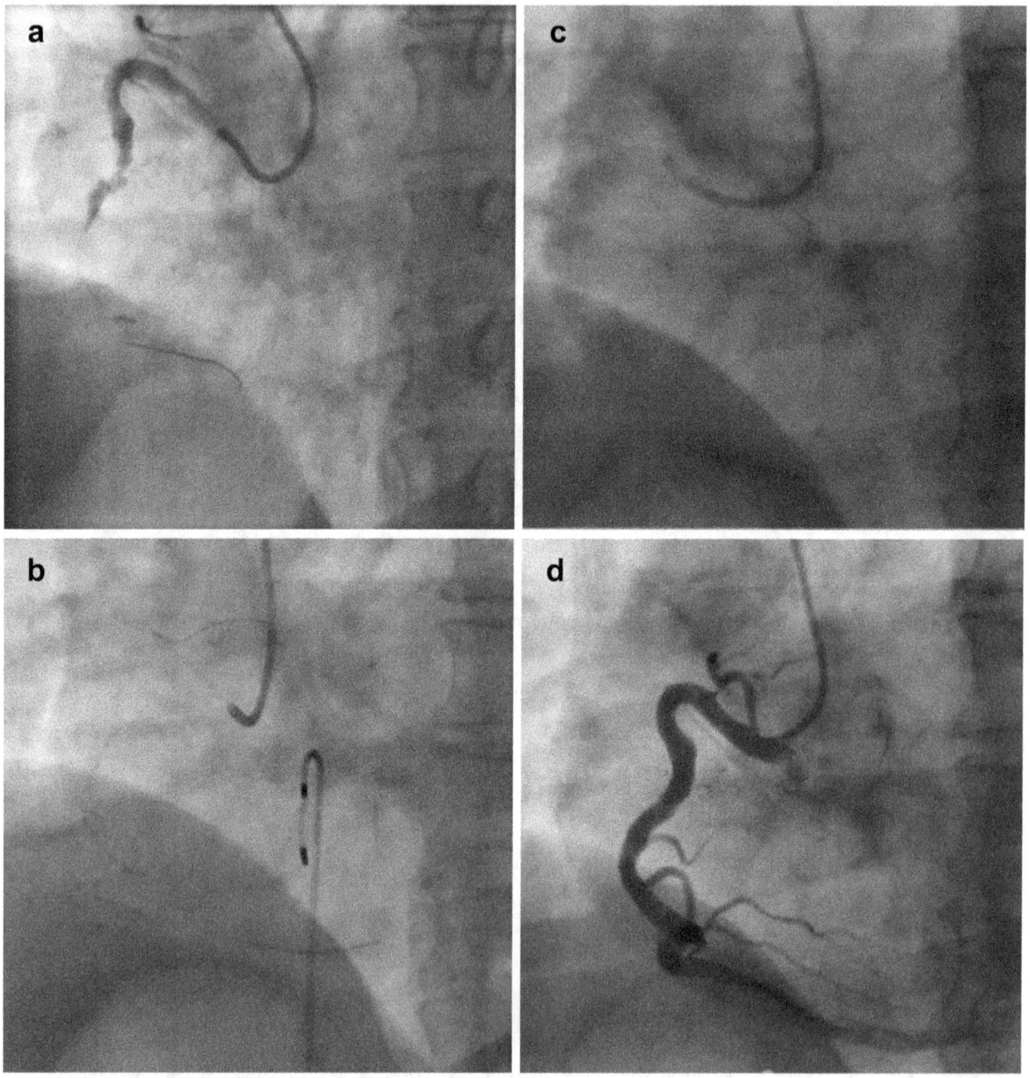

Fig. 7.11 (**a**) A case with inferior ST elevation myocardial infarction. Coronary angiography showed tortuous right coronary artery with total occlusion. An Amplatz left guiding catheter had insufficient backup force. A guidewire passed but no balloon passed. (**b**) A 7Fr guiding catheter with anchor balloon technique supported balloon pass. However, a stent could not pass the lesion due to insufficient backup force of the guiding catheter. (**c**) A 6Fr Ikari L 3.5 with power position engaged well into right coronary artery. (**d**) Final angiographic result after delivery of the stent which had passed easily due to the high backup force of the power position

In our center, a young operator tried PPCI using 7Fr Ikari L with an anchor balloon technique (Fig. 7.11b) used to further engage the guide catheter more deeply. The balloon passed the lesion, and TIMI3 flow was achieved. The thrombus was allowed to dissolve over a few days, and he was brought back for relook angiography and stenting. This time the procedure was performed using a 6Fr Ikari L guide. In the normal position, it was not possible to pass the lesion with a stent. However, in the power position (Fig. 7.11c), a stent easily passed the lesion because of the strong backup force with excellent final result (Fig. 7.11d).

7.6.3 Summary

The Ikari left guide is a useful time-saving measure for patients undergoing PPCI. Moreover, in expert hands, the power position can offer greater support than possible with conventional guides, especially in the RCA.

References

1. Hofmann R, et al. Oxygen therapy in suspected acute myocardial infarction. N Engl J Med. 2017;377(13):1240–9.
2. Valgimigli M, et al. Radial versus femoral access in patients with acute coronary syndromes undergoing invasive management: a randomised multicentre trial. Lancet. 2015;385(9986):2465–76.
3. Chase AJ, et al. Association of the arterial access site at angioplasty with transfusion and mortality: the M.O.R.T.A.L study (mortality benefit of reduced transfusion after percutaneous coronary intervention via the arm or leg). Heart. 2008;94(8):1019–25. https://doi.org/10.1136/hrt.2007.136390. Epub 2008 Mar 10
4. Seto AH, et al. Real-time ultrasound guidance facilitates transradial access. JACC Cardiovasc Interv. 2015;8(2):283–91.
5. Kiemeneij F. Left distal transradial access in the anatomical snuffbox for coronary angiography (ldTRA) and interventions (ldTRI). EuroIntervention. 2017;13:851–7.
6. Ikari Y, Nagaoka M, Kim JY, Morino Y, Tanabe T. The physics of guiding catheters for the left coronary artery in transfemoral and transradial interventions. J Invasive Cardiol. 2005;17:636–41.
7. Ikari Y, Ochiai M, Hangaishi M, Ohno M, Taguchi J, Hara K, Isshiki T, Tamura T, Yamaguchi T. Novel guide catheter for left coronary intervention via a right upper limb approach. Catheter Cardiovasc Diagn. 1998;44:244–7.
8. Youssef AA, Hsieh YK, Cheng CI, Wu CJ. A single transradial guiding catheter for right and left coronary angiography and intervention. EuroIntervention. 2008;3:475–81.
9. Ikari Y, Masuda N, Matsukage T, Ogata N, Nakazawa G, Tanabe T, Morino Y. Backup force of guiding catheters for the right coronary artery in transfemoral and transradial interventions. J Invasive Cardiol. 2009;21:570–4.
10. Chow J, Tan CH, Tin AS, Ong SH, Tan VH, Goh YS, Gan HW, Tan KS, Lingamanaicker J. Feasibility of transradial coronary angiography and intervention using a single Ikari left guiding catheter for ST elevation myocardial infarction. J Interv Cardiol. 2012;25:235–44.
11. Torii S, Fujii T, Murakami T, Nakazawa G, Ijichi T, Nakano M, Ohno Y, Shinozaki N, Yoshimachi F, Ikari Y. Impact of a single universal guiding catheter on door-to-balloon time in primary transradial coronary intervention for ST segment elevation myocardial infarction. Cardiovasc Interv Ther. 2017;32:114–9.

Dual Antiplatelet and Glycoprotein Inhibitors in Emergency PCI

8

Alan Yean Yip Fong and Hwei Sung Ling

8.1 Introduction

Platelet inhibition remains the core pharmacotherapy component in patients undergoing emergency or primary percutaneous coronary interventions (PCI). This can be achieved using a number of intravenous and oral preparations. Intravenous (iv) antiplatelets include various glycoprotein IIb/IIIa (GPIIb/IIIa) inhibitors and the only available intravenous P_2Y_{12} inhibitor, cangrelor. Available oral agents include aspirin and various P_2Y_{12} inhibitors or their analogues. These are usually used in combination with the intention to maintain dual antiplatelet therapy (DAPT) for a period of time (generally up to 12 months) after the index PCI procedure.

Understanding and appropriate use of antiplatelet agents are vital in optimizing clinical outcomes of patients with acute coronary syndromes, particularly in the emergency setting where the patient may be naïve to all pharmacological agents. In this review, an overview on antiplatelet therapy for patient needing emergency PCI is described, including evidence from important clinical trials and suggested antiplatelet therapy regimens by published clinical practice guidelines.

8.2 Aspirin

Aspirin (acetylsalicylic acid) (≥75 mg daily) permanently inhibits platelet-dependent cyclooxygenase 1 (COX-1) enzyme and consequently preventing synthesis of and thromboxane A_2 (TXA_2), which is a powerful promoter of platelet aggregation [1]. At higher doses, aspirin inhibits COX-2 which offers analgesic and

A. Y. Y. Fong (✉)
Sarawak Heart Centre, Kota Samarahan, Malaysia
e-mail: alanfong@crc.gov.my

H. S. Ling
Sarawak General Hospital, Kuching, Malaysia

T. J. Watson et al. (eds.), *Primary Angioplasty*,
https://doi.org/10.1007/978-981-13-1114-7_8

antipyretic effects by blocking production of prostaglandin. Aspirin in a broad range of patients has been shown to offer clinically important benefits on protection from coronary artery disease (CAD). This predominantly appears related to antiplatelet effects, although the drug may also play a role in reducing atherosclerosis by blocking COX-dependent vasoconstrictors and prevent oxidation of low density lipoprotein. Importantly, aspirin has become a central component of the antiplatelet regimen both for patients with established CAD and those undergoing PCI procedures.

8.2.1 Evidence of Aspirin in Myocardial Infarction and PCI

Major studies indicating a central role for aspirin in patients with acute MI and undergoing emergency revascularization include:

- International Study of Infarct Survival (ISIS-2) [2]
- This study was performed in the thrombolysis era but demonstrated a headline 23% reduction of mortality rate among patients with MI with a near to 50% reduction of nonfatal reinfarction or stroke.

- Meta-analysis of aspirin usage for prevention of stroke, myocardial infarction, and death among high-risk patients [3]
- This study from the Antithrombotic Trialists' Collaboration showed a 53% reduction of death and vascular events in those underwent coronary angioplasty.

- Aspirin in prevention of restenosis after PCI [4]
  This study showed that in addition to protection from stent thrombosis, aspirin offered a significant reduction of stent restenosis rate after PCI.

8.2.2 Aspirin Dosing

Consensus with regard to dosing of aspirin before and after PCI (including primary PCI) has been established and recommended as follows [5]:

- Loading (prior to PCI)
  Tablet 300–325 mg stat dose—if not on chronic aspirin therapy, at least 2 h before PCI
  Tablet 81–325 mg stat dose—if already on chronic aspirin therapy
- Maintenance therapy (post PCI)
  Tablet 75–162 mg OD—to continue indefinitely

8.3 P_2Y_{12} Inhibitors

The P_2Y_{12} receptor plays a key role in the platelet activation process. Adenosine diphosphate (ADP) interacts with the platelet P_2Y_{12} receptor stimulating activation of the glycoprotein IIb/IIIa (GPIIb/IIIa) receptor. In turn, activation of the GP2b3a receptor results in enhanced platelet degranulation and thromboxane production, driving platelet aggregation [6].

Various P_2Y_{12} inhibitors are available. Clopidogrel and prasugrel are thienopyridine prodrugs that must undergo cytochrome P450-mediated conversion to the active metabolite which then covalently bond to the P_2Y_{12} receptor, thus inhibiting platelet activation. In contrast, ticagrelor and cangrelor are direct-acting platelet inhibitors which do not need activation. These agents are thus more potent and have more rapid onset of action.

8.3.1 Evidence for P_2Y_{12} Inhibitor in MI and PCI

- **CURE (PCI-CURE)** [7]
- This trial showed a significant reduction of cardiovascular death and myocardial infarction post PCI using clopidogrel.

- **TRITON-TIMI 38** [8]
- This trial showed a significant reduction of cardiovascular death, nonfatal myocardial infarction, and stroke using prasugrel among patients with high-risk ACS undergoing PCI. Of note, patients with prior stroke, transient ischemic attack (TIA), age > 75, and weight < 60 kg had no net benefit.

- **PLATO** [9]
- This trial showed a reduction of composite death from vascular causes, MI, and stroke with use of ticagrelor. Of note, patients with prior stroke, TIA which led to net harm, age > 75, and weight < 60 kg had no net benefit.

8.3.2 P_2Y_{12} *Inhibitor Dosing*

- Clopidogrel
  Loading (prior to PCI)
    Tablet 150–300 mg stat dose
  Maintenance therapy
    Tablet 75–100 mg OD
- Prasugrel
  Loading (prior to PCI)
    Tablet 60 mg stat dose
  Maintenance therapy
    Tablet 10 mg OD
    Tablet 5 mg OD (if body weight < 60 kg)
- Ticagrelor
  Loading (prior to PCI).
    Tablet 180 mg stat dose
  Maintenance therapy
    Tablet 90 mg BD

8.4 Glycoprotein IIb/IIIa Inhibitors

GPIIb/IIIa inhibitors directly target the platelet glycoprotein IIb/IIIa (GPIIb/IIIa) receptor. This receptor is the most abundant integrin found on the surface of platelets and is composed of two separate subunits, α_{IIb} (GPIIb) and β_3 (GPIIIa). GPIIb/IIIa inhibitors prevent binding of primarily fibrinogen, but various other ligands also, hence, inhibit the aggregation of platelets [10]. Various agents are available: Abciximab is a monoclonal antibody. Eptifibatide is a synthetic cyclic heptapeptide. Tirofiban is a nonpeptidal antagonist to glycoprotein IIb/IIIa receptor.

8.4.1 Evidence for GPIIb/IIIa Inhibitors in MI and PCI

– **Guidance on the Use of Glycoprotein IIb/IIIa Inhibitors in the Treatment of Acute Coronary Syndrome** [10]

Review of multiple trials showed statistically significant benefit in GPIIb/IIIa treatment groups in terms of composite outcome of death, subsequent MI, and revascularization.

– **Evaluation of 7e3 for Prevention of Ischemic Complication (EPIC)** [11]

Usage of abciximab during coronary angioplasty after presentation with high-risk unstable angina showed significant reduction in composite death, nonfatal MI, repeat coronary artery bypass grafting (CABG), repeat PCI for recurrent ischemia, or requirement for a coronary stent after balloon angioplasty.

– **Platelet Glycoprotein IIb/IIIa in Unstable Angina: Receptor Suppression Using Integrilin Therapy (PURSUIT)** [12]

Usage of eptifibatide in patient with ST changes and MI (but not persistent ST elevation) together with aspirin and intravenous heparin, via infusion for up to 96 h, significantly reduces composite of death and nonfatal myocardial infarction within 30 days from index event.

– **The Platelet Receptor Inhibition in Ischemic Syndrome Management in Patients Limited by Unstable Signs and Symptoms (PRISM PLUS)** [13]

Usage of tirofiban with heparin infusion in patient with acute myocardial infarction for up to 72 h showed significant decrease of 7 days to 30 days composite death, recurrent myocardial infarction.

8.4.2 Dosing

- Abciximab
  Bolus of 0.25 mg/kg intravenous
  Infusion at 0.125 μg/kg/min (maximum 10ug/min) for 12 h

- Eptifibatide
  Double bolus of 180 μg/kg intravenous (given at 10-min interval)
  Infusion 2.0 μg/kg/min for up to 18 h
- Tirofiban
  Bolus of 25 μg/kg over 3 min
  Infusion at 0.15 μg/kg/min for up to 18 h
  DAPT and glycoprotein IIb/IIIa inhibitor in emergency PCI

8.5 Recommended Treatment Algorithms from Consensus Guidelines [14, 15]

1. A potent, faster onset and superior clinical efficacy P_2Y_{12} inhibitor (prasugrel or ticagrelor) is recommended ideally prior to (or at least at the time of) PCI.
2. Ticagrelor is recommended as P_2Y_{12} inhibitor of choice on top of aspirin in patients with ACS.
3. Ticagrelor should not be used in patient with previous intracranial hemorrhage or ongoing bleeds or on oral anticoagulants.
4. Prasugrel should not be used in patient with previous intracranial hemorrhage, previous ischemic stroke or transient ischemic attack, or ongoing bleeds or on oral anticoagulants. Prasugrel is generally not recommended in patient >75 years old or weighing <60 kg.
5. In cases prasugrel is used for patient >75 years old or weighing <60 kg, a dose of 5 mg OD should be used.
6. When none of the ticagrelor or prasugrel can be used, clopidogrel can be the choice of P_2Y_{12} inhibitor.
7. Switching from clopidogrel to either ticagrelor or prasugrel in acute setting need not consider prior clopidogrel timing and dosing (Fig. 8.1).

	PRECISE-DAPT score[18]	DAPT score[15]
Time of use	At the time of coronary stenting	After 12 months of uneventful DAPT
DAPT duration strategies assessed	Short DAPT (3-6 months) vs. Standard/long DAPT (12-24 months)	Standard DAPT (12 months) vs. Long DAPT (30 months)
Score calculation[2]	HB ≥12 11.5 11 10.5 ≤10 WBC ≤5 8 10 12 14 16 18 ≥20 Age ≤50 60 70 80 ≥90 CrCl ≥100 80 60 40 20 0 Prior Bleeding No Yes Score points 0 2 4 6 8 10 12 14 16 18 20 22 24 26 28 30	Age ≥75 −2 pt 65 to <75 −1 pt <65 0 pt Cigarette smoking +1 pt Diabetes mellitus +1 pt MI at presentation +1 pt Prior PCI or prior MI +1 pt Paclitaxel-eluting stent +1 pt Stent diameter <3 mm +1 pt CHF or LVEF <30% +2 pt Vein graft stent +2 pt
Score range	0 to 100 points	−2 to 10 points
Decision making cut-of suggested	Score ≥25 → Short DAPT Score <25 → Standard/long DAPT	Score ≥2 → Long DAPT Score <2 → Standard DAPT
Calculator	www.precisedaptscore.com	www.daptstudy.org

Fig. 8.1 Switching of P_2Y_{12} inhibitor product in acute setting [13]

8. Switching in between ticagrelor and prasugrel or from either one to clopidogrel in acute setting requires 24-h lapse since the last dose (Fig. 8.1).
9. Bleeding risk can be assessed using risk model, e.g., PRECISE-DAPT and DAPT score. Bleeding risk decides duration of DAPT (Fig. 8.2).
10. Suggested duration of DAPT (Fig. 8.3):
    (a) Acute coronary syndrome receiving PCI
    - At least 12 months of DAPT (aspirin and a P_2Y_{12} inhibitor) is recommended.
    - Six months of DAPT should be considered if there is high bleeding risk; with emerging data for abbreviated DAPT with certain stents, even earlier cessation may be possible.
    - Extension of DAPT >12 months may be considered if no bleeding complication during initial treatment.

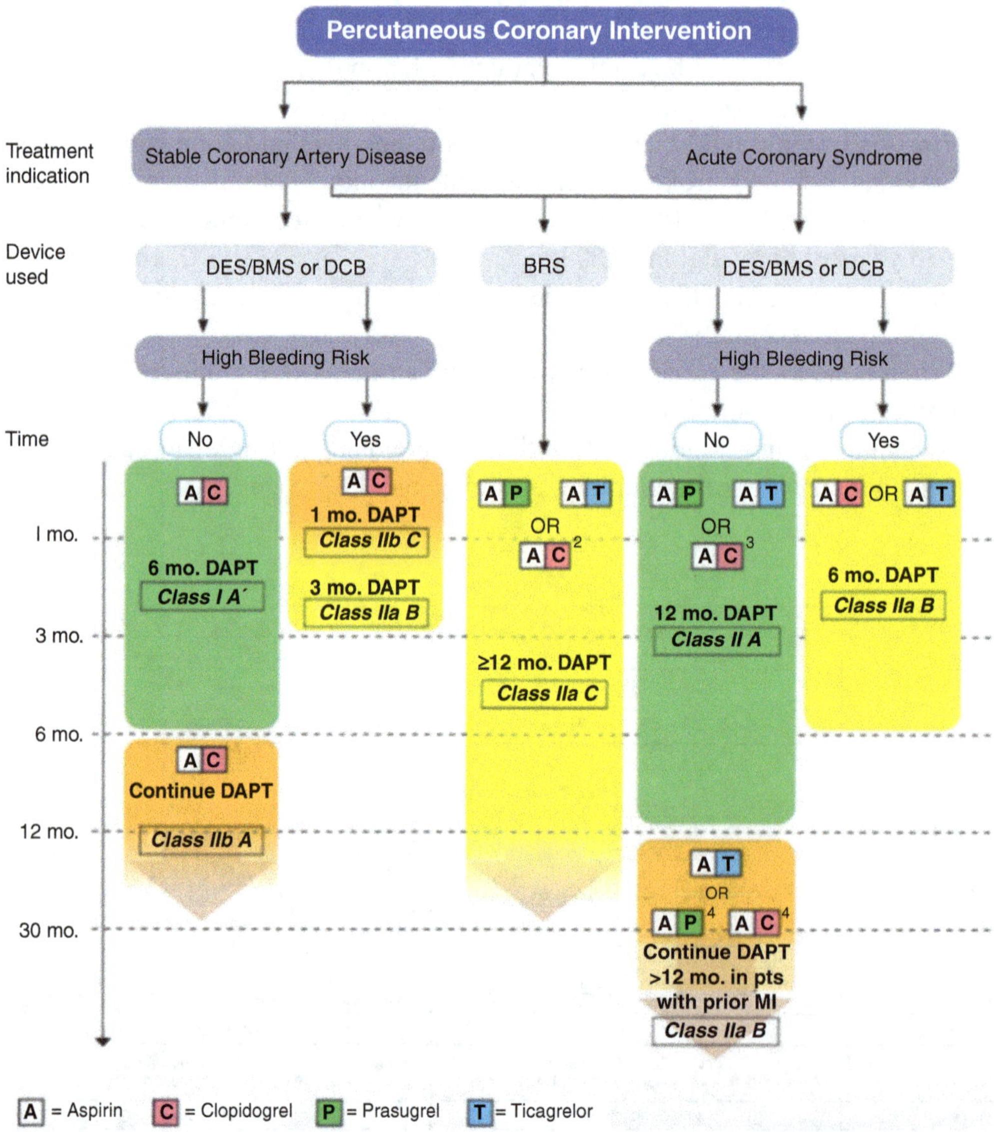

Fig. 8.2 Bleeding risk assessment before deciding duration of dual antiplatelet therapy [14]

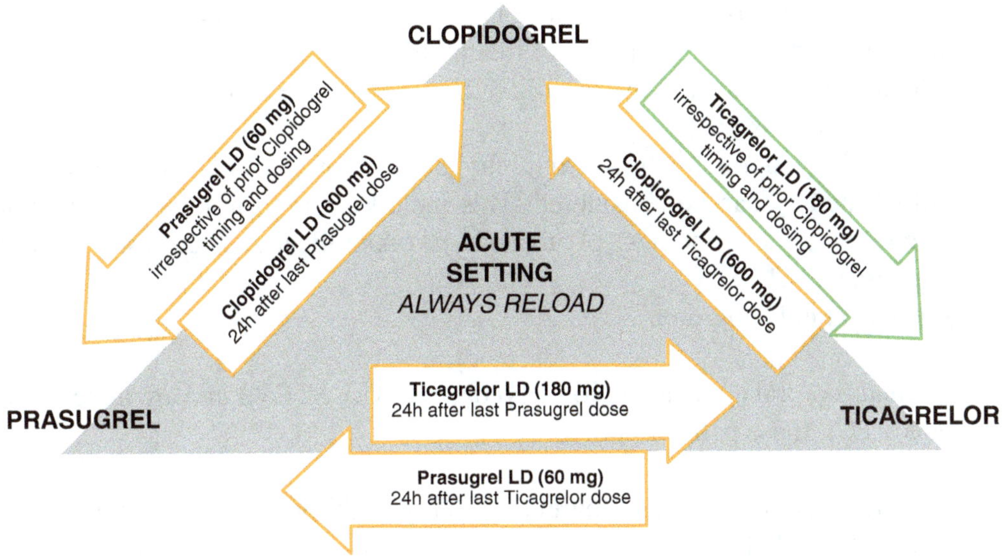

Fig. 8.3 Recommended duration of DAPT in patient undergoing PCI [14]

   (b) Benefits and risks of extended DAPT (18–36 months)
      - Absolute decrease in risk of instent thrombosis, myocardial infarction, and major adverse cardiac events by 1–2%.
      - Absolute increase in bleeding complications by 1%.
      - More benefits are seen in patient with ACS rather stable IHD.

11. Types of stent and its duration:
   (a) Shorter duration (3–6 months) may be reasonable in patients treated with newer-generation stents as compared to first generation. Emerging data may permit even shorter duration; trials are awaited.
12. DAPT dose in chronic kidney disease:
   (a) Stages 1–3
      - EGFR >30 mL/min/1.73 m^2

        Aspirin: Loading at 150–300 mg orally, followed by maintenance 75 mg–100 mg/day
        Clopidogrel: Loading at 300–600 mg orally, followed by 75 mg/day
        Ticagrelor: Loading at 180 mg orally, followed by 90 mg BD/day
        Prasugrel: Loading at 60 mg orally, followed by 10 mg/day
   (b) Stage 4
      - EGFR 15–30 mL/min/1.73 m^2

        No dose adjustment
   (c) Stage 5
      - EGFR <15 mL/min/1.73 m^2

        Aspirin: No dose adjustment
        Clopidogrel: No information available
        Ticagrelor and prasugrel: NOT recommended

13. Glycoprotein IIb/IIIa inhibitor usage in prehospital or upstream settings has not shown extra benefits on efficacy of treatment.
14. Selective downstream usage of GPIIb/IIIa inhibitors reduces cost of treatment and bleeding risk [15].
15. Usage of glycoprotein IIb/IIIa inhibitor during coronary catheterization as a bailout therapy can be considered. This includes large thrombus, slow or no reflow, or other findings of thrombotic complications during coronary angiogram [16].
16. Special patient subgroup.

In patients on oral anticoagulation who present with STEMI and are undergoing emergency PCI, these patients should:

(a) Loading of aspirin and clopidogrel (the P_2Y_{12} inhibitor of choice, 600 mg loading dose) should be done.
(b) Also receive additional parenteral anticoagulation.
(c) Chronic oral anticoagulation therapy should not be stopped during admission.
(d) Gastric protection with a proton pump inhibitor is recommended.
(e) Triple therapy (oral anticoagulation, aspirin, and clopidogrel) should be considered for 6 months after STEMI.
(f) Oral anticoagulation plus aspirin or clopidogrel should be considered for an additional 6 months; after which, it is then indicated to maintain oral anticoagulation.
(g) For patients with atrial fibrillation as the indication for anticoagulation, rivaroxaban in combination with clopidogrel and without aspirin may be a reasonable choice.
(h) The use of ticagrelor or prasugrel is not recommended as part of a triple therapy regimen with aspirin and oral anticoagulation.

8.6 Summary

- DAPT is an important periprocedural pharmacotherapy in patient receiving PCI.
- DAPT, aspirin, and a P_2Y_{12} inhibitor are to be loaded orally as soon as diagnosis of ACS was made.
- Choice of P_2Y_{12} inhibitor includes prasugrel, ticagrelor, and clopidogrel.
- Duration of DAPT treatment after emergency PCI depends on bleeding risk assessment and types of stents used.
- Extra attention in cases with bioresorbable vascular scaffold, which requires at least 12 months of DAPT regardless of bleeding risk.
- Glycoprotein IIb/IIIa inhibitor usage depends on treating physician justification as no conclusive evidence of its routine use in emergency PCI.

References

1. Patrono C, Bachmann F, Baigent C, Bode C, De Caterina R, Charbonnier B, et al. Expert consensus document on the use of antiplatelet agents: the task force on the use of antiplatelet agents in patients with atherosclerotic cardiovascular disease of the European Society of Cardiology. Eur Heart J. 2004;25(2):166–81.
2. Randomised trial of intravenous streptokinase, oral aspirin, both, or neither. among 17,187 cases of suspected acute myocardial infarction: ISIS-2. ISIS-2. (Second International Study of Infarct Survival) Collaborative Group. Lancet 1988;2(8607):349–60.
3. Antithrombotic Trialists' Collaboration, Trialists A. Collaborative meta-analysis of randomised trials of antiplatelet therapy for prevention of death, myocardial infarction, and stroke in high risk patients. BMJ 2002;324(7329):71–86. http://view.ncbi.nlm.nih.gov/pubmed/11786451
4. Schwartz L, Bourassa MG, Lesperance J, Aldridge HE, Kazim F, Salvatori VA, et al. Aspirin and dipyridamole in the prevention of restenosis after percutaneous transluminal coronary angioplasty. N Engl J Med. 1988;318(26)
5. Levine GN, Bates ER, Blankenship JC, Bailey SR, Bittl JA, Cercek B, et al. 2011 ACCF/AHA/SCAI guideline for percutaneous coronary intervention a report of the American College of Cardiology Foundation/American Heart Association Task Force on Practice Guidelines and the Society for Cardiovascular Angiography and Interventions. Circulation. 2011;124(23)
6. Wallentin L. P_2Y_{12} inhibitors: differences in properties and mechanisms of action and potential consequences for clinical use. Eur Heart J. 2009;30(16):1964–77.
7. Mehta SR, Yusuf S, Peters RJ, et al. Effects of pretreatment with clopidogrel and aspirin followed by long-term therapy in patientsundergoing percutaneous coronary intervention: the PCI-CURE study. Lancet. 2001;358:527–33.
8. Montalescot G, Wiviott SD, Braunwald E, Murphy SA, Gibson CM, McCabe CH, Antman EM, RITON-TIMI 38 Investigators. Prasugrel compared with clopidogrel in patients undergoing percutaneous coronary intervention for ST-elevation myocardial infarction (TRITON-TIMI 38): double-blind, randomised controlled trial. Lancet. 2009;373:723–31.
9. Cannon CP, Harrington RA, James S, Ardissino D, Becker RC, Emanuelsson H, Husted S, Katus H, Keltai M, Khurmi NS, Kontny F, Lewis BS, Steg PG, Storey RF, Wojdyla D, Wallentin L, inhibition PLAT, Investigators p O. Comparison of ticagrelor with clopidogrel in patients with a planned invasive strategy for acute coronary syndromes (PLATO): a randomised double-blind study. Lancet. 2010;375:283–93.
10. Guidance on the use of glycoprotein IIb/IIIa inhibitors in the treatment of acute coronary syndromes. Technology appraisal guidance [TA47]. Published date: 05 September 2002; Last updated: 01 March 2010. https://www.nice.org.uk/guidance/ta47.
11. The EPIC Investigators. Use of a monoclonal antibody directed against the platelet glycoprotein IIb/IIIa receptor in high-risk coronary angioplasty. N Engl J Med. 1994;330:956–61.
12. Boersma E, Pieper KS, Steyerberg EW, Wilcox RG, Chang WC, Lee KL, Akkerhuis KM, Harrington RA, Deckers JW, Armstrong PW, Lincoff AM, Califf RM, Topol EJ, Simoons ML. Predictors of outcome in patients with acute coronary syndromes without persistent ST-segment elevation. Results from an international trial of 9461 patients. The PURSUIT Investigators. Circulation. 2000;101:2557–67.
13. PRISM-PLUS Study Investigators. Inhibition of the platelet glycoprotein IIb/IIIa receptor with tirofiban in unstable angina and non-Q-wave myocardial infarction: Platelet Receptor Inhibition in Ischemic Syndrome Management in Patients Limited by Unstable Signs and Symptoms (PRISM-PLUS) Study Investigators. N Engl J Med. 1998;338:1488–97.
14. Levine GN, Bates ER, Bittl JA, Brindis RG, Fihn SD, Fleisher LA, et al. 2016 ACC/AHA guideline focused update on duration of dual antiplatelet therapy in patients with coronary artery disease: a report of the American College of Cardiology/American Heart Association task force on clinical practice guidelines. J Am Coll Cardiol [internet]. 2016;68(10):1082–115. https://doi.org/10.1016/j.jacc.2016.03.513.

15. Ibanez B, James S, Agewall S, Antunes MJ, Bucciarelli-Ducci C, Bueno H, et al. 2017 ESC guidelines for the management of acute myocardial infarction in patients presenting with ST-segment elevation. Eur Heart J. 2017;70(12):1082. http://academic.oup.com/eurheartj/article/doi/10.1093/eurheartj/ehx393/4095042/2017-ESC-Guidelines-for-the-management-of-acute
16. De Luca G, Navarese EP, Cassetti E, Verdoia M, Suryapranata H. Meta-analysis of randomized trials of glycoprotein IIb/IIIa inhibitors in high-risk acute coronary syndromes patients undergoing invasive strategy. Am J Cardiol. 2011;107(2):198–203. https://doi.org/10.1016/j.amjcard.2010.08.063.

9 Anticoagulants and Primary PCI

Fahim H. Jafary

9.1 Introduction

Percutaneous coronary interventions (PCI) mandate usage of anticoagulants to facilitate a successful and safe procedure. This chapter reviews commonly used anticoagulant regimens used for PCI with tailored guidance for the acute setting, in particular primary PCI for ST-elevation myocardial infarction (STEMI).

9.2 Rationale for the Use of Anticoagulant Therapy

PCI involves a variety of events that cumulatively increase the risk of intra and post procedure thrombosis. These include balloon-induced injury and dissection with exposure of the subendothelial tissue to blood, activation of platelets and the coagulation cascade and implantation of a potentially thrombogenic foreign body (stent) in the coronary circulation. These effects are, of course, more pronounced during PCI for acute coronary syndromes (ACS) where the thrombotic milieu is already "hot" at the outset. Therefore, anticoagulation with antiplatelet and antithrombotic therapy during PCI is considered obligatory. Of note, no placebo-controlled trials of antithrombotic therapy in PCI have ever been conducted, nor will there ever be such a trial. Indeed, the 2017 European Society of Cardiology (ESC) guidelines [1] give anticoagulation (antithrombotic therapy) a class I indication for routine use during STEMI PCI.

F. H. Jafary
Tan Tock Seng Hospital, Singapore, Singapore
e-mail: fahim_haider_jafary@ttsh.com.sg

T. J. Watson et al. (eds.), *Primary Angioplasty*,
https://doi.org/10.1007/978-981-13-1114-7_9

9.3 Classes of Anticoagulant

Several classes of anticoagulant regimens are available. Each of these is discussed in detail below.

9.3.1 Unfractionated Heparin and STEMI

Unfractionated heparin (UFH) has been available since the 1930s, and there is, therefore, an extensive generational physician experience with this drug in a variety of clinical settings. Derived from porcine intestine, a bag of UFH contains a heterogeneous mix of polysaccharides with a wide variety of molecular weights (Table 9.1). Only a third of the UFH molecules are biologically active as a result of possessing a key pentasaccharide sequence that is able to bind to antithrombin (AT) [2]. UFH attaches to AT to form a tertiary complex that binds to and inhibits

Table 9.1 Comparative chart of characteristics of various anticoagulants used in the primary PCI setting

Drug	UFH	LMWH	Fondaparinux	Bivalirudin
Molecular weight (kDa)	3–30 (mean 15)	2–10	1.7	2.2
Action	Binds to AT, inhibits IIa and Xa	Binds to AT, inhibits Xa	Binds to AT, inhibits Xa	Directly binds to thrombin
Xa:IIa ratio	1:1	4:1	Pure Xa	Pure IIa
Plasma proteins binding	Extensive	Low	None	
T ½ after dose	Variable (dose dependent)[a]			25 min
PCI dose	70–100 U/kg (no GPI planned) 50–70 U/kg IV (GPI planned). Target to therapeutic ACT	0.5 mg/kg IV bolus		0.75-mg/kg IV bolus, then 1.75-mg/kg/h infusion
Activates platelets	+++	+	–	–
HIT	0.5%	<0.1%	Negligible	Negligible
Monitoring	ACT[b]	Anti Xa levels ?ACT	Anti Xa levels[c]	ACT[d]
Reversal	Protamine	Protamine (partial)	None	None

AT antithrombin, *ACT* activated clotting time, *HIT* heparin-induced thrombocytopenia
[a]Half-life increases with dose
[b]ACT reflects therapeutic effect
[c]No point-of-care options
[d]ACT does *not* reflect therapeutic effect, only reflects delivery of drug

both factor Xa and as IIa (thrombin), thereby inhibiting production and action of thrombin. As UFH inhibits both molecules, its anti Xa:IIa activity ratio is 1:1. In contrast, low molecular weight heparins (LMWH) by virtue of their predominantly shorter chains are only able to bind to AT and hence have primarily anti-Xa activity (Table 9.1).

Some well-known limitations of UFH include its inability to penetrate and bind to clot-bound thrombin, extensive binding by plasma proteins which limit bioavailability, an inherent platelet-activating effect of heparin and complex pharmacokinetics which make the anticoagulation response to a given dose somewhat unpredictable [2]. Despite these limitations unfractionated heparin remains the most widely used antithrombotic agent during PCI, and both the ACCF/AHA [3] and ESC [1] guidelines give UFH a class I recommendation in primary PCI.

There are no comparative dosing trials of UFH in primary PCI and dosing recommendations are somewhat arbitrary. The 2017 ESC guidelines [1] recommend an UFH dose of 70–100 IU/kg intravenous bolus when no glycoprotein IIb/IIIa inhibitor is planned and 50–70 IU/kg bolus with planned glycoprotein IIb/IIIa inhibitor use. It remains unclear whether STEMI patients, given the ongoing thrombotic milieu, should receive the higher end of the dose spectrum of UFH.

9.3.2 Low-molecular Weight Heparins and STEMI

Unlike UFH, LMWH consist of a relatively more homogeneous mix of molecules and have better bioavailability and longer half-life. As a result, LMWH have the advantage of more predictable and consistent anticoagulation compared to UFH. Although extensively studied in the ACS population, there is limited data in the context of STEMI. In the randomized ATOLL trial [4], 910 STEMI patients were randomized to an intravenous bolus of 0.5 mg/kg enoxaparin or standard dose UFH. Although the trial had a strong trend towards benefit favouring enoxaparin (17% relative risk reduction; $p = 0.068$), it failed to meet the primary endpoint. Moreover, it should be recognized that this was an open label trial, and while a per-protocol analysis that excluded 13% of the study group (for protocol violations) suggested that enoxaparin was statistically superior to UFH, this can be regarded as hypothesis generating at best. Furthermore, > 70% of the study population received a glycoprotein IIb/IIIa inhibitor; therefore it is difficult to extrapolate the data to patients not receiving additional glycoprotein IIb/IIIa inhibitor therapy. Nevertheless, these results do imply that enoxaparin is at least as safe as UFH in the primary PCI setting. The ACCF/AHA guidelines make no recommendations on enoxaparin, but the 2017 ESC guidelines [1] give it a class IIa recommendation (level of evidence A) (Table 9.2). Both the ACCF/AHA [3] and ESC guidelines recommend against the use of fondaparinux, a synthetic pentasaccharide LMWH, during primary PCI given a higher risk of ischemic events and catheter thrombosis in the OASIS-6 trial [5].

Table 9.2 Summary of major societal guidelines on the use of various antithrombotic agents in primary PCI

Drug	ACCF/AHA		ESC	
	Rec.	LOA:	Rec.	LOA
UFH	I	C	I	C
Enoxaparin	No recommendation		IIa	A
Fondaparinux	III	B	III	B
Bivalirudin	I	B	IIa I[a]	A C

ACCF/AHA American College of Cardiology Foundation/American Heart Association, *ESC* European Society of Cardiology, *Rec* recommendation, *LOA* level of evidence
[a]In patients with heparin-induced thrombocytopenia

Table 9.3 Summary of randomized trials of bivalirudin vs. heparin in primary PCI

Trial	Year	Treatment	Control	Radial	MACE	Bleeding	ST
HORIZONS-AMI [13]	2007	Bival + pGPI	Heparin + GPI	6%	↓	↓	↑
EUROMAX[14]	2013	Bival[a]	Heparin	~50%	↓	↓	↑
HEAT-PPCI [15]	2014	Bival	Heparin	80%	↑	No diff	↑
BRIGHT [16]	2015	Bival[a]	Heparin or heparin + GPI	78%	No diff	↓	No diff
VALIDATE-SWEDEHEART[17]	2017	Bival[a]	Heparin	90%	No diff	No diff	No diff

Bival bivalirudin, *pGPI* provisional GP IIb/IIIa inhibitor, *MACE* major adverse cardiac events, *ST* stent thrombosis
[a]Bivalirudin infusion continued post PCI

9.3.3 Direct Thrombin Inhibitors and STEMI

The most widely studied and used direct thrombin inhibitor (DTI) is bivalirudin. Bivalirudin binds reversibly to the catalytic site of thrombin and acts as a competitive inhibitor. Unlike heparins, bivalirudin can bind to clot-bound thrombin, is not bound by plasma proteins and, therefore, has excellent bioavailability. Bivalirudin also blocks thrombin-induced platelet aggregation. The dosing schedule of bivalirudin for STEMI patients undergoing PCI is outlined in Table 9.1. Despite its numerous theoretical advantages, recent randomized trials have failed consistently to demonstrate unequivocal superiority of bivalirudin over unfractionated heparin in the STEMI setting (Table 9.3). The studies do suggest a lowered risk of major bleeding, driven at least partially by reduced access site bleeding. Of note, several trials suggested an increased risk of early stent thrombosis (possibly ameliorated by prolonging the bivalirudin infusion post PCI).

Given the lack of superiority and significantly higher costs, the role of bivalirudin in STEMI remains questionable. This is of particular importance in the current era of using more potent P2Y12 inhibitors (e.g. ticagrelor and prasugrel) and transradial access (which all but eliminates access site bleeding). Society guidelines are somewhat discordant, with the ACCF/AHA guidelines [3] awarding bivalirudin a class IB recommendation in STEMI, while the more updated 2017 ESC guidelines [1] give it a IIa recommendation unless there is a history of heparin-induced thrombocytopenia (class Ib).

9.4 Monitoring of Intensity of Anticoagulation in the Cardiac Catheterization Laboratory

9.4.1 Unfractionated Heparin

The anticoagulation response of UFH is variable and unreliable. Therefore, monitoring the level of anticoagulation using a point-of-care testing device is inherently attractive. The most widely used test to measure the anticoagulant effect of high doses of heparin (levels at which the aPTT would be "immeasurable") is the activated clotting time (ACT) which has a linear dose-response to heparin concentrations in the very high 1–5 U/mL range and is available as a point-of-care assay. That said, there is lack of robust data to suggest that ACT testing and monitoring is necessary and beneficial. Several studies have questioned the relationship between ACT levels achieved and ischemic complications [6, 7]. Despite its limitations, ACT remains widely used in the cardiac catheterization laboratory to gauge the intensity of heparinization. Indeed, the ACCF/AHA guidelines [3] give monitoring ACT levels and titrating UFH dosing during primary PCI a class I recommendation, though the ESC guidelines are silent on the subject. The ACCF/AHA/SCAI PCI guidelines [8] recommend titrating UFH dosing to target ACT levels (Table 9.4) although these "targets" are largely based on consensus and experience rather than systematic study.

Table 9.4 Effect of various antithrombotic drugs on activated clotting time

Drug	Xa:IIa activity	Effect on ACT	Target ACT (s)
UFH	1:1	Linear ↑	GPI, 300–350 (Hemochron), 250–300 (HemoTech) No GPI, 200–250 (any device)
Enoxaparin	4:1	Modest ↑	None defined[a]
Fondaparinux	Pure Xa	No effect	No recommendation
Bivalirudin	Pure IIa	Disproportionate ↑	No recommendation[b]

UFH unfractionated heparin, *ACT* activated clotting time, *GPI* glycoprotein IIb/IIIa inhibitor
[a]See text for recommendations
[b]ACT levels do not correlate with therapeutic efficacy; only an indicator of drug delivery

9.4.2 Low Molecular Weight Heparin

Monitoring anticoagulation with enoxaparin is difficult because the ACT does not follow a linear dose-response unlike with UFH. The most definitive assay of enoxaparin's anticoagulant effect (measuring anti factor Xa activity) is not a readily available laboratory or point-of-care assay. Nevertheless, enoxaparin does moderately prolong the ACT, and several authors have suggested a role of ACT testing to guide enoxaparin therapy in the cardiac catheterization laboratory. One group has proposed a target ACT of 175 s for PCI performed with and 200 s for PCI performed without a glycoprotein IIb/IIIa inhibitor [9]. They also propose that every additional 0.1 mg/kg bolus of intravenous enoxaparin may be expected to increase the ACT by 10 s [10]. Of note, this has not been systematically studied for outcomes and remains a rough guide at most.

9.4.3 Bivalirudin

Bivalirudin raises the ACT usually in the "super therapeutic" range (often >300 s). However, studies with bivalirudin have reproducibly demonstrated no relationship between ACT levels and either bleeding or ischemic complications, quite in contrast to heparin. Thus, it may be reasonable to check an ACT once following the bolus of bivalirudin to confirm that the drug was delivered, thereby avoiding inadvertent failure of drug administration (e.g. intravenous line occlusion and other errors which may easily occur in the emergency setting). However, there is no role of sequentially testing ACT for the above-mentioned reasons. It is important to note, though, that the pivotal bivalirudin trials gave an additional dose of 0.3 mg/kg bolus if the post bolus ACT was <225 s. However, the ACCF/AHA or ESC guidelines do not specifically recommend this practice.

9.5 Approach to the Patient Who Has Received Anticoagulation Prior to Primary PCI

Although relatively unusual for a patient to receive parental anticoagulation prior to arrival to the cardiac catheterization laboratory for primary PCI, historically, some emergency room (ER) physicians have routinely administered UFH in the ER to STEMI patients. Also, in a "rescue" or "salvage" PCI setting, a patient may have received full-dose thrombolytic therapy prior to arriving to the laboratory. Furthermore, a situation may arise in which a patient admitted with an acute coronary syndrome "heats up" and progresses to STEMI despite receiving some sort of anticoagulation therapy. Table 9.5 shows the therapeutic options for the patient who arrives to the cardiac catheterization laboratory with anticoagulant therapy on board. Table 9.6 summarizes the approach to dosing if prior therapy has been administered.

Table 9.5 Therapeutic options for anticoagulation during primary PCI based on pretreatment status

Pretreatment	Therapeutic options during primary PCI
None	UFH Enoxaparin Bivalirudin
UFH[a]	UFH Bivalirudin
Enoxaparin	Enoxaparin[a]
Fondaparinux	UFH
GPI	UFH—check ACT and adjust dose (see Table 9.1)
Thrombolytic[b]	UFH—check ACT and adjust dose

UFH unfractionated heparin, *GPI* glycoprotein IIb/IIIa inhibitors
[a]No good "formula" to convert dosing of UFH to enoxaparin and vice versa
[b]Salvage" PCI setting

Table 9.6 Dosing of anticoagulation therapy in the cardiac catheterization laboratory in patients receiving anticoagulation prior to arrival

Drug	On treatment	Not on treatment
UFH	Check ACT on arrival "Top-up" UFH according to ACT	70–100 U/kg (no GPI planned) 50–70 U/kg IV (GPI planned). Target to therapeutic ACT
Enoxaparin	Last SC dose <8 h—no additional[a] Last SC dose >8 h—additional bolus 0.3 mg/kg IV bolus	0.5 mg/kg IV bolus
Fondaparinux	70–100 U/kg (no GPI planned) 50–70 U/kg IV (GPI planned) Target to therapeutic ACT [18]	
Bivalirudin	0.5 mg/kg bolus; ↑ drip to 1.75 mg/kg/h	0.75 mg/kg bolus; 1.75 mg/kg/h drip

ACT activated clotting time, *UFH* unfractionated heparin, *SC* subcutaneous, *GPI* glycoprotein IIb/IIIa inhibitor
[a]If patient received <2 doses, assume no steady state and administer additional bolus

As a rule of thumb, if a patient has been on therapy, then a "booster" dose of the anticoagulant is recommended. On the other hand, if a patient has received no prior therapy, then the full dose of the anticoagulant should be administered. It is important to note that "on therapy" for these purposes assumes a steady state of the drug. For enoxaparin, which is commonly used in the acute coronary syndrome setting, this means at least two doses have been administered. Hence if a patient arrives to the cardiac catheterization laboratory after receiving one dose of enoxaparin in the ward, it is safer to administer an additional dose of enoxaparin (Table 9.6). Note that no good "formula" exists to switch previous therapy with UFH to enoxaparin and vice versa when a patient arrives to the cardiac catheterization laboratory.

9.6 Role of Anticoagulation Following Successful PCI

By and large, anticoagulation should be stopped after a successful procedure. Data suggests that extending the anticoagulation with post procedure UFH or LMWH does not reduce ischemic complications but does increase bleeding risks [11, 12]. Therefore barring some compelling indication (very high thrombus burden or left ventricular thrombus) UFH or LMWH should not be continued after primary PCI. Similarly routine ACT check post procedure likely has little cumulative value other than to determine when the access sheath may be removed in the case of femoral access. In the case of bivalirudin, trials have suggested an increased risk of acute stent thrombosis following drug cessation at the end of the procedure (Table 9.3). This may be related to the very short half-life of the drug with a rapid wash-out. Prolonging the infusion may help mitigate that risk, although the data shows mixed results.

9.7 Summary

Anticoagulation with an antithrombotic drug is considered mandatory during PCI. UFH remains the most widely used antithrombotic agent during primary PCI and ideally should be dosed to a target therapeutic ACT. Enoxaparin may be a reasonable alternative in primary PCI, although advantage for this over heparin is debatable. Bivalirudin has many theoretical advantages over the heparins; however, trials in the primary PCI setting have failed to show superiority of bivalirudin for ischemic events, although bleeding events (driven partially by access site bleeding) are reduced. Furthermore, acute stent thrombotic events may be increased with bivalirudin, and consequently use of this drug is less widespread. Anticoagulation dosing in the cardiac catheterization laboratory needs to be tailored according to prior therapy and titrated (at least in the case of UFH) either empirically or to a therapeutic ACT where monitoring is available.

References

1. Ibanez B, James S, Agewall S, et al. 2017 ESC guidelines for the management of acute myocardial infarction in patients presenting with ST-segment elevation: the task force for the management of acute myocardial infarction in patients presenting with ST-segment elevation of the European Society of Cardiology (ESC). Eur Heart J. 2018;39(2):119–77.
2. De Caterina R, Husted S, Wallentin L, et al. Parenteral anticoagulants in heart disease: current status and perspectives (section II). Position paper of the ESC Working Group on thrombosis-task force on anticoagulants in heart disease. Thromb Haemost. 2013;109(5):769–86.
3. O'Gara PT, Kushner FG, Ascheim DD, et al. 2013 ACCF/AHA guideline for the management of ST-elevation myocardial infarction: executive summary: a report of the American College of Cardiology Foundation/American Heart Association Task Force on practice guidelines. Circulation. 2013;127(4):529–55.

4. Montalescot G, Zeymer U, Silvain J, et al. Intravenous enoxaparin or unfractionated heparin in primary percutaneous coronary intervention for ST-elevation myocardial infarction: the international randomised open-label ATOLL trial. Lancet. 2011;378(9792):693–703.
5. Yusuf S, Mehta SR, Chrolavicius S, et al. Effects of fondaparinux on mortality and reinfarction in patients with acute ST-segment elevation myocardial infarction: the OASIS-6 randomized trial. JAMA. 2006;295(13):1519–30.
6. Brener SJ, Moliterno DJ, Lincoff AM, Steinhubl SR, Wolski KE, Topol EJ. Relationship between activated clotting time and ischemic or hemorrhagic complications: analysis of 4 recent randomized clinical trials of percutaneous coronary intervention. Circulation. 2004;110(8):994–8.
7. Chew DP, Bhatt DL, Lincoff AM, et al. Defining the optimal activated clotting time during percutaneous coronary intervention: aggregate results from 6 randomized, controlled trials. Circulation. 2001;103(7):961–6.
8. Levine GN, Bates ER, Blankenship JC, et al. 2011 ACCF/AHA/SCAI guideline for percutaneous coronary intervention: executive summary: a report of the American College of Cardiology Foundation/American Heart Association Task Force on Practice Guidelines and the Society for Cardiovascular Angiography and Interventions. Circulation. 2011;124(23):2574–609.
9. Cavusoglu E, Lakhani M, Marmur JD. The activated clotting time (ACT) can be used to monitor enoxaparin and dalteparin after intravenous administration. J Invasive Cardiol. 2005;17(8):416–21.
10. Marmur JD, Bullock-Palmer RP, Poludasu S, Cavusoglu E. Avoiding intelligence failures in the cardiac catheterization laboratory: strategies for the safe and rational use of dalteparin or enoxaparin during percutaneous coronary intervention. J Invasive Cardiol. 2009;21(12):653–64.
11. Riaz IB, Asawaeer M, Riaz H, et al. Optimal anticoagulation duration of unfractionated and low molecular weight heparin in non-ST elevation acute coronary syndrome: a systematic review of the literature. Int J Cardiol. 2014;177(2):461–6.
12. Ducrocq G, Steg PG, Van 't Hof A, et al. Utility of post-procedural anticoagulation after primary PCI for STEMI: insights from a pooled analysis of the HORIZONS-AMI and EUROMAX trials. Eur Heart J Acute Cardiovasc Care. 2017;6(7):659–65.
13. Stone GW, Witzenbichler B, Guagliumi G, et al. Bivalirudin during primary PCI in acute myocardial infarction. N Engl J Med. 2008;358(21):2218–30.
14. Steg PG, Van 't Hof A, Hamm CW, et al. Bivalirudin started during emergency transport for primary PCI. N Engl J Med. 2013;369(23):2207–17.
15. Shahzad A, Kemp I, Mars C, et al. Unfractionated heparin versus bivalirudin in primary percutaneous coronary intervention (HEAT-PPCI): an open-label, single centre, randomised controlled trial. Lancet. 2014;384(9957):1849–58.
16. Han Y, Guo J, Zheng Y, et al. Bivalirudin vs heparin with or without tirofiban during primary percutaneous coronary intervention in acute myocardial infarction: the BRIGHT randomized clinical trial. JAMA. 2015;313(13):1336–46.
17. Erlinge D, Koul S, Eriksson P, et al. Bivalirudin versus heparin in non-ST and ST-segment elevation myocardial infarction-a registry-based randomized clinical trial in the SWEDEHEART registry (the VALIDATE-SWEDEHEART trial). Am Heart J. 2016;175:36–46.
18. Alfonso F. Comments on the 2017 ESC guidelines for the Management of Acute Myocardial Infarction in patients presenting with ST-segment elevation. Rev Esp Cardiol. 2017;70(12):1039–45.

Management of Intracoronary Thrombus 10

Janarthanan Sathananthan, Timothy J. Watson, Dale Murdoch, Christopher Overgaard, Deborah Lee, Deanna Khoo, and Paul J. L. Ong

10.1 Introduction

Partial or complete occlusion of the infarct-related artery (IRA) with intracoronary thrombus (ICT) is the pathognomonic hallmark of patients presenting with ST-elevation myocardial infarction (STEMI). Thrombus burden can be highly variable, but its presence is associated with worse outcomes, including lower procedural success, increased abrupt vessel closure and an increased frequency of major in-hospital complications including death and recurrent myocardial infarction (MI). ICT poses a unique series of challenges, but appropriate management is an essential prerequisite for successful primary percutaneous coronary intervention (PPCI). This can largely be achieved using a combination of pharmacological and mechanical approaches prior to coronary stent insertion.

In this chapter, we discuss the causes, sequelae and treatment of intracoronary thrombus specific to patients presenting with STEMI.

J. Sathananthan (✉)
St. Pauls Hospital, Vancouver, BC, Canada

T. J. Watson
HSC Medical Center, Menara HSC, Kuala Lumpur, Malaysia

D. Murdoch
Department of Cardiology, The Prince Charles Hospital, Brisbane, QLD, Australia

The University of Queensland, St. Lucia, QLD, Australia

C. Overgaard
Cardiac Catheterization Laboratories and Coronary Intensive Care Unit, Toronto General Hospital, University Health Network, Toronto, ON, Canada

D. Lee · D. Khoo · P. J. L. Ong
Tan Tock Seng Hospital, National Healthcare Group, Singapore

T. J. Watson et al. (eds.), *Primary Angioplasty*,
https://doi.org/10.1007/978-981-13-1114-7_10

10.2 Pathophysiology of Intracoronary Thrombus Formation

In the majority of cases, the nidus for thrombogenesis is erosion of an underlying atherosclerotic plaque and subsequent exposure of thrombogenic subendothelial matrix and plaque to circulating platelets [1]. Plaque rupture initiates the coagulation cascade in one of two distinct but ultimately synergistic pathways (Fig. 10.1). In the first pathway, platelet glycoprotein VI binds directly with collagen exposed by the denuded endothelium. Concurrently platelet glycoprotein Ib-V-IX interacts with collagen-bound von Willebrand factor (vWf). This process triggers platelet activation, adherence and accumulation to the vessel wall leading to formation of 'white' thrombi. In contrast, the second pathway leads to formation of 'red' thrombi where tissue factor initiates a proteolytic cascade which leads to generation of thrombin which in turn converts fibrinogen to fibrin while also triggering activation and accumulation of platelets through release of various agonists including adenosine, thromboxane A_2 and serotonin. These agents activate other platelets, thereby amplifying the thrombogenic process. Coronary thrombus consists of platelets, erythrocytes, inflammatory cells and fibrin. The thrombin-generating process leads to denser, more fibrin-rich thrombus which becomes progressively more difficult to disrupt (both pharmacologically and mechanically) with time [2–5].

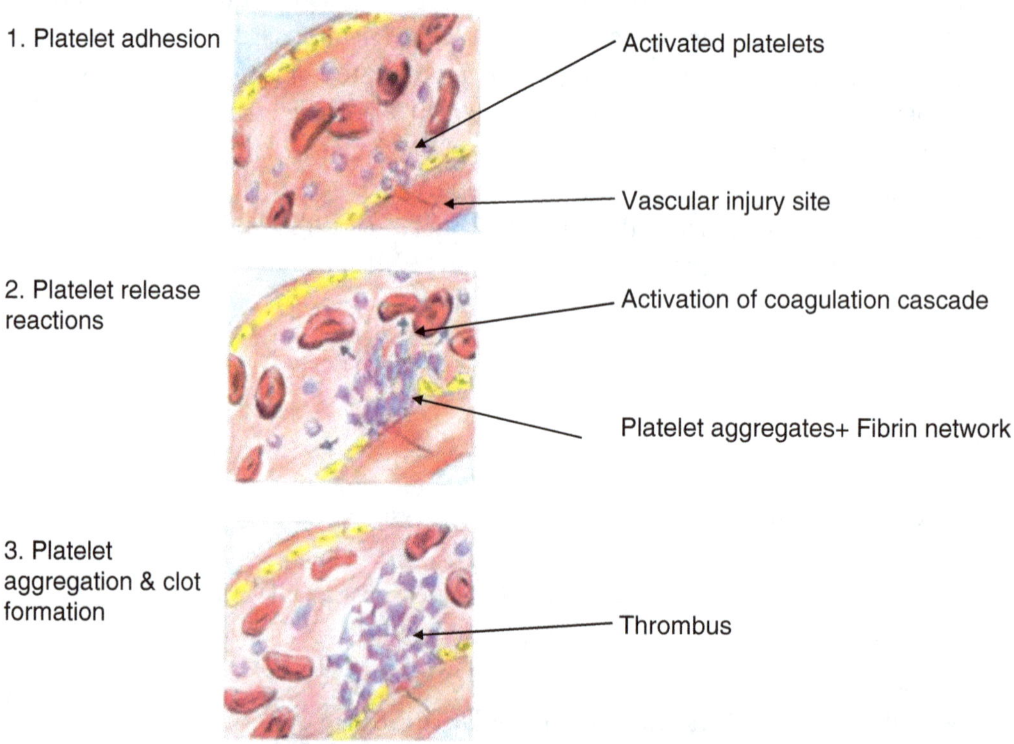

Fig. 10.1 Intracoronary effects of coagulation cascade. [Courtesy of Miss Christina YS Wong]

The more friable the thrombus burden is at the time of PCI, the more susceptible it is to mechanical intervention. However, particularly with late presentations, thrombus can also be resistant to coronary devices, including balloons and aspiration catheters. Thrombus variability relates to the two types of fibrin fibres that are deposited at the time of thrombogenesis, including thin dense fibres (which are poorly dissolved by thrombolytic agents and mechanical devices) and thick fibrin fibres (which are more susceptible to treatment).

10.2.1 Grading Coronary Thrombus

Grading tools are useful to quantify the thrombus burden in patients presenting with STEMI. The TIMI (thrombolysis in myocardial infarction) thrombus grading scale (Fig. 10.2) is commonly used and is a simple numerical scale ranging from grade 0 (no thrombus) to grade 5 (very large thrombus that completely occludes vessel flow) [6, 7]. The scale is subject to variability in interpretation and can be simplified to a binary system: low-grade thrombus (TIMI 1–3) and high-grade thrombus (TIMI 4–5) [8]. Visual grading tools also tend to underestimate thrombus size compared to other tools such as intracoronary imaging.

TIMI Thrombus Grade

0. No cine-angiographic characteristics of thrombus present
1. Possible thrombus present. Angiography shows characteristics such as reduced contrast density, haziness, irregular lesion contour, or a smooth convex meniscus at the site of total occlusion suggestive but not diagnostic of thrombus
2. Thrombus present, small size: definite thrombus with greatest dimensions less than or equal to half vessel diameter
3. Thrombus present, moderate size: definite thrombus but with greatest linear dimension greater than half but less than 2 vessel diameters
4. Thrombus present, large size: as in grade 3 but with the largest dimension greater than or equal to 2 vessel diameters
5. Total occlusion

Fig. 10.2 TIMI thrombus grade

10.2.2 Intracoronary Thrombus and Clinical Outcomes

The presence of ICT during acute coronary syndromes often results in suboptimal coronary reperfusion and worse clinical outcomes [7, 9, 10]. The effect of thrombus on the microvascular circulation can be quantified using degree of ST-segment resolution or the myocardial blush grade [11]. The myocardial blush grade is used as a marker of a perfusion in the capillary level at the tissue level. Both the degree of ST-segment resolution and myocardial blush grade have been shown to be independent markers of mortality [12].

Use of a grading tool allows a consistent method for thrombus assessment and correlation to clinical outcomes. Importantly they can also aid in management decisions prior to and during PCI. The presence of ICT and distal embolization to the microcirculation can lead to persistent chest pain, electrocardiogram changes and distal vessel occlusion. Even if normal epicardial flow is achieved, distal embolization and microvascular obstruction are associated with increased infarct size, reduced ventricular function and worse survival. Due to the negative clinical consequences of incomplete thrombus resolution, it is essential that interventional cardiologists consider strategies to prevent and treat ICT during STEMI.

10.3 Management

The extent of ICT observed during PPCI correlates strongly with both procedural success and clinical outcome. Due to the complex nature of intracoronary thrombogenesis, a multi-faceted and systematic approach is required to achieve successful thrombus dissolution. This includes arrest of the coagulation cascade (usually achieved using pharmacotherapy), flow restoration (usually through mechanical techniques) and occasionally with the use of thrombus extraction tools. Thrombus extraction may theoretically limit distal embolization of thrombus, thereby preventing microvascular obstruction and incomplete microvascular reperfusion.

10.3.1 Pharmacological Interventions

Comprehensive review of pharmacological interventions utilized during PPCI is available in Chaps. 8 and 9. Due to the self-propagating nature of thrombogenesis, early and effective pharmacological interventions to inhibit this process are key. At point of initial STEMI diagnosis, patients should receive a loading dose of aspirin (e.g. 300 mg or institutional practice) and a P_2Y_{12} antagonist (e.g. clopidogrel 600 mg, prasugrel 60 mg or ticagrelor 180 mg) [13–15]. In some healthcare systems, community STEMI diagnosis may occur, and early administration of these oral antiplatelet agents may be feasible [16]. More commonly, administration occurs in the emergency department; with shorter transfer times to the cardiac catheterization laboratory, this could lead to suboptimal platelet inhibition during the PPCI procedure [17]. Such considerations are important, particularly for the immediate peri-PCI period in a freshly stented patient who is naïve to antiplatelet therapy and in cases where thrombus burden is significant. This has led to development of rapid-onset intravenous P_2Y_{12} antagonists (e.g. cangrelor), which may prove useful as a bridge until the maximal antiplatelet effect of oral agents is realized [18]. An intravenous P_2Y_{12} agent may also be advantageous in STEMI patients that are intubated or unable to have oral agents. However, these agents are not broadly available.

Peri-procedural anticoagulation is generally achieved using unfractionated heparin or in some catheter laboratories using low-molecular weight heparin (e.g. enoxaparin), factor Xa inhibition (e.g. fondaparinux) or a reversible direct thrombin inhibitor (bivalirudin) [19, 20]. Each strategy has individual merit and choice is therefore largely determined by operator/unit preference or cost. The progressive shift from transfemoral to transradial intervention amongst patients with STEMI has vastly reduced vascular access complications such as bleeding and improved procedural safety [21, 22]. Consequently, the purported advantage of agents such as bivalirudin that reduce bleeding to improve clinical outcomes may be less marked [23].

In our opinion, peri-procedural anticoagulation is best achieved in keeping with the standard protocol each laboratory uses for PCI in stable patients without need for modified protocols. In most instances, this is likely to be adjusted dose heparin (70–100 international units/Kg) titrated to maintain an activated coagulation time (ACT) of >300 s. There is variability between catheterization laboratories regarding routine ACT assessment during PCI. We recommend that in cases with high burden of ICT, assessment of ACT may be useful to ensure that patients have had a therapeutic response to anticoagulation and may need additional heparin as required. Additionally, given the concern regarding efficacy of oral antiplatelet agents in pharmacologically naïve patients, a repeat ACT check at intervals and at procedure completion (with top-up heparin if required) may be prudent, although this strategy has not been proven in published trials to date.

Various ancillary pharmacological therapies have been utilized to treat distal embolization as a consequence of intracoronary thrombus formation. These agents include calcium channel blockers, adenosine, nicorandil, glycoprotein IIb/IIIa inhibitors, vasodilators and nitroprusside. Calcium channel blockers may inhibit platelet aggregation and have a direct effect on calcium flux through the sarcolemmal membrane that could protect injured myocytes [24, 25]. Adenosine affects intracellular calcium and inhibits neutrophil accumulation, superoxide generation [26, 27]. Nicorandil, an ATP-dependent potassium channel opener, can prevent reperfusion injury and protect cardiac myocytes [28–30]. Glycoprotein IIB/IIIA inhibitors have also been used in cases of no reflow and inhibit platelet aggregation [31, 32]. Each of these agents has variable success and none has been proven to be superior to another. Additionally, whether to administer these agents, pre- or post-stent deployment is also undetermined. The clinical benefit of each of these individual agents on epicardial flow and myocardial salvage continues to be limited.

Intracoronary thrombolytic prior to aspiration thrombectomy could also be considered in selective cases. The DISSOLUTION trial compared intracoronary thrombolytic delivered via microcatheter and aspiration thrombectomy with aspiration thrombectomy alone. Patients treated with upfront thrombolytic had high rate of TIMI 3 flow and higher proportion of patients with myocardial blush grade of 2/3. Patients also had greater volume of aspirate compared to aspiration thrombectomy alone [33]. Further study is needed with larger clinical trials.

10.4 Thrombectomy

Although PPCI has been established as the dominant reperfusion strategy for the treatment of STEMI, the benefit of this approach can sometimes be limited. Mechanisms that may explain this limited benefit have included delays in time from symptom onset to reperfusion, reperfusion injury following vessel recanalization and distal embolization of thrombus. This lead to the development of thrombus removal with the concept that prevention of distal embolization might improve outcomes of primary PCI.

10.4.1 Thrombectomy Systems

Thrombectomy catheters while bulky confer benefits of better thrombus aspiration. Various systems exist that have different mechanisms of action which include rheolytic, fragmentation and manual thrombectomy. Rheolytic involves using high-velocity jets of saline which creates negative pressure through a Venturi effect. The AnjioJet is an example of a rheolytic system [34]. This device has lost its appeal after trials demonstrated an increased mortality with no difference in infarct size or resolution of ST segments [35, 36]. Manual or 'aspiration' thrombectomy has been studied in large randomized controlled trials and emerged as the preferred method of thrombus removal primary due to its simplicity and ease of use.

Aspiration thrombectomy initially showed promise with benefit seen from early smaller randomized trials. These studies demonstrated the feasibility and potential benefit of thrombus extraction on indices of myocardial perfusion and ST segment resolution at time of PPCI. Infarct size was found to be less in patients undergoing thrombectomy before stenting compared with controls undergoing stenting without prior thrombectomy [37, 38]. These initial favourable studies lead to considerable uptake of routine manual thrombectomy during primary PCI. The advantages cited were improved reperfusion with less need for predilatation and arguably improved myocardial blush. Mechanistically, the postulated benefits of aspiration thrombectomy were less distal embolization and prevention of reperfusion injury. However, the large randomized TOTAL trial did not show any benefit for use of routine thrombectomy, and of concern there was a signal for harm with increased risk of stroke in the thrombectomy arm of the study [39–41]. The mechanism of stroke is likely due to aspiration back of clot and subsequent embolization to the brain.

In patient presenting with acute coronary syndrome and preexisting thrombus as a consequence of plaque rupture, routine thrombectomy is not recommended. While manual thrombectomy has a theoretical and intuitive basis for incremental value, results from pivotal trials and "real-world" registries of manual thrombectomy have not consistently demonstrated benefit over standard PCI [42]. Current European Society of Cardiology guidelines do not recommend routine use of thrombus aspiration. There may potentially be a benefit of selective thrombectomy. Patients who have very large thrombus may benefit, but this has not been robustly proven with randomized controlled evidence [43]. A recent meta-analysis of the three randomized trials showed a trend towards less cardiovascular death with aspiration thrombectomy compared to PCI. Of concern, there was also increased stroke or transient ischaemic attack despite a benefit in mortality. The pathophysiology is likely multifactorial and more complex, warranting further study. Additionally, thrombectomy may be helpful in cases where thrombus develops during PCI and after post-stent deployment. Aspiration thrombectomy may aid restoration of flow and help guide subsequent PCI.

10.4.2 Suggested Technique for Manual Thrombectomy

While routine aspiration thrombectomy is not advocated, there may be some patients that may benefit. In selected cases where a decision is made to proceed with thrombectomy, we suggest the following technique using the commonly available aspiration thrombectomy catheter.

- Ensure the guiding catheter is well engaged at all times.
- Start aspiration in the guiding catheter and make multiple passes until syringe is full.
- Continue to switch syringes as needed.
- Ensure a new syringe is placed with full negative pressure at time of removal of aspiration catheter. Prior to removal of the aspiration catheter, a small contrast test injection is advised to check that the guide is engaged.
- After removal of the aspiration catheter, we suggest allowing the guide catheter to bleed back or to aspirate through the side port of the manifold or autoinjector to ensure any clots that remain in the guide catheter are cleared prior to taking any further angiographic images.

Fastidious technique may reduce the likelihood of any subsequent stroke occurring.

10.5 Other Causes of Intracoronary Thrombus Formation in STEMI Patients

It is important to appreciate other causes of ICT that can occur in patients presenting with STEMI. While most patients present with ICT due to plaque rupture, patients can also present with STEMI and ICT due to embolism, vasospasm, spontaneous coronary artery dissection, coagulation disorders, trauma and endothelial dysfunction. In some cases, the underlying coronary artery is normal.

In cases where there is suspicion of another cause of STEMI other than plaque rupture, intracoronary imaging can be very helpful. In some cases, such as embolism, aspiration thrombectomy can aid restoration of vessel flow. Use of intravascular imaging with IVUS or OCT is very important to exclude underlying coronary artery disease. If the underlying vessel is normal, then stenting may not be required. In some causes such as spontaneous coronary artery dissection, diagnostic angiography and medical treatment only may be the optimal therapy for most cases. While intracoronary imaging can be used in cases of SCAD, routine use is not advocated as there is a risk of acute vessel closure with any further manipulation of the vessel.

10.6 Stenting Strategy

Large thrombus burden at time of primary PCI can lead to challenges with stent sizing, stent apposition and final TIMI flow, which can in turn increase the risk of stent thrombosis. While not recommended routinely, aspiration thrombectomy can be useful in cases of large thrombus burden to allow visualization of the vessel and appropriate stent sizing [43]. During PPCI judicious use of nitroglycerin is recommended to limit vasoconstriction which is common during STEMI due to inflammation and higher circulating catecholamines. Drug-eluting stents are recommended for PPCI. Some novel mesh-covered stents such as the MGuard stent which by design aim to prevent thrombus distal embolization have been trialled in small trials but have not been proven beneficial for routine use [44, 45].

10.6.1 Deferred Stenting

Primary PCI and stenting is the current recommended treatment for patients presenting with STEMI. This allows restoration of flow in the infarct artery and reduces reocclusion and restenosis. Implantation of a stent in a highly thrombotic milieu at the time of initial presentation with STEMI can be associated with risk of distal embolization and increased peri-procedural events. Furthermore, despite appropriate administration of antiplatelet agents, patients are often taken to the catheterization laboratory before these agents have achieved their desired therapeutic effect. One strategy to overcome this issue is 'deferred stenting', a practice that is not recommended routinely for all STEMI patients [46]. In selected cases, with high thrombus burden that are haemodynamically stable, deferred stenting may offer a therapeutic option. All patients should proceed urgently to the catheterization laboratory, and flow may need to be restored with a wire or gentle predilatation with a balloon. If high burden of thrombus is seen, deferred stenting with an interim period of adjunctive antiplatelet/anti thrombotic therapy may be useful to reduce the thrombus load and minimize complications (such as no-reflow) at time of stenting [47, 48].

10.7 Conclusion

Intracoronary thrombus during STEMI is common and can lead to worse clinical outcomes. While there is no gold-standard therapy to deal with ICT, there are a combination of both pharmacological and mechanical therapies that can be utilized. Importantly, aspiration thrombectomy should not be used routinely in STEMI cases but may be helpful in selected cases at the discretion of the operator. The management of intracoronary thrombus at time of STEMI continues to remain a therapeutic challenge, but an awareness and aggressive management of ICT can lead to improved outcomes.

10.8 Case Report: Heavy Thrombus Load in Primary PCI

Janarthanan Sathananthan, Dale Murdoch, and Christopher Overgaard

10.8.1 History

A 42-year-old man with risk factors of type 2 diabetes and hypertension presented with a 6-h history of central chest pain and inferior ST segment elevation to a non-PCI capable hospital. He was loaded with aspirin 325 mg and ticagrelor 180 mg and transferred to a hospital capable of primary PCI. At time of presentation to the catheterization laboratory, he had ongoing chest discomfort and was bradycardic but haemodynamically stable.

10.8.2 Management

Arterial access was obtained via the transradial route. Intravenous heparin was administered at a dose of 100 IU/kg. Diagnostic coronary angiography showed a critical occlusion in the right coronary artery with a significant ICT burden and TIMI 1 flow. Using a Judkins right guiding catheter, the right coronary artery was wired with a Balance Middle Weight coronary wire. Given the significant burden of ICT, a bolus dose and infusion of glycoprotein IIb/IIIa inhibitor were then administered. Following this, aspiration thrombectomy was performed to aid in restoration of vessel flow to prevent the need for balloon predilatation. Aspiration thrombectomy restored flow in the right coronary artery, but there was distal embolization of thrombus to the posterolateral vessel. Further aspiration thrombectomy was performed restoring flow and the culprit lesion was stented with a long drug-eluting stent. After stent deployment, there was evidence of no-reflow phenomenon. Repeated doses of intracoronary nitroglycerin and adenosine were administered. Subsequent angiographic pictures showed restoration of TIMI 3 flow and normal myocardial blush grade (Fig. 10.3). A left ventriculogram showed normal left ventricular function.

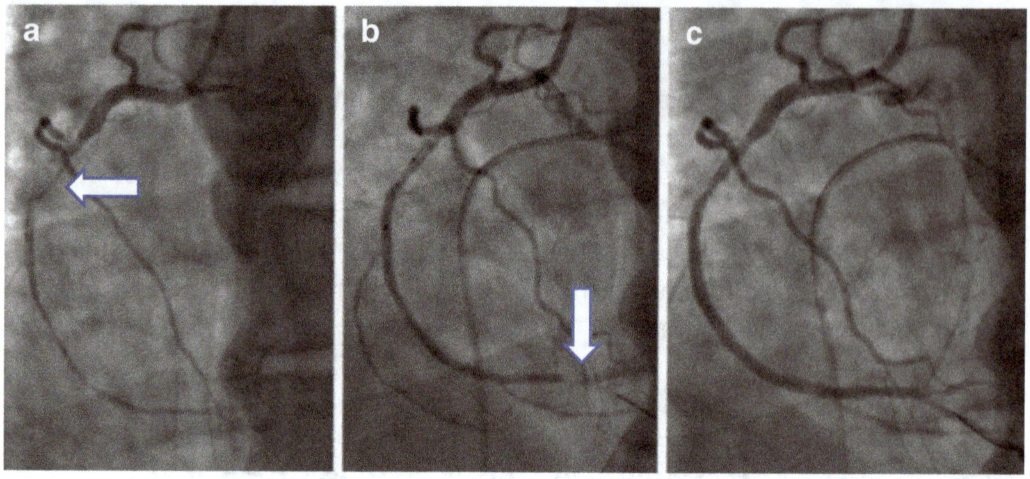

Fig. 10.3 Case example of intracoronary thrombus management during an inferior STEMI. (**a**) Initial diagnostic angiogram showing critical right coronary lesion with large thrombus (white arrow) at lesion. (**b**) Angiographic picture following aspiration thrombectomy with evidence of distal thrombus embolization to the posterolateral branch. (**c**) Angiographic picture following further thrombectomy and dose of glycoprotein IIb/IIIa inhibitor. (**d**) Final angiographic picture following stent deployment and doses of intracoronary adenosine and nitroglycerin to treat no reflow

10.8.3 Outcome

Following PPCI the patient's chest pain resolved. He had an uncomplicated recovery on the coronary care unit. Transthoracic echocardiography also showed normal left ventricular function. This case highlights that with judicious attention to the management of ICT, use of both pharmacological and percutaneous techniques can be used to successfully deal with ICT.

10.9 Acute STEMI with Extensive Thrombus: An Illustrative Case

Deborah Lee, Deanna Khoo, and Paul JL Ong

10.9.1 Introduction

Intracoronary thrombus poses a considerable challenge during percutaneous coronary intervention (PCI) and is associated with risk of no reflow, less intra-procedural success and increased in-hospital complications including myocardial infarction (MI) and death [49]. Many of these events are a direct result of distal embolization and microvascular obstruction. Consequently, various strategies to reduce thrombus burden have been explored. These include pharmacological thrombolysis, covered stents and thrombectomy—performed by manual aspiration or mechanical thrombus disruption. However, these strategies become a great challenge in the setting of large thrombus load. The use of stent retrievers for thrombus removal in acute ischaemic stroke has been shown to be safe and effective [39]. We describe the use of the Solitaire thrombus retrieval system (Medtronic MN, USA) in a patient with MI and heavy thrombus burden which was refractory to treatment by conventional means.

10.9.2 Case Report

A 54-year-old male smoker presented to the emergency department with a 2-day history of intermittent chest pain and anterior ST depression. He was loaded with aspirin 300 mg and ticagrelor 180 mg and referred for emergent cardiac catheterization.

Coronary angiography demonstrated the culprit to be an occluded distal left circumflex (LCx) artery (Fig. 10.4). During the procedure, he received enoxaparin and two boluses of intravenous eptifibatide. The occlusion was crossed easily with a Sion Blue wire (Asahi Intecc, JP) following which balloon angioplasty was performed with a 1.25 mm and then 2.0 mm compliant balloons inflated to nominal pressure. Although flow improved, a large intracoronary thrombus was now evident. Manual aspiration thrombectomy was performed with multiple runs of a 6F Eliminate catheter (Terumo, JP) which only managed to retrieve small fragments of thrombus. As flow in the LCx had been restored, we opted for a strategy of deferred stenting 48 h later after completion of an eptifibatide infusion and ongoing therapeutic enoxaparin.

At repeat angiography, the thrombus burden was largely unchanged (Fig. 10.5). Having failed both aspiration thrombectomy and pharmacological thrombolysis, thrombectomy was attempted with a 2–4 mm × 20 mm Solitaire thrombus retrieval

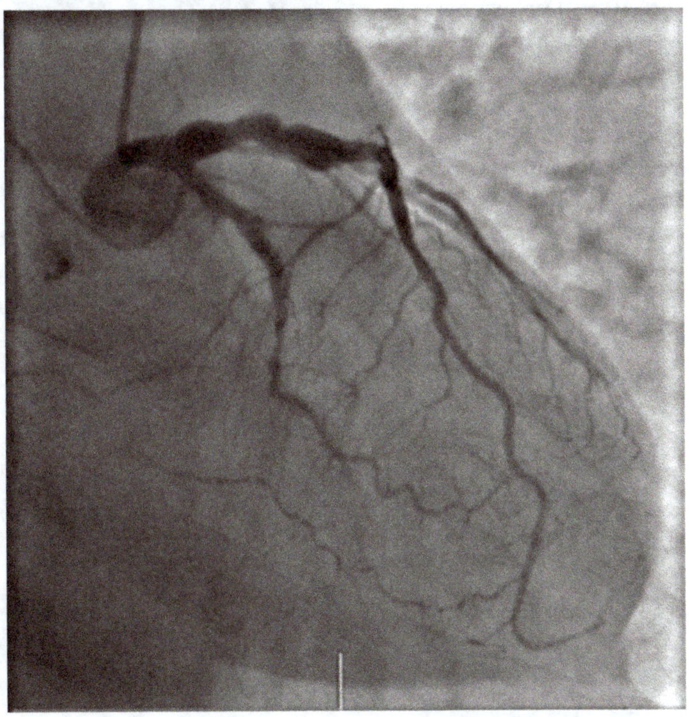

Fig. 10.4 Coronary angiogram of left coronary system. Note occlusion of the left circumflex artery

device. The left main was engaged with a 6F BL 3.5 guide catheter (Terumo), and a Sion Blue wire was advanced into the distal LCx, across the thrombus. A microcatheter was advanced through the wire and positioned distal to the thrombus. The self-expanding Solitaire was then loaded inside the microcatheter and deployed across the thrombus (Fig. 10.6). The device was left expanded for 5 min, following which it was carefully retrieved together with the microcatheter under continuous

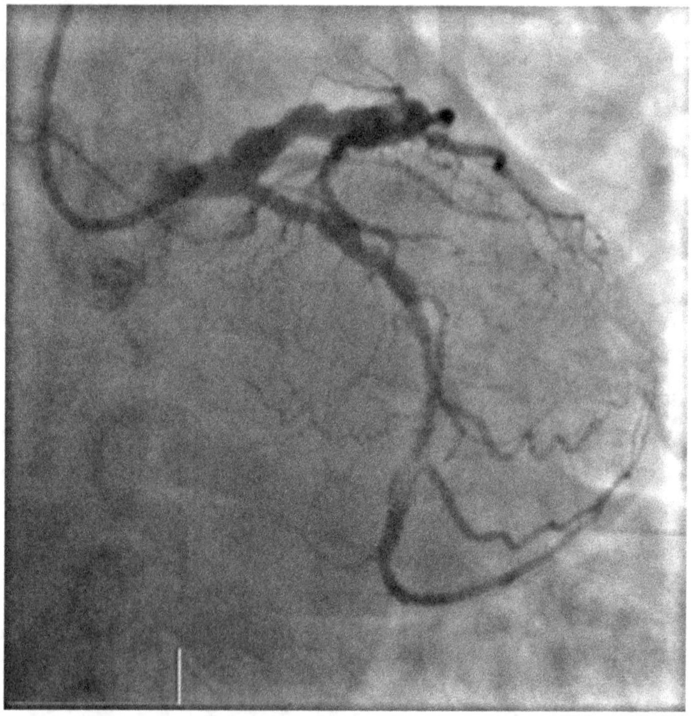

Fig. 10.5 Coronary angiogram after eptifibatide infusion. Note presence of large organized thrombus (arrow)

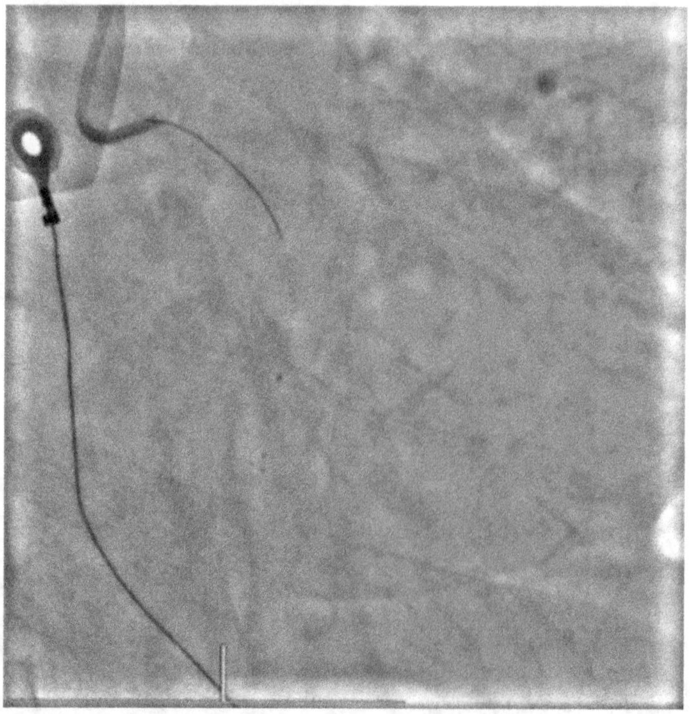

Fig. 10.6 Deployment of Solitaire device. Note the three dots visible at distal tip of Solitaire device. The microcatheter is still visible and will be used to partially collapse the proximal OD of the Solitaire and permit safe withdrawal

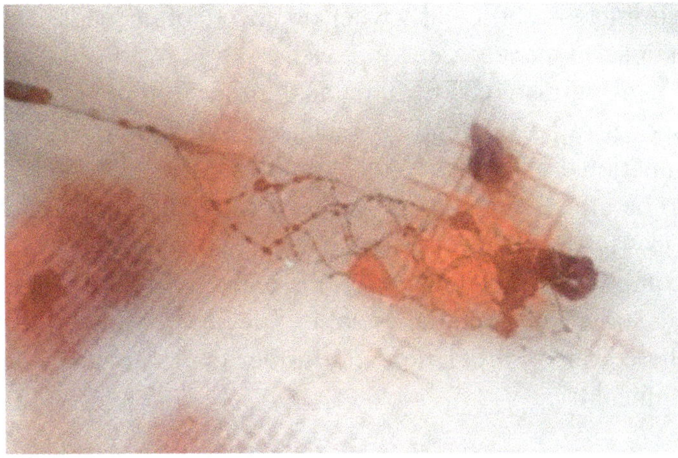

Fig. 10.7 Removal of Solitaire device. Note large thrombus entrapped within the struts of the device

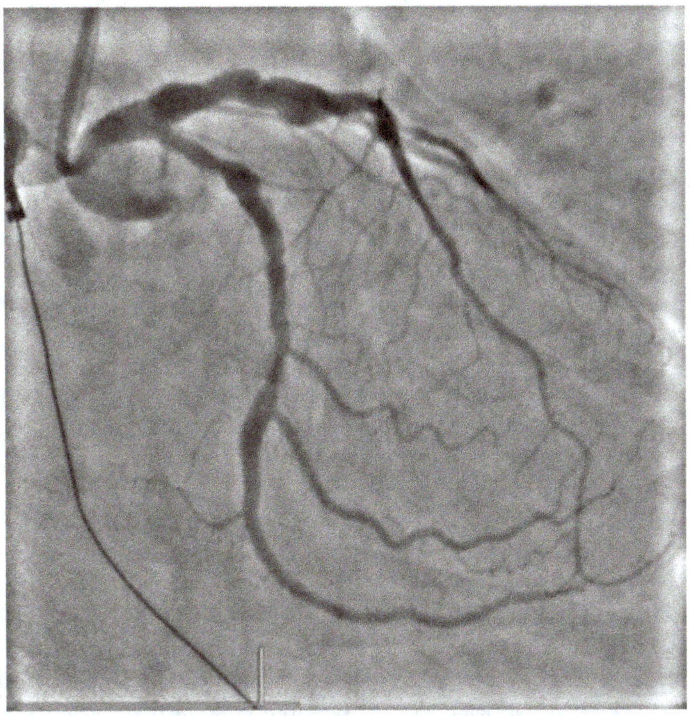

Fig. 10.8 Coronary angiogram post thrombus retrieval. Note that the thrombus has largely been retrieved and the entirety of the circumflex artery is now widely patent

aspiration through the guide catheter. Device inspection showed successful retrieval of a large thrombus (Fig. 10.7). A TIMI three distal flow was accomplished (Fig. 10.8). The procedure was completed with a BioMatrix 3.5 × 33 mm stent (Biosensor) being deployed across the culprit lesion. The patient was discharged stable 2 days later and has remained symptom-free ever since.

10.9.3 Discussion

Aspiration thrombectomy for ST-elevation MI is no longer considered routine due to no effect on clinical outcomes and association with stroke [39], thus in favour of a balloon strategy to restore coronary flow. However, in cases of persistent coronary thrombus—particularly when organized often leads to adverse sequelae and requires a tailored management approach.

In contrast to STEMI, manual thrombectomy in acute ischaemic stroke has been shown to be safe and is associated with improved recanalization rates and better functional outcomes [50]. Thrombus retrieval systems such as the Solitaire appear to be effective and are now class I guideline recommendation [51]. This device is easy to deliver even through tortuous cerebral vasculature; nonetheless reported complications include vessel dissection and thrombus embolization [52]. This case illustrates the potential use of this device to successfully retrieve the thrombus from the coronary circulation and further exploration of this strategy is warranted in a clinical trial.

References

1. Nabel EG, Braunwald E. A tale of coronary artery disease and myocardial infarction. N Engl J Med. 2012;366(1):54–63.
2. Furie B, Furie BC. Mechanisms of thrombus formation. N Engl J Med. 2008;359(9):938–49.
3. Davies MJ. The pathophysiology of acute coronary syndromes. Heart. 2000;83(3):361–6.
4. Falk E, Shah PK, Fuster V. Coronary plaque disruption. Circulation. 1995;92(3):657–71.
5. Topol EJ, Yadav JS. Recognition of the importance of embolization in atherosclerotic vascular disease. Circulation. 2000;101(5):570–80.
6. Gibson CM, de Lemos JA, Murphy SA, Marble SJ, McCabe CH, Cannon CP, et al. Combination therapy with abciximab reduces angiographically evident thrombus in acute myocardial infarction: a TIMI 14 substudy. Circulation. 2001;103(21):2550–4.
7. Sianos G, Papafaklis MI, Daemen J, Vaina S, van Mieghem CA, van Domburg RT, et al. Angiographic stent thrombosis after routine use of drug-eluting stents in ST-segment elevation myocardial infarction the importance of thrombus burden. J Am Coll Cardiol. 2007;50(7):573–83.
8. Niccoli G, Spaziani C, Marino M, Pontecorvo ML, Cosentino N, Bacà M, et al. Effect of chronic aspirin therapy on angiographic thrombotic burden in patients admitted for a first ST-elevation myocardial infarction. Am J Cardiol. 2010;105(5):587–91.
9. Fokkema ML, Vlaar PJ, Svilaas T, Vogelzang M, Amo D, Diercks GF, et al. Incidence and clinical consequences of distal embolization on the coronary angiogram after percutaneous coronary intervention for ST-elevation myocardial infarction. Eur Heart J. 2009;30(8):908–15.
10. Napodano M, Ramondo A, Tarantini G, Peluso D, Compagno S, Fraccaro C, et al. Predictors and time-related impact of distal embolization during primary angioplasty. Eur Heart J. 2009;30(3):305–13.
11. Sharma V, Jolly SS, Hamid T, Sharma D, Chiha J, Chan W, et al. Myocardial blush and microvascular reperfusion following manual thrombectomy during percutaneous coronary intervention for ST elevation myocardial infarction: insights from the TOTAL trial. Eur Heart J. 2016;37(24):1891–8.
12. Stone GW, Peterson MA, Lansky AJ, Dangas G, Mehran R, Leon MB. Impact of normalized myocardial perfusion after successful angioplasty in acute myocardial infarction. J Am Coll Cardiol. 2002;39(4):591–7.
13. Patrono C. Aspirin as an antiplatelet drug. N Engl J Med. 1994;330(18):1287–94.
14. Wallentin L, Becker RC, Budaj A, Cannon CP, Emanuelsson H, Held C, et al. Ticagrelor versus clopidogrel in patients with acute coronary syndromes. N Engl J Med. 2009;361(11):1045–57.
15. Wessler JD, Stant J, Duru S, Rabbani L, Kirtane AJ. Updates to the ACCF/AHA and ESC STEMI and NSTEMI guidelines: putting guidelines into clinical practice. Am J Cardiol. 2015;115(5 Suppl):23A–8A.

16. Montalescot G, van 't Hof AW. Prehospital ticagrelor in ST-segment elevation myocardial infarction. N Engl J Med. 2339;371(24):2014.
17. Ernst NM, Suryapranata H, Miedema K, Slingerland RJ, Ottervanger JP, Hoorntje JC, et al. Achieved platelet aggregation inhibition after different antiplatelet regimens during percutaneous coronary intervention for ST-segment elevation myocardial infarction. J Am Coll Cardiol. 2004;44(6):1187–93.
18. Bhatt DL, Stone GW, Mahaffey KW, Gibson CM, Steg PG, Hamm CW, et al. Effect of platelet inhibition with cangrelor during PCI on ischemic events. N Engl J Med. 2013;368(14):1303–13.
19. Stone GW, Mehran R, Goldstein P, Witzenbichler B, Van 't Hof A, Guagliumi G, et al. Bivalirudin versus heparin with or without glycoprotein IIb/IIIa inhibitors in patients with STEMI undergoing primary percutaneous coronary intervention pooled patient-level analysis from the HORIZONS-AMI and EUROMAX trials. J Am Coll Cardiol. 2015;65(1):27–38.
20. Yusuf S, Mehta SR, Chrolavicius S, Afzal R, Pogue J, Granger CB, et al. Effects of fondaparinux on mortality and reinfarction in patients with acute ST-segment elevation myocardial infarction: the OASIS-6 randomized trial. JAMA. 2006;295(13):1519–30.
21. Routledge H, Sastry S. Radial versus femoral access for acute coronary syndromes. Curr Cardiol Rep. 2015;17(12):117.
22. Jolly SS, Yusuf S, Cairns J, Niemelä K, Xavier D, Widimsky P, et al. Radial versus femoral access for coronary angiography and intervention in patients with acute coronary syndromes (RIVAL): a randomised, parallel group, multicentre trial. Lancet. 2011;377(9775):1409–20.
23. Shahzad A, Kemp I, Mars C, Wilson K, Roome C, Cooper R, et al. Unfractionated heparin versus bivalirudin in primary percutaneous coronary intervention (HEAT-PPCI): an open-label, single Centre, randomised controlled trial. Lancet. 2014;384(9957):1849–58.
24. Pomerantz RM, Kuntz RE, Diver DJ, Safian RD, Baim DS. Intracoronary verapamil for the treatment of distal microvascular coronary artery spasm following PTCA. Catheter Cardiovasc Diagn. 1991;24(4):283–5.
25. Kaplan BM, Benzuly KH, Kinn JW, Bowers TR, Tilli FV, Grines CL, et al. Treatment of no-reflow in degenerated saphenous vein graft interventions: comparison of intracoronary verapamil and nitroglycerin. Catheter Cardiovasc Diagn. 1996;39(2):113–8.
26. Micari A, Belcik TA, Balcells EA, Powers E, Wei K, Kaul S, et al. Improvement in microvascular reflow and reduction of infarct size with adenosine in patients undergoing primary coronary stenting. Am J Cardiol. 2005;96(10):1410–5.
27. Movahed MR, Baweja G. Distal administration of very high doses of intracoronary adenosine for the treatment of resistant no-reflow. Exp Clin Cardiol. 2008;13(3):141–3.
28. Sakata Y, Kodama K, Ishikura F, Komamura K, Hasegawa S, Hirayama A. Disappearance of the 'no-reflow' phenomenon after adjunctive intracoronary administration of nicorandil in a patient with acute myocardial infarction. Jpn Circ J. 1997;61(5):455–8.
29. Matsuo H, Watanabe S, Watanabe T, Warita S, Kojima T, Hirose T, et al. Prevention of no-reflow/slow-flow phenomenon during rotational atherectomy—a prospective randomized study comparing intracoronary continuous infusion of verapamil and nicorandil. Am Heart J. 2007;154(5):994.e1–6.
30. Ito H, Taniyama Y, Iwakura K, Nishikawa N, Masuyama T, Kuzuya T, et al. Intravenous nicorandil can preserve microvascular integrity and myocardial viability in patients with reperfused anterior wall myocardial infarction. J Am Coll Cardiol. 1999;33(3):654–60.
31. de Lemos JA, Antman EM, Gibson CM, McCabe CH, Giugliano RP, Murphy SA, et al. Abciximab improves both epicardial flow and myocardial reperfusion in ST-elevation myocardial infarction. Observations from the TIMI 14 trial. Circulation. 2000;101(3):239–43.
32. Neumann FJ, Blasini R, Schmitt C, Alt E, Dirschinger J, Gawaz M, et al. Effect of glycoprotein IIb/IIIa receptor blockade on recovery of coronary flow and left ventricular function after the placement of coronary-artery stents in acute myocardial infarction. Circulation. 1998;98(24):2695–701.
33. Greco C, Pelliccia F, Tanzilli G, Tinti MD, Salenzi P, Cicerchia C, et al. Usefulness of local delivery of thrombolytics before thrombectomy in patients with ST-segment elevation myocardial infarction undergoing primary percutaneous coronary intervention (the delivery of throm-

bolytics before thrombectomy in patients with ST-segment elevation myocardial infarction undergoing primary percutaneous coronary intervention [DISSOLUTION] randomized trial). Am J Cardiol. 2013;112(5):630–5.

34. Migliorini A, Stabile A, Rodriguez AE, Gandolfo C, Rodriguez Granillo AM, Valenti R, et al. Comparison of AngioJet rheolytic thrombectomy before direct infarct artery stenting with direct stenting alone in patients with acute myocardial infarction. The JETSTENT trial. J Am Coll Cardiol. 2010;56(16):1298–306.
35. Ali A, Cox D, Dib N, Brodie B, Berman D, Gupta N, et al. Rheolytic thrombectomy with percutaneous coronary intervention for infarct size reduction in acute myocardial infarction: 30-day results from a multicenter randomized study. J Am Coll Cardiol. 2006;48(2):244–52.
36. Parodi G, Valenti R, Migliorini A, Maehara A, Vergara R, Carrabba N, et al. Comparison of manual thrombus aspiration with rheolytic thrombectomy in acute myocardial infarction. Circ Cardiovasc Interv. 2013;6(3):224–30.
37. Svilaas T, Vlaar PJ, van der Horst IC, Diercks GF, de Smet BJ, van den Heuvel AF, et al. Thrombus aspiration during primary percutaneous coronary intervention. N Engl J Med. 2008;358(6):557–67.
38. Lagerqvist B, Fröbert O, Olivecrona GK, Gudnason T, Maeng M, Alström P, et al. Outcomes 1 year after thrombus aspiration for myocardial infarction. N Engl J Med. 2014;371(12):1111–20.
39. Jolly SS, Cairns JA, Yusuf S, Meeks B, Pogue J, Rokoss MJ, et al. Randomized trial of primary PCI with or without routine manual thrombectomy. N Engl J Med. 2015;372(15):1389–98.
40. Jolly SS, Cairns JA, Yusuf S, Rokoss MJ, Gao P, Meeks B, et al. Outcomes after thrombus aspiration for ST elevation myocardial infarction: 1-year follow-up of the prospective randomised TOTAL trial. Lancet. 2016;387(10014):127–35.
41. Bhindi R, Kajander OA, Jolly SS, Kassam S, Lavi S, Niemelä K, et al. Culprit lesion thrombus burden after manual thrombectomy or percutaneous coronary intervention-alone in ST-segment elevation myocardial infarction: the optical coherence tomography sub-study of the TOTAL (ThrOmbecTomy versus PCI ALone) trial. Eur Heart J. 2015;36(29):1892–900.
42. Jolly SS, James S, Džavík V, Cairns JA, Mahmoud KD, Zijlstra F, et al. Thrombus aspiration in ST-segment-elevation myocardial infarction: an individual patient meta-analysis: Thrombectomy Trialists collaboration. Circulation. 2017;135(2):143–52.
43. Ibanez B, James S, Agewall S, Antunes MJ, Bucciarelli-Ducci C, Bueno H, et al. 2017 ESC guidelines for the management of acute myocardial infarction in patients presenting with ST-segment elevation: The Task Force for the management of acute myocardial infarction in patients presenting with ST-segment elevation of the European Society of Cardiology (ESC). Eur Heart J. 2017;39(2):119–77.
44. Stone GW, Abizaid A, Silber S, Dizon JM, Merkely B, Costa RA, et al. Prospective, randomized, multicenter evaluation of a polyethylene terephthalate micronet mesh-covered stent (MGuard) in ST-segment elevation myocardial infarction: the MASTER trial. J Am Coll Cardiol. 2012;60(19):1975–84.
45. Gracida M, Romaguera R, Jacobi F, Gómez-Hospital JA, Cequier A. The MGuard coronary stent: safety, efficacy, and clinical utility. Vasc Health Risk Manag. 2015;11:533–9.
46. Qiao J, Pan L, Zhang B, Wang J, Zhao Y, Yang R, et al. Deferred versus immediate stenting in patients with ST-segment elevation myocardial infarction: a systematic review and meta-analysis. J Am Heart Assoc. 2017;6(3):pii: e004838.
47. De Maria GL, Alkhalil M, Oikonomou EK, Wolfrum M, Choudhury RP, Banning AP. Role of deferred stenting in patients with ST elevation myocardial infarction treated with primary percutaneous coronary intervention: a systematic review and meta-analysis. J Interv Cardiol. 2017;30(3):264–73.
48. Carrick D, Oldroyd KG, McEntegart M, Haig C, Petrie MC, Eteiba H, et al. A randomized trial of deferred stenting versus immediate stenting to prevent no- or slow-reflow in acute ST-segment elevation myocardial infarction (DEFER-STEMI). J Am Coll Cardiol. 2014;63(20):2088–98.

49. Singh M, Berger PB, Ting HH, et al. Influence of coronary thrombus on outcome of percutaneous coronary angioplasty in the current era (the Mayo Clinic experience). Am J Cardiol. 2001;88:1091–6.
50. Davalos A, Pereira VM, Chapot R. Retrospective multicenter study of solitaire FR for revascularization in the treatment of acute ischemic stroke. Stroke. 2012;43:2699–705.
51. Jauch EC, Saver JL, et al. Guidelines for the early Management of Patients with Acute Ischemic Stroke. Stroke. 2013;44:870–947.
52. Elgendy IY, Kumbhani DJ, et al. Mechanical thrombectomy for acute ischaemic stroke: a meta-analysis of randomized trials. JACC. 2015;66:2498–505.

Is There a Role for Bare-Metal Stents in Current STEMI Care?

11

Mark Hensey, Janarthanan Sathananthan, Wahyu Purnomo Teguh, and Niall Mulvihill

11.1 Introduction

Early attempts at percutaneous coronary intervention (PCI) using balloon angioplasty were largely hampered by technical limitations. Although balloon angioplasty was moderately successful at relieving an obstruction, the procedure frequently resulted in dissections which, if uncontrolled, often led to abrupt vessel closure. Furthermore, while acute luminal gain could be impressive, a combination of elastic recoil and smooth muscle hyper-proliferation often negated the benefits of an acceptable immediate angiographic result. Elastic recoil could occur minutes to hours post-procedure resulting in acute myocardial infarction (AMI) and need for emergent coronary artery bypass grafting (CABG). This led to a pivotal development in the history of PCI with introduction of the metallic stent, which drove rapid improvements in short- and long-term procedural safety and efficacy. Stent design has been a remarkable area of technological advances with pivotal milestones including evolution of metallic architecture and introduction of the drug-eluting stent (DES). Although DES is now considered the default option for most PCI, bare-metal stents (BMS) still represent a sizeable proportion of stent procedures in some countries and in some settings may have arguable advantage. In this chapter we aim to review contemporary evidence for the use of BMS in modern interventional practice.

M. Hensey (✉) · J. Sathananthan
Saint Paul's Hospital, Vancouver, BC, Canada
e-mail: mhensey@providencehealth.bc.ca

W. P. Teguh
Ulin General Hospital, South Kalimantan, Indonesia

N. Mulvihill
Saint Vincent's University Hospital, Dublin, Ireland

T. J. Watson et al. (eds.), *Primary Angioplasty*,
https://doi.org/10.1007/978-981-13-1114-7_11

11.2 Bare-Metal Stents

The introduction of BMS in the mid-1980s allowed PCI procedures to rapidly enter mainstream clinical practice. Early BMS were crude, being largely constructed of relatively thick 316 L stainless steel and needed to be cut to length, and then crimped onto the delivery balloon catheter. However, once successfully in situ, these devices were able to effectively maintain vessel patency and thereby largely prevent the abrupt vessel closure and elastic recoil which had hampered balloon only procedures. Consequently, PCI was to become safer and more efficacious. As technology improved further, particularly with pre-cut and pre-crimped stents delivered using a monorail system, PCI was to rapidly evolve into the preferred mode of revascularization for selected patients due to the minimal invasive nature of the procedure coupled with rapid recovery.

Early BMS had important limitations, related to both device design and to biocompatibility. This led to the emergence of neo-intimal hyperplasia and neo-atherosclerosis as factors which could preclude optimal long-term outcomes and result in in-stent restenosis (ISR). With time, it was learned that reduced strut thickness lessened the localized inflammatory responses that may both hinder endothelialization and drive ISR. This led to improved stent architecture and a shift from 316 L stainless steel to cobalt chromium, thereby permitting a marked reduction in strut thickness without loss of radial strength, while also facilitating improved delivery and conformability. Clinical studies demonstrated that the reduction in stent strut thickness resulted in improved delivery, conformability and reduced incidence of ISR.

11.3 Drug-Eluting Stents

One the most important milestones in interventional cardiology in recent decades was development of the DES. Initially these were developed by coating standard BMS with an anti-proliferative agent (e.g. sirolimus) which was bonded to the stent using a polymer which also served to regulate drug release. The anti-proliferative agent effectively led to localized arrest of the smooth muscle cell proliferation cycle around the implanted device and thereby limited propensity to ISR. With cardiologists eager to avoid ISR, DES technology rapidly entered mainstream practice and quickly became the default stent choice, with device implants both on and off label.

However an important downside to first-generation DES rapidly emerged related to delayed and incomplete neo-endothelialization around the stent struts. In early-generation DES, this led to observations of increased rates of stent thrombosis as compared to BMS. This resulted in the Food and Drug Administration (FDA) issuing an advisory warning regarding the risk of late stent thrombosis after DES. Consequently, this led to an immediate decline in DES usage. Progress to tackle these deficiencies was rapidly developed. Pharmacologically, more potent antiplatelet agents were brought to market with increased duration of dual antiplatelet therapy (DAPT). Meanwhile stent technological advances included thinner struts, improvements in anti-proliferative drugs, use of new polymers with increased biocompatibility or biodegradability and more recently polymer-free stents and the concept of a bioresorbable vascular scaffold (BVS) which over time is completely reabsorbed. Although in theory BVS offer advantage over both BMS and DES due to lack of permanent metallic structure, initial results have not met expectations with higher stent thrombosis and target-vessel MI rates resulting in some early platforms being withdrawn from clinical use. Research and development is ongoing, but currently BVS cannot be recommended for use during primary PCI and will not be discussed further in this chapter.

11.3.1 Anti-proliferative Drugs

Once the issues of ISR and stent thrombosis associated with use of stents were identified, several agents including gold, carbon and heparin were coated onto stents to try and improve biocompatibility, reduce inflammation and prevent thrombosis. None of these agents were shown to have any significant beneficial effects, and thus other solutions were clearly required.

The use of the anti-proliferative agents sirolimus and paclitaxel showed significant reductions in ISR compared to BMS and was utilized in first-generation DES. Sirolimus is an immunosuppressive compound that acts by receptor inhibition of the mammalian target of rapamycin (mTOR) resulting in the cell-cycle progression and consequently inhibits cell proliferation. Paclitaxel is an oncological agent that inhibits cell proliferation by disturbing cellular microtubule organization. The use of the 'limus' drugs has been shown to be superior to other anti-proliferative agents, and newer agents such as zotarolimus, everolimus and the more lipophilic biolimus are used in most current-generation DES with similar efficacy.

11.3.2 Polymers

Initial DES technology required the incorporation of anti-proliferative drugs into permanent synthetic polymers. These polymers however increase local inflammatory response and reduced endothelialization and were thought to be a key flaw in early designs driving propensity to stent thrombosis and mandating longer duration of DAPT. More biocompatible and even biodegradable polymers have now been developed. These cause less inflammation and hence permit more rapid and complete endothelial coverage. More recently, polymer-free DES have also been developed. These use the concept of drug storage 'wells' or surface etching to load the drug but allow rapid dissolution of the anti-proliferative agent without use of a polymer giving the benefits of the pharmacology with the early endothelialization offered by BMS.

Current-generation DES have reduced ISR rates to incredibly low levels while improving the safety profile of the devices and thus have become the 'gold standard' for definitive PCI in the majority of patients. This is supported by numerous randomized controlled trials, meta-analyses and real-world data showing improved safety and efficacy with new-generation DES. Nonetheless, some still argue that there remains a role for BMS in contemporary clinical practice. A number of important issues remain and in the context of primary PCI for STEMI.

Potential Advantages of BMS

- More rapid endothelialization allowing abbreviated DAPT
  - Safety in high bleeding risk patients
  - Safety in elderly patients
  - Safe with concomitant need for anticoagulation (e.g. atrial fibrillation)
- Reduced cost
  - Price sensitive healthcare models

11.4 DES vs. BMS for Primary PCI

Primary PCI is established as the optimal treatment strategy for STEMI patients with the use of coronary stenting achieving far superior reperfusion at lower risk compared to fibrinolysis. The use of BMS has been shown to be superior to balloon angioplasty alone, and several studies have subsequently shown advantage of DES over BMS. However, the supposed advantage of DES is predominantly driven by reduced need for long-term revascularization rather than immediate post-infarct survival. Newer-generation DES have largely been shown to be superior to first-generation stents for a broad range of indications with similar outcomes between most contemporary devices.

The EXAMINATION (everolimus-eluting stents versus bare-metal stents in ST-segment elevation myocardial infarction) trial investigated the use of everolimus-eluting stents (Xience V, Abbott Vascular) versus BMS (Multi-Link Vision, Abbott Vascular) in an all-comer STEMI population. 1498 patients were randomized in a 1:1 fashion, and 2-year analysis found that EES had a trend towards a reduction in the primary endpoint, namely, the combined endpoint of all-cause death, recurrent MI and any revascularization from 17.3% in BMS to 14.4% ($p = 0.11$). Rate of target lesion revascularization (TLR) was significantly lower in the EES group at 2.9% vs. 5.6% ($p = 0.009$) as was definite or probable stent thrombosis (0.8% vs. 2.1%; $p = 0.03$ and 1.35 vs. 2.8%; $p = 0.04$, respectively). Recently published 5-year follow-up results showed a significant reduction in the primary endpoint (21% vs. 26%; $p = 0.033$) with use of EES, mainly driven by the reduction of all-cause mortality by EES as compared to BMS (9% vs. 12%; $p = 0.047$). TLR was also significantly reduced although there was no difference in rates of stent thrombosis at 5 years.

COMFORTABLE AMI (the effect of biolimus-eluting stents with biodegradable polymer vs. bare-metal stents on cardiovascular events among patients with AMI) compared a biolimus DES (BioMatrix, Biosensors) with a biodegradable polymer

(BES) with BMS in 1161 patients presenting with STEMI. Major adverse cardiac events (MACE) were reduced in BES (4.3%) vs. BMS (8.7%) at 1 year ($p = 0.004$). This reduction was driven by a reduction in target-vessel-related re-infarction (0.5% vs. 2.7%, $p = 0.01$) and ischaemia-driven TLR (1.6% vs. 5.7%, $p < 0.001$) in BES as compared to BMS. At 2-year follow-up, TLR continued to be reduced in the BES group (3.1% vs. 8.2%; $p < 0.001$) and cardiac death or target-vessel MI was also reduced (4.2% vs. 7.2%, $p = 0.036$). A combined analysis of EXAMINATION and COMFORTABLE AMI demonstrated a reduction in both stent thrombosis and target-vessel MI with the use of DES over BMS.

The Norwegian coronary stent trial (NORSTENT) examined the use of DES versus BMS in 9013 patients undergoing PCI (26.3% with STEMI) over a 3-year period. Patients were randomized in a 1:1 fashion to BMS or DES (82.9% everolimus-eluting stents and 13.1% zotarolimus-eluting stents). The primary outcome was a composite of death from any cause and nonfatal MI. After 6 years of follow-up, there was no difference found in the primary outcome between the groups (16.6% in the DES group vs. 17.1% in the BMS group; $p = 0.66$), which is reassuring given the ongoing use of BMS. There was however, in line with previous studies, a reduction in repeat revascularization (16.5% in DES vs. 19.8% in BMS; $p < 0.001$). There was also a reduction in the rate of definite stent thrombosis with DES (0.8% vs. 1.2%; $p = 0.0498$).

In light of these and other studies, it can be said that in the general STEMI population, the use of current-generation DES is preferable to BMS. This is driven by the reduction in target-vessel revascularization and myocardial infarction. There are some special specific issues however, which require review.

11.4.1 Stent Thrombosis

Although an infrequent occurrence, stent thrombosis (ST) is the most feared complication of stent implantation. ST can present immediately after stent implant or sometimes even many years later. Mode of presentation is highly variable but can include sudden (cardiac) death and STEMI. Worryingly ST has an extremely high mortality rate of up to 50% in some series—far in excess of that seen with STEMI due to de novo lesions. The explanation for the disparate mortality rate remains unclear. Nonetheless, avoidance of ST is of paramount importance, and the interventional cardiologist must always be mindful of the various factors that may predispose to this malignant process during any PCI procedure.

Purported mechanisms for ST are predominantly considered either mechanical, related to platelet activity, or a combination of both. The former includes stent malapposition, stent under-expansion, stent edge dissection, longer stent length and small stent calibre. In contrast, factors related to platelet function are represented by failure to adequately inhibit platelet adhesion/aggregation. This may include aspirin or thienopyridine 'non-responders' and, when these drugs have been erroneously omitted or withheld due to prescribing error, poor compliance, bleeding complications or need for emergent surgical interventions. Acute coronary syndrome (ACS) as a clinical entity at the time of the index procedure is also frequently cited as an independent predictor of stent thrombosis.

The timing of stent thrombosis differs between the types of stents. During the first months, it may occur after both BMS and DES implantation. However, beyond 1 year, it is more frequently observed after first-generation DES implantation. It was long assumed that this related to suboptimal endothelialization due to presence of the antimitotic agent or localized inflammation from ongoing presence of non-biocompatible polymers. Although autopsy and experimental studies have shown delayed healing to be more common with DES, new-generation DES have consistently shown a reduction in ST as compared to BMS, both short and long term. Therefore the risk of stent thrombosis is no longer a reason to advocate the use of BMS over DES.

11.4.2 DAPT Duration

The most common convincing reason for the use of BMS is to allow shorter durations of DAPT. This may be because of concerns of a high bleeding risk, poor compliance or the need for urgent/semi-urgent surgery. In a recent survey looking at the reasons for the decision to use BMS over DES at 31 European centres, concerns with patient DAPT compliance were the main reason for using BMS (39%). Concerns regarding compliance should be dealt with in a multidisciplinary fashion with assessment of a patient's psychosocial status and patient education being of utmost importance. In high-risk anatomy, despite likely technical success of PCI, plain balloon angioplasty as a temporary reperfusion measure followed by coronary artery bypass may need to be considered.

The addition of more potent antiplatelet agents (e.g. prasugrel, ticagrelor) and studies demonstrating cardiovascular benefits of longer DAPT duration have resulted in the need for individualized DAPT decision-making with bleeding risk having to be balanced against the risk of further cardiovascular events. Tools such as the DAPT and PRECISE-DAPT scores can be used to guide the decision-making process. One study has shown safety of a <15 days of DAPT post PCI with BMS. However, in general, a minimum of 1-month DAPT is advised post BMS and 6 months post DES (for elective PCI).

Current guidelines advise the use of DAPT for 12 months post PCI for acute coronary syndromes, independent of the type of stent used. These guidelines however are largely based on the results of old studies with use of first-generation stents, and a number of recent studies have challenged these guidelines. The recent DAPT-STEMI trial assessed the efficacy of 6 vs. 12 months of DAPT in STEMI with the use of a zotarolimus-eluting stent in 1496 patients with the 6-month strategy reaching non-inferiority. Shorter DAPT regimes have also been investigated with several trials demonstrating safety of DES use with a 3-month DAPT regimen. Two studies have specifically examined very short DAPT strategies.

The ZEUS trial investigated the use of a zotarolimus-eluting stent (Endeavor, Medtronic) versus BMS with a short DAPT duration strategy in 1606 patients who were deemed uncertain for DES use on the basis of bleeding, thrombotic or restenosis risk criteria. 19% of the patients in the study were treated for STEMI and the median DAPT duration was 32 days. There was a reduction in the primary endpoint of MACE in the ZES group (17.5% vs. 22.1%; HR 0.76; 95% CI 0.61–0.95; $p = 0.011$) with lower MI (2.9% vs. 8.1% $p < 0.001$) and target-vessel revascularization (TVR) rates (5.9% vs. 10.7%; $p = 0.001$). Definite or probable stent thrombosis was also significantly reduced (2.0% vs. 4.1%; $p = 0.019$). The Endeavor stent has now been replaced by the newer-generation Resolute stent which has thinner struts and a more biocompatible polymer which theoretically should offer additional protection, although this has not been demonstrated in a randomized controlled trial.

A polymer-free and carrier-free drug-coated stent (DCS) that transfers umirolimus (biolimus A9) (BioFreedom, Biosensors) was compared to BMS (Gazelle, Biosensors) with a 1-month DAPT strategy in the LEADERS-FREE trial in 2466 high bleeding risk patients. 22.8% of the study population was treated for STEMI. 2-year follow-up demonstrated superiority of DCS over BMS with a reduction of a combined endpoint of cardiac death, MI or stent thrombosis (12.6% vs. 15.3%; HR 0.80; CI 0.64–0.99; $p = 0.039$). Clinically driven TLR was also significantly lower in the DCS (5.6% vs. 10.3%; $p < 0.001$). Recently published 2-year outcomes showed sustained benefits of DCS vs. BMS with a lower rates of the primary endpoint (13% vs. 21.5%, HR 0.57; 95% CI 0.39–0.85; $p = 0.005$) and TLR (7.4% vs. 10.4%; HR 0.45; 95% CI 0.24–0.83; $p = 0.009$). Stent thrombosis rates also tended to be lower with DCS (1.2% vs. 3.2%, HR 0.39; 95% CI 0.12–1.25; $p = 0.1$).

In summary, the requirement for a shortened duration of DAPT is no longer a robust reason to justify the use of BMS over DES with growing evidence that the use of DES is in fact superior (Fig. 11.1). Future trials are likely to add to the current evidence base.

11.4.3 Atrial Fibrillation

Atrial fibrillation (AF) is a common comorbidity in the setting of STEMI, estimated to occur in up to 20% of patients, and it is associated with a significant increase in mortality. The most important management issue in AF is the prevention of embolic events with anticoagulation. Traditionally this was achieved by the use of warfarin; however, the use of non-vitamin K antagonist oral anticoagulants (NOACs) is now recommended as first-line treatment for anticoagulation for AF. The addition of antiplatelet agents for the treatment of STEMI in patients with AF, or conversely the addition of anticoagulation for the treatment of AF in patients post-STEMI, significantly increases the risk of major bleeding. As part of a strategy to reduce duration of triple therapy with DAPT and an anticoagulant, the use of BMS for PCI in the setting of AF has been advocated; however this is no longer the accepted strategy due to evidence of the safety of shorter or indeed absence of the so-called triple therapy.

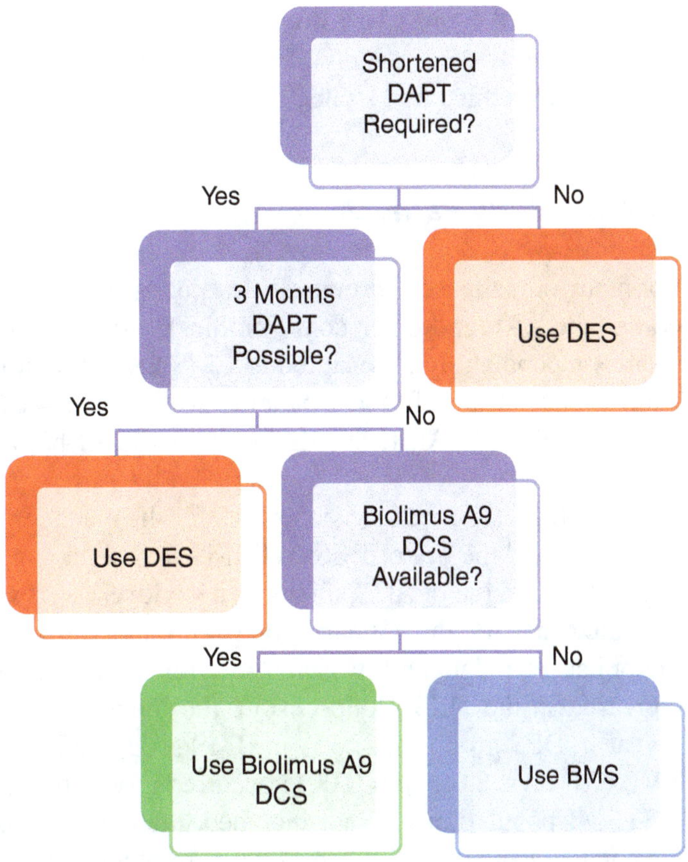

Fig. 11.1 Simplified flow chart for choice of stent with shortened DAPT

The WOEST (what is the optimal antiplatelet and anticoagulant therapy in patients with oral anticoagulation and coronary stenting) trial investigated the use of triple therapy (aspirin, clopidogrel and warfarin) versus double therapy (plavix and warfarin) in 573 patients undergoing PCI. Among the patient population, 28% had PCI for ACS and 31% of patients received BMS. The rate of bleeding episodes was significantly reduced in patients who received double therapy without any increase in thrombotic or cerebrovascular complications. In fact a composite endpoint of death, MI, stroke, TVR and stent thrombosis was lower in the double-therapy group (11.1% vs. 17.6%; HR 0.6; 95% CI 0.38–0.94; $p = 0.025$).

The use of NOACs in post-PCI regimens was examined in depth in the PIONEER-AF trial. Patients undergoing PCI with AF (either BMS or DES) were randomized to one of three pharmacological strategies; rivaroxaban 15 mg o.d. plus single P2Y12 inhibitor, low-dose rivaroxaban (2.5 mg b.d.) plus DAPT or warfarin and DAPT. 12% of the population included presented with STEMI and 31.8% received BMS. Both of the rivaroxaban regimens were associated with lower risk of clinically significant bleeding than the warfarin arm with no increase in cardiovascular or thromboembolic events. The use of other NOACs with similar shortened or less aggressive regimens is currently under investigation with results expected soon.

The evidence supporting the safety of shortened, or absence of, triple therapy in post-PCI patients with AF means that there is no compelling reason to use BMS in patients with AF and with broader indications for anticoagulation (paired with development of safer agents), combination of NOAC with a P2Y12 inhibitor is likely to be the favoured strategy.

11.4.4 Elderly Patients

For many of the reasons previously outlined (high bleeding risk, concerns regarding compliance, AF and other comorbidities), elderly patients have been traditionally seen as a population more suited to BMS use. In addition, they are often excluded from clinical trials. Elderly patients were not excluded in EXAMINATION or COMFORTABLE AMI, but the average age in both studies was approximately 60 years old.

The XIMA (Xience or vision stents for the management of angina in the elderly) trial compared the use of EES and BMS in 800 patients ≥80 years of age undergoing PCI for angina or ACS, and patients with STEMI were excluded. Results demonstrated that for the primary composite endpoint of death, MI, stroke, TVR or major haemorrhage, DES was non-inferior to BMS. Rates of haemorrhage were not increased in the DES group despite the longer use of DAPT (94% on DAPT at 1 year in DES group vs. 32.2% in BMS group). MI (8.7% vs. 4.3%; $p = 0.01$) and TVR (7.0% vs. 2.0%; $p = 0.001$) occurred more often in the BMS group. Although a STEMI population was not included, the data is reassuring in regard to similar advantages gained by the use of DES in elderly patients as seen in trials with a younger cohort.

The SENIOR (drug-eluting stents in elderly patients with coronary artery disease) trial investigated the use of DES vs. BMS in 1200 patients over the age of 75 undergoing PCI; 10.6% were treated for STEMI and DAPT duration was shortened—1 month in stable patients and 6 months in those presenting with ACS. The use of a bioabsorbable polymer DES (Synergy, Boston Scientific) was associated with a 29% reduction in the composite primary endpoint of all-cause mortality, MI stroke and revascularization at 1 year. Consistent with other studies, the benefit was driven by a 71% reduction in ischaemia-driven TLR. Bleeding and stent thrombosis rates in both groups were low.

As demonstrated there is growing evidence that the use of BMS in elderly patients, including in the setting of STEMI, is no longer a recommended strategy.

11.4.5 Cost

Reduced cost is a common reason cited for the use of BMS over DES in PCI. Although upfront costs may be reduced, the increase in use of DES has reduced this gap. A number of studies on the cost-effectiveness of using DES as opposed to BMS have shown that although periprocedural costs are higher, long-term cost-effectiveness is achieved due to the lower rates of future cardiovascular events with the use of new-generation DES. However cost-benefit analyses are not universally applicable to every healthcare environment, but we believe that in general stent cost cannot be used to justify use of BMS in STEMI.

11.5 Summary and Recommendations

In the present era, given generally excellent clinical outcomes, it is widely accepted that current-generation DES should be the default consideration for all patients undergoing PCI including primary PCI. Although theoretical advantages of BMS are often cited, current-generation DES not only appear to be more efficacious but also safer than BMS in a broad range of patients and clinical presentations. This likely now includes patients at high bleeding risk or where DAPT may need to be prematurely discontinued. However BMS use is likely to be continued in certain healthcare systems predominantly due to cost analyses. Recent data has shown that modern BMS have good long-term outcomes in regard to mortality and nonfatal MI but at the expense of increased revascularization.

Recommendations

- New-generation DES should be the stent of choice for PCI including in STEMI presentations.
- If a shortened DAPT regime is required, the use of DES is still preferable with safety of a 3-month strategy established.
- If very short DAPT duration is required (1 month), then the use of a polymer-free biolimus A9-coated stent, if available, is preferable to BMS, although other contemporary platforms are currently under investigation in this setting.
- BMS should not be used for complex anatomical subsets with higher rates of ISR.

11.6 Case Report: Primary PCI with Direct Stenting in Patient with Inferior Myocardial Infarction

Wahyu Purnomo Teguh

11.6.1 Introduction

A 66-year-old male came to the hospital with continuing central chest pain of 3-h duration, accompanied by diaphoresis and dyspnoea. His risk factors were hypertension and dyslipidaemia. The ECG showed an inferior ST-elevation myocardial infarction (STEMI) with complete heart block (Fig. 11.2). His blood pressure was

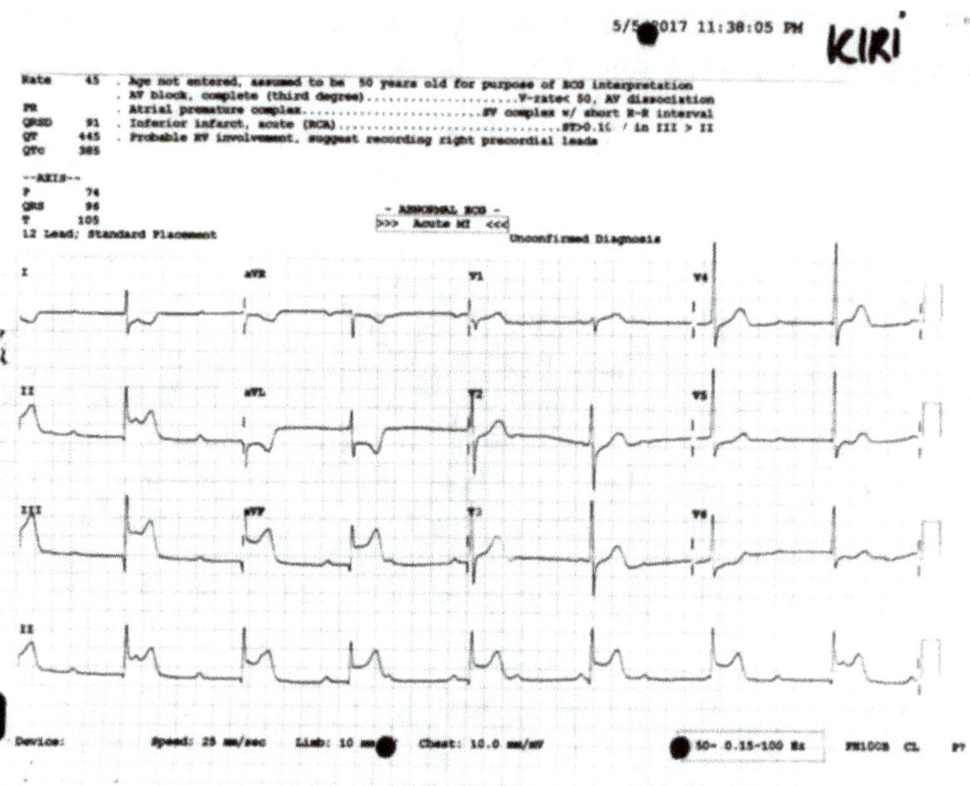

Fig. 11.2 12-lead ECG. Note complete heart block and inferior ST elevation

80/60 mmHg. He was loaded with Aspirin 300 mg and clopidogrel 300 mg, given fluid boluses to support his BP and brought to the catheter laboratory for primary PCI (PPCI).

A temporary pacemaker wire was delivered to the right ventricle through the right femoral vein. Primary PCI was performed through right radial approach. A diagnostic TIG catheter was engaged to left coronary artery, and images were taken demonstrating that this was unobstructed (Fig. 11.3).

A JR 3.5 guide catheter was then delivered to right coronary artery but failed to engage adequately. The patient had VF requiring defibrillation two times at 200 joules with successful restoration of circulation. The guide was switched to an AL 0.75 which engaged well. Angiography revealed a 99% stenosis in the mid-right coronary artery (RCA), which was somewhat ectatic (Fig. 11.4). A Sion Blue was used to cross the lesion. Direct stenting was then done with a Promus Element Plus 3.5 × 20 mm, inflated at 14 ATM for 13 s (Fig. 11.5). Post dilatation was performed with a non-compliant 4 mm balloon up to 16 ATM. The final angiogram showed no dissection, TIMI flow III, residual stenosis 0% (Fig. 11.6).

Our patient was transferred to the coronary care unit for observation and discharged after 4 days. He remains well at subsequent outpatient review.

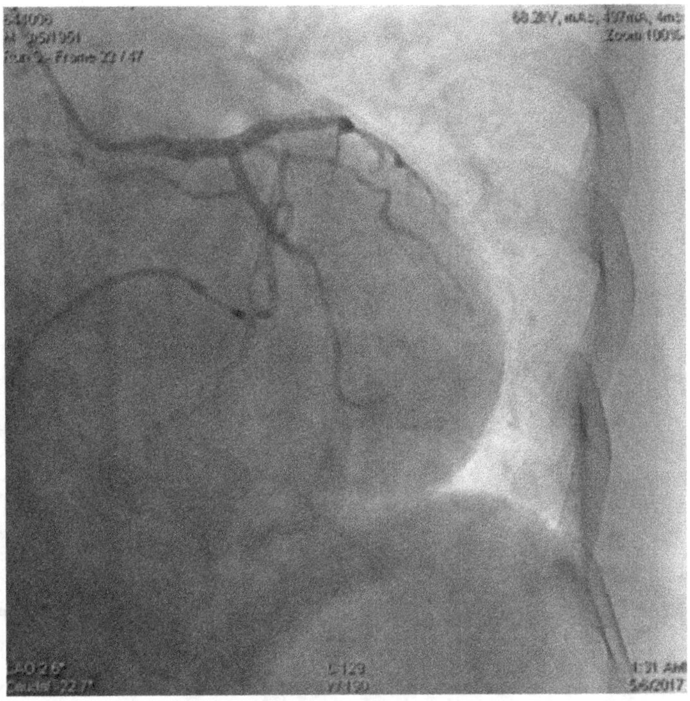

Fig. 11.3 Coronary angiogram of left coronary artery which was unobstructed. Note temporary pacing wire in situ

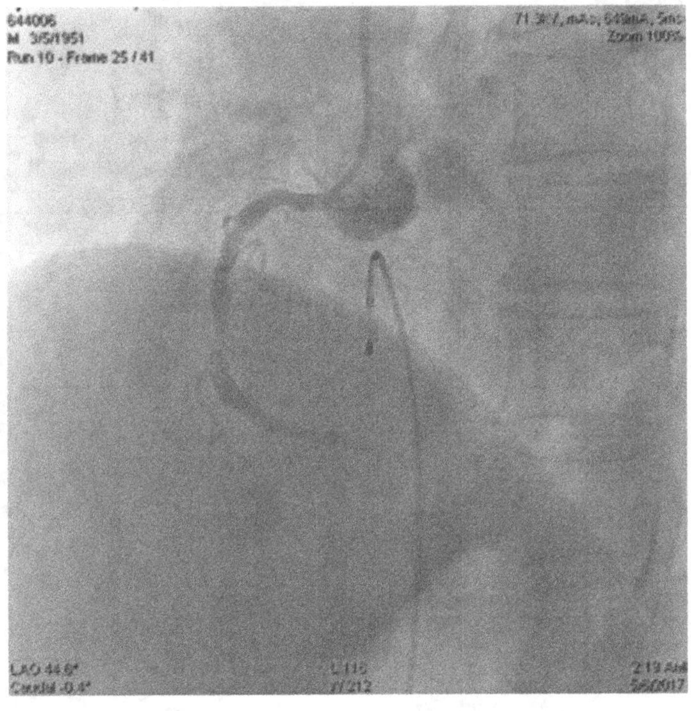

Fig. 11.4 AL 0.75 engaged to RCA. Coronary angiogram of right coronary artery. Note 99% lesion in mid RCA

This case illustrates the utility of contemporary DES platforms. Coronary artery calibre can easily be misjudged, particularly in primary PCI; however many contemporary platforms allow for significant oversizing without disruption of stent architecture, polymer or drug release kinetics. Moreover, even in a large-calibre vessel, the benefit of a DES in terms of reduction of ISR and improving long-term outcomes particularly among diabetic patients cannot be disregarded.

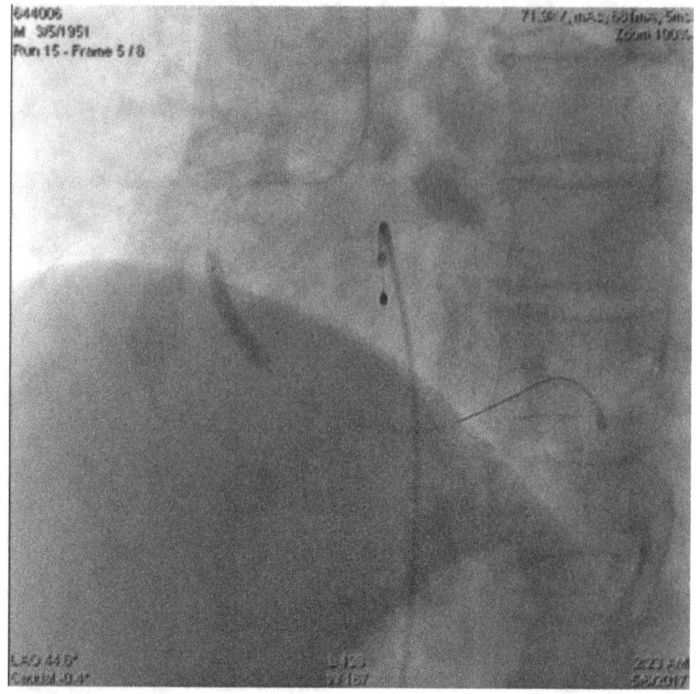

Fig. 11.5 Direct stenting, Promus Element Plus 3.5 × 20 mm, 14 ATM, 13 s, note minimal residual wasting

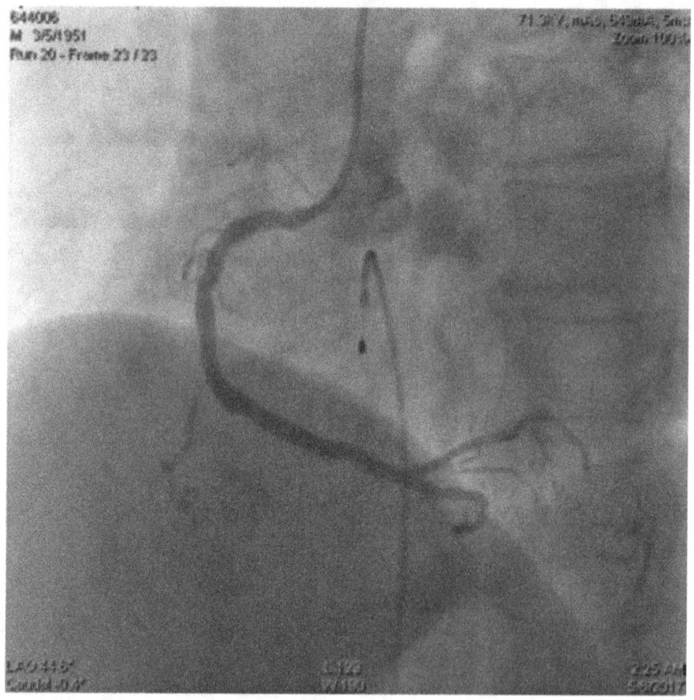

Fig. 11.6 Final angiographic images demonstrating excellent stent expansion and TIMI-3 flow

Further Readings

Bonaa KH, Mannsverk J, Wiseth R, Aaberge L, Myreng Y, Nygard O, et al. Drug-eluting or bare-metal stents for coronary artery disease. N Engl J Med. 2016;375(13):1242–52.

Ibanez B, James S, Agewall S, Antunes MJ, Bucciarelli-Ducci C, Bueno H, et al. 2017 ESC guidelines for the management of acute myocardial infarction in patients presenting with ST-segment elevation: the task force for the management of acute myocardial infarction in patients presenting with ST-segment elevation of the European Society of Cardiology (ESC). Eur Heart J. 2018;39(2):119–77.

Raber L, Kelbaek H, Ostojic M, Baumbach A, Heg D, Tuller D, et al. Effect of biolimus-eluting stents with biodegradable polymer vs bare-metal stents on cardiovascular events among patients with acute myocardial infarction: the COMFORTABLE AMI randomized trial. JAMA. 2012;308(8):777–87.

Sabate M, Brugaletta S, Cequier A, Iniguez A, Serra A, Hernadez-Antolin R, et al. The EXAMINATION trial (Everolimus-eluting stents versus bare-metal stents in ST-segment elevation myocardial infarction): 2-year results from a multicenter randomized controlled trial. JACC Cardiovasc Interv. 2014;7(1):64–71.

Valgimigli M, Bueno H, Byrne RA, Collet JP, Costa F, Jeppsson A, et al. 2017 ESC focused update on dual antiplatelet therapy in coronary artery disease developed in collaboration with EACTS: the task force for dual antiplatelet therapy in coronary artery disease of the European Society of Cardiology (ESC) and of the European Association for Cardio-Thoracic Surgery (EACTS). Eur Heart J. 2018;39(3):213–60.

12 Drug-Coated Balloons in STEMI

Upul Wickramarachchi, Hee Hwa Ho, and Simon Eccleshall

12.1 Introduction

The management of ST-elevation myocardial infarction (STEMI) has evolved significantly with the introduction of new pharmacological therapies as well as interventional procedures and devices. The GISSI and ISIS-2 studies showed a mortality benefit of streptokinase over standard therapy (heparin ± oral anticoagulation)/placebo which lead to the widespread use of streptokinase in the late 1980s [1, 2]. The use of recombinant tissue plasminogen activator (rt-PA) was shown to be more beneficial than streptokinase in the TIMI and GUSTO trials [3, 4]. Results of other studies such as CLARITY and COMMIT paved the way for addition of clopidogrel to the drug regime which further reduced mortality [5, 6].

Primary percutaneous coronary intervention (PPCI) became the preferred choice of treatment for acute STEMI, with balloon angioplasty (BA) showing an improvement in mortality (or the combined endpoint of mortality and MI) over thrombolysis in a number of studies [7, 8]. Subsequently, bare-metal stent (BMS) implantation in STEMI showed a reduction in target vessel revascularizations (TVR) in comparison with BA but without a reduction in death or MI in the Stent PAMI and CADILLAC trials [9, 10]. The percentage of vessels with TIMI III flow was numerically higher in the BA group as compared to the BMS group, while mortality and MI rates were numerically but not statistically lower [9]. When stenting (BMS) was compared with thrombolysis as in the STAT study, the results were similar with stenting showing a reduction in TVR but no reduction in death or MI [11]. When both first- and second-generation drug-eluting stents (DES) were compared to BMS in the setting

U. Wickramarachchi · S. Eccleshall (✉)
Norfolk and Norwich University Hospital, Norwich, UK
e-mail: simon.eccleshall@nnih.nhs.uk

H. H. Ho
Tan Tock Seng Hospital, Singapore, Singapore

T. J. Watson et al. (eds.), *Primary Angioplasty*,
https://doi.org/10.1007/978-981-13-1114-7_12

of an acute STEMI, target vessel/lesion revascularization rates were shown to be lower with DES, but yet again no reduction in death or MI was shown [12–15]. Brodie et al. in a single-center study of 2195 patients over a follow-up period of 16 years showed long-term target vessel MI, and stent or lesion thrombosis was significantly higher with both BMS and DES as compared to BA (after landmark analysis at 1 year) [16]. Thus, although stent implant is often considered as definitive treatment for PPCI by securing the vessel lumen, this may not always provide optimal longer-term outcomes.

12.2 Drug-coated Balloons

There has been great interest recently in the concept of angioplasty with minimal or no permanent implant, by way of using either absorbable polymer DES or scaffolds. Drug-coated balloon-only (DCB-only) PCI has emerged as an alternative therapeutic option to treat coronary artery disease (CAD) and has the additional benefit of implanting no material with the exception of the necessary anti-restenotic drug. DCBs are semi-compliant balloons with a chemotherapeutic drug (commonly paclitaxel) incorporated with an excipient to facilitate the drug transfer upon inflation of the balloon. Paclitaxel is the drug of choice in most commonly available DCBs because of its highly lipophilic properties allowing rapid delivery into the vessel wall and sustained antiproliferative effect despite its short contact time with the vessel wall [17].

The SeQuent Please (B Braun, Melsungen AG, Germany), Pantera Lux (Biotronik, Berlin, Germany), and In.Pact Falcon (Medtronic, CA, USA) have the most published data supporting their efficacy and safety. The best long-term results of DCB are achieved with a DCB-only approach as compared to DCB plus BMS. DCB-only PCI is associated with a lower late lumen loss and lower target vessel revascularization.

12.3 Evidence for DCB Angioplasty in PPCI

Several studies have reported their experience of using DCB without stenting in the PPCI setting. Vos et al. carried out a pilot study involving 100 patients presenting with acute STEMI using the paclitaxel-coated Pantera Lux™. Cardiogenic shock and intubated out of hospital arrests were excluded. 59% had DCB-only PCI, with the rest requiring BMS implantation due to dissections of type C or greater (National Heart, Lung, and Blood Institute (NHLBI) classification). A 12-month follow-up revealed cardiac death in 2%, MI 0%, and target lesion revascularization rate of 3% in this selected group. TIMI III flow was achieved in 96% of patients [18].

Ho et al. reported their preliminary experience with paclitaxel-coated balloon (SeQuent Please) in the PPCI setting for 89 patients. 70% had TIMI 0 flow pre-procedure, and TIMI III flow was achieved in 98% patients. Glycoprotein IIb/IIIa inhibitors were used in 80%, and thrombus aspiration was carried out in 56%. DCB-only PCI was carried out in 96%, while the other 4% had bail out stenting for significant acute recoil or dissections. They reported a death rate of 4.5%, MI 0%, and TLR/TVR of 0% at 30 days [19].

Nijhoff et al. in a subgroup analysis from the DEBAMI trial showed that there was no difference in major adverse cardiac events in 40 patients treated with DCB-only PPCI in comparison with BMS only, BMS + DCB, and paclitaxel-eluting stent implantation at 6 months follow-up [20].

Wickramarachchi et al. in an abstract published at EuroPCR, 2017 in Paris, reported their experience in the use of DCB-only PPCI in an all-comer cohort of 253 patients. 4% of patients were in cardiogenic shock, and 6.7% were out of hospital cardiac arrests. 91% had DCB-only PCI. A 30-day mortality was only 2.4% and mortality for 379 days was 6.3%. For a mean follow-up period of 261 days, MI and TLR rates were 2.6% and 3.3%, respectively [21].

These publications suggest that DCB-only PPCI is a safe alternative to standard stent implantation in this high-risk group. We advocate this approach for several compelling reasons:

12.3.1 No Mortality Benefit with Stents

The use of BA in PPCI has been superseded by routine stenting in the contemporary era due to the reduction of TVR as mentioned before. However, DCB therapy addresses the issue of restenosis with its drug delivery reducing neointimal hyperplasia. An improvement of the quality in angiography and the use of potent antiplatelet therapy have reduced acute vessel closure rates. Currently, there are no studies showing a mortality benefit of stent implantation over balloon-only angioplasty or, in a majority of studies, a reduction of recurrent MI in this setting.

12.3.2 Risk of Stent Thrombosis

Studies have shown that the cumulative frequency of stent thrombosis (ST) following stenting with both BMS and DES for STEMI continues to increase beyond 1 year and that the frequency of very late ST may be higher with early-generation DES [16]. Moreover, the rate of stent thrombosis in patients undergoing PPCI can be high (ranging from 1 to 3% in contemporary trials). Patients with AMI have higher rates of stent-specific adverse events when compared to those with stable CAD. This could be related to coronary vasoconstriction and the presence of thrombus at culprit lesion site leading to suboptimal stent sizing and subsequent stent mal-apposition.

12.3.3 Inadequate Time to Know Patient's History

Time pressure to open the occluded artery promptly in PPCI (shorter door-to-balloon times) may result in inadequate time to know patient's full medical history. Routine stenting as per guidelines may therefore not be appropriate in some patients.

It remains a challenge to decide whether the patient is a candidate for a prolonged course of DAPT at the time of the PPCI. DES should be avoided in the presence of elevated bleeding risk, need for invasive or surgical procedures in the near future, and financial/social barriers that may limit patient compliance.

12.3.4 Avoidance of Long Stents in PPCI

DCB maybe a good alternative to treat diffuse lesions in PPCI as outcomes remain relatively unfavorable for stent-based coronary intervention especially those with de novo long CAD. Even in the DES era, studies have shown that the TLR rates can range from 6 to 28% for such lesion subsets with higher rates of instent restenosis for paclitaxel DES. Longer stent length is also recognized as predisposing factor for ST.

12.4 Technical Tips and Tricks with DCB-Only Angioplasty in Primary PCI

We recommend following the German consensus guidelines but with additional steps when successfully performing DCB-only PPCI [22].

12.4.1 Lesion Preparation

We recommend *aspiration thrombectomy* when faced with a high thrombus burden, i.e., TIMI thrombus grade 3 or more, aiming to reduce the thrombus burden to TIMI thrombus grade of 2 or less. A thrombus-laden lesion is more likely to hamper effective drug delivery to the vessel wall.

This should be followed by *mandatory pre-dilatation* of the lesion using semi- or non-compliant balloons with a balloon to vessel ratio of 0.8 to 1.0. This should be done *carefully and slowly* with enough pressure only to fully inflate the balloon (usually 6–8 atm). Liberal use of *intracoronary nitrates* is recommended as this helps accurate vessel sizing. We have a *low threshold for the use of glycoprotein IIb/IIIa inhibitors* in treating lesions with high thrombus burden. Also, acquisition runs after pre-dilatation should be of a slightly longer duration to carefully look for evidence of vessel-threatening dissections, in particular any contrast hang-up or accumulation within a dissection plane indicating a NHLBI type C dissection and possible early vessel closure due to intramural hematoma formation.

Coronary dissections are an inevitable result of BA, but most are microdissections that cannot be seen on angiography and are of no clinical significance. However, abrupt vessel closure remains one of the most fearful complications of BA usually associated with NHLBI dissection grades of type C and above. With a good knowledge of the different NHLBI grades of coronary dissection, careful selection of those patients suitable for DCB-only angioplasty is possible [23]. Ho et al. in their study reported no abrupt closure of the culprit artery. Only 4% of patients required bailout stenting for significant recoil/dissections of type C and above. Wickramarachchi U et al. reported acute vessel closure rate of 0.75% requiring bailout stenting and an overall bailout stenting rate of only 9%. The incidence of abrupt closure is also significantly reduced in the current era of more potent anti-platelet use.

12.4.2 Drug Delivery

If there are no dissections of more than NHLBI type C, TIMI III flow, and not more than 30% residual stenosis, drug delivery should be considered with the deployment of the DCB. DCB diameter should be the diameter of the largest balloon used to pre-dilate the lesion. *The DCB should be used only for drug delivery* and not for further angioplasty. It is good practice to check the guide catheter and wire position and ensure the O-ring is fully open before start delivering the DCB. Care should be taken not to touch the DCB prior to introduction. We recommend following manufacturer's instructions for use to ensure adequate drug delivery. This will include maximum transit time to the lesion and balloon inflation times. In the case of a coronary dissection of type C or above after DCB use, we recommend bailout stenting with a second-generation DES rather than a BMS [24]. Figure 12.1 summarizes the key steps.

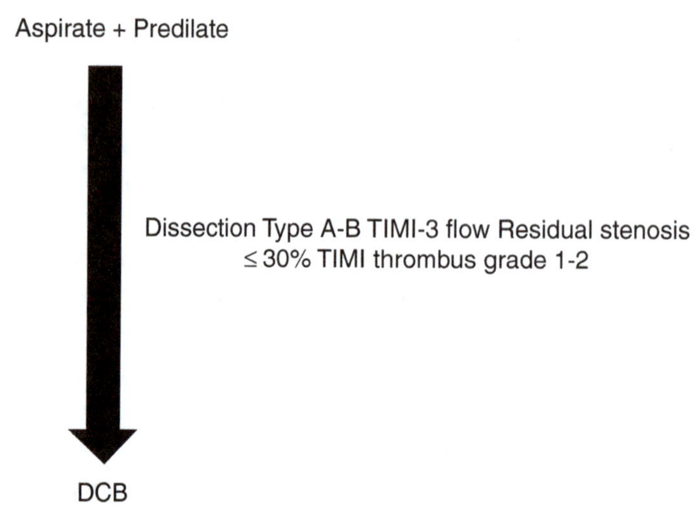

Fig. 12.1 Proposed protocol for optimal use of DCB
The lesion should be aspirated if there is presence of intracoronary thrombus. The lesion should then be carefully pre-dilated. After check angiography, where there is TIMI-3 flow, dissection of grades A to B, residual stenosis of less than 30%, and TIMI thrombus grade no worse than grade 1–2, it is reasonable to proceed with DCB therapy. Alternatively, insertion of an intracoronary stent is likely to be required

12.5 Conclusion

In conclusion, the use of DCB as primary therapy in primary PCI represents a novel approach in treating STEMI patients. This approach is possible with appropriate patient selection and by performing two key preconditioning steps, namely, aspiration thrombectomy for lesions with high thrombus burden and careful lesion preparation. A randomized controlled trial (REVELATION) is underway to assess the safety and efficacy of a DCB-only strategy versus DES in primary PCI [25]. However, we would recommend performing DCB-only angioplasty in stable patients first, preferably with proctoring before treating such high-risk patient groups.

12.6 Primary PCI of RCA with Drug-Coated Balloon Angioplasty

Upul Wickramarachchi, Hee Hwa Ho, and Simon Eccleshall

12.6.1 History

A 47-year-old male smoker presented with inferior ST-elevation myocardial infarction (STEMI).

12.6.2 Baseline Coronary Angiography

The right coronary artery (RCA) showed 95% stenosis in mid-segment (culprit lesion site) and 70% diffuse stenosis in distal segment (Fig. 12.2).

12.6.3 Procedure

A 6 Fr sheath was inserted into the right radial artery, and the RCA was engaged with a 6 Fr Ikari left 3.5 guiding catheter.

A Runthrough NS guidewire was advanced into the right posterior descending artery. As there was minimal thrombus, aspiration thrombectomy was not performed. The mid- and distal RCA lesions were pre-dilated with a 2.5 × 15 mm balloon.

As POBA results were satisfactory (Fig. 12.3) and RCA lesions were diffuse in nature, we decided to treat these segments with drug-coated balloon (DCB).

Distal RCA was treated with a SeQuent Please Neo DCB 2.5 × 30 mm (inflated at 12 atm for 50 s) (Fig. 12.4).

Mid-RCA was treated with a SeQuent Please Neo DCB 2.75 × 30 mm (inflated at 12 atm for 45 s) (Fig. 12.5).

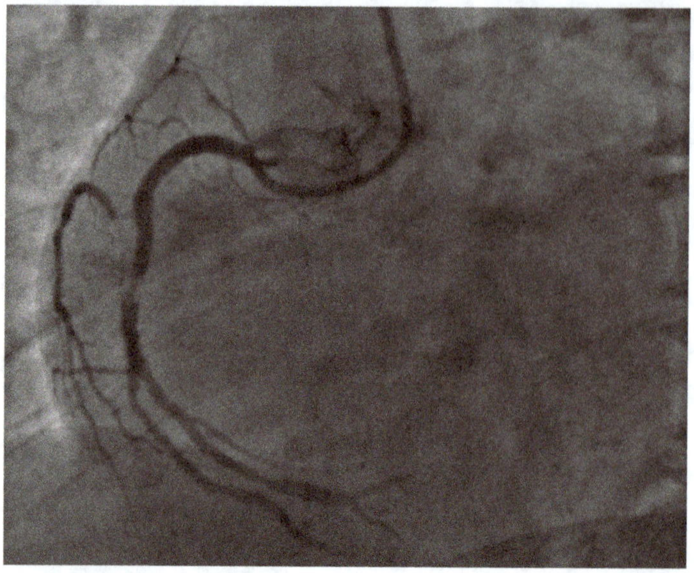

Fig. 12.2 Baseline RCA angiography

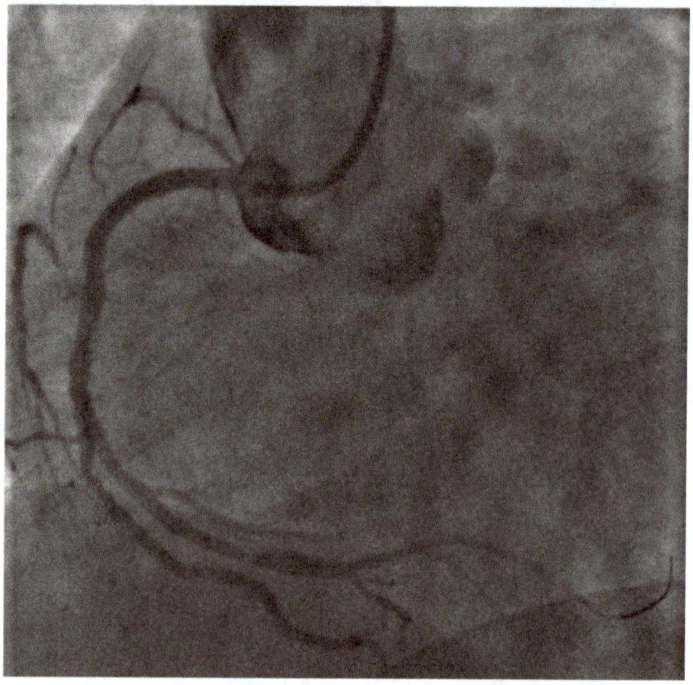

Fig. 12.3 RCA after balloon angioplasty

Final angiographic results were satisfactory (Fig. 12.6) with TIMI 3 flow restored at the end of the procedure. There was residual stenosis of 30% with no obvious dissection.

12.6.4 Restudy Angiogram

Restudy angiogram (Fig. 12.7) 9 months later showed widely patent RCA with positive remodeling observed in mid-RCA.

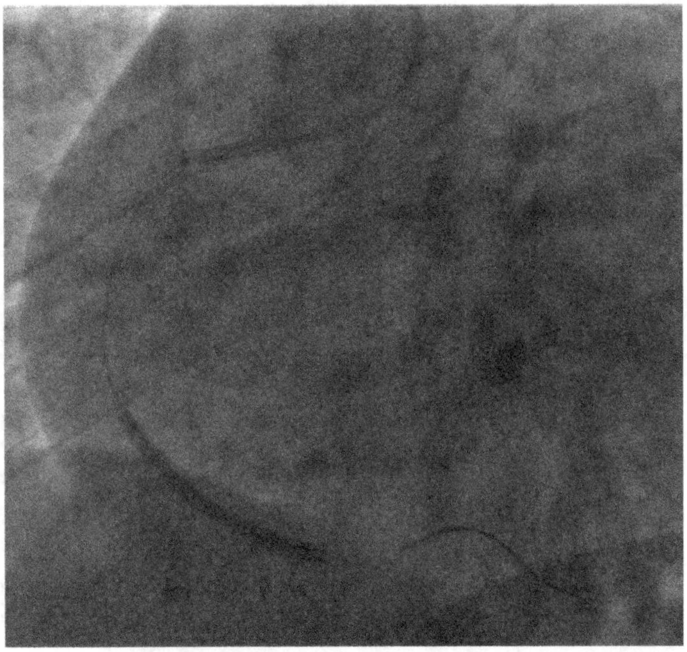

Fig. 12.4 Distal RCA treated with a DCB 2.5 × 30 mm

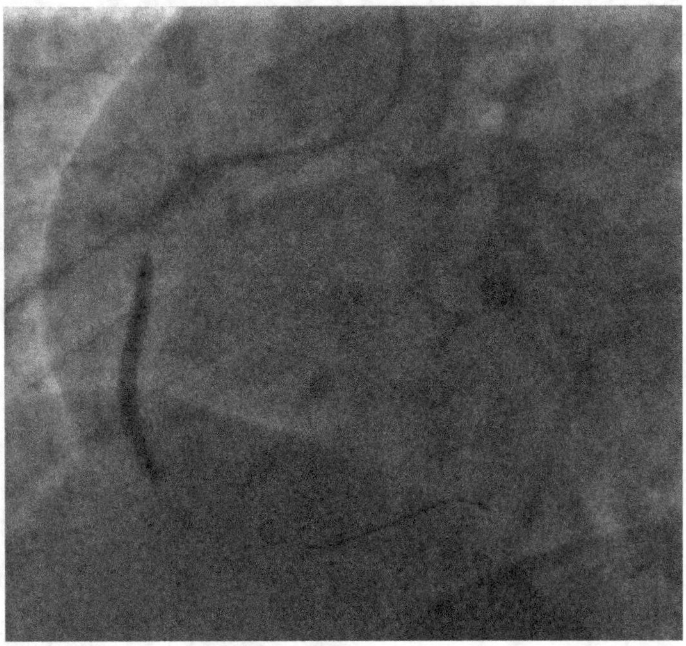

Fig. 12.5 Mid-RCA treated with a DCB 2.75 × 30 mm

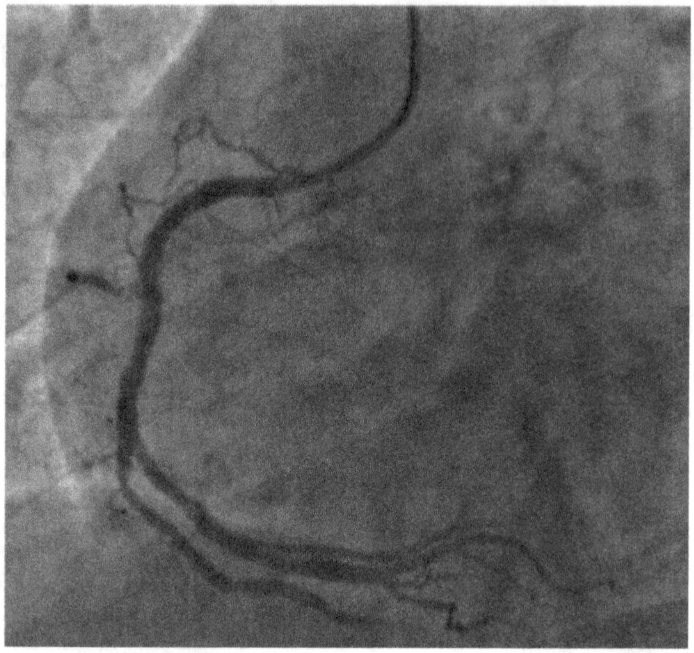

Fig. 12.6 Final RCA angiography after DCB angioplasty

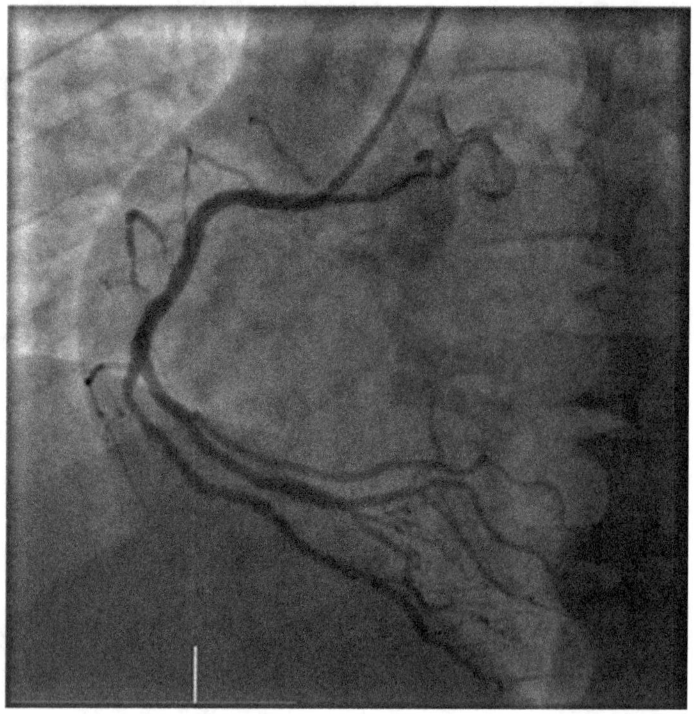

Fig. 12.7 Restudy RCA angiography

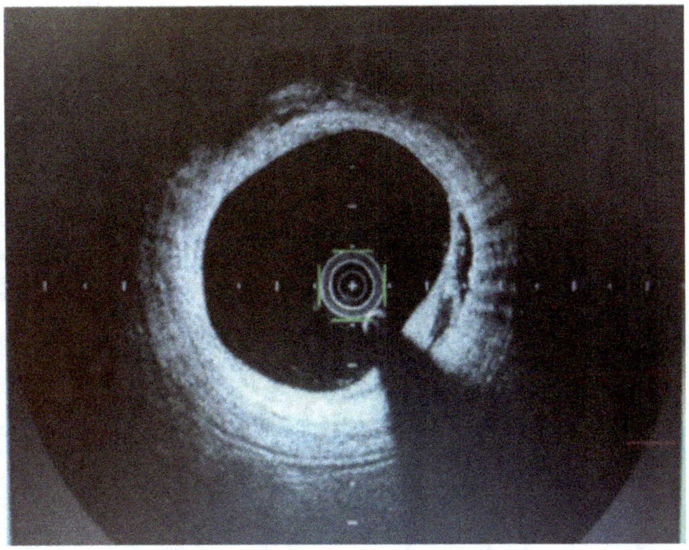

Fig. 12.8 OCT image of mid RCA

Optical coherence tomographic (OCT) imaging study (Fig. 12.8) showed a nicely healed plaque at mid-RCA (culprit lesion site).

Case illustration 2: Pre-, immediate-, and post-DCB-only PCI and follow-up angiography at 22 months of a 60-year-old male presenting with an anterior STEMI

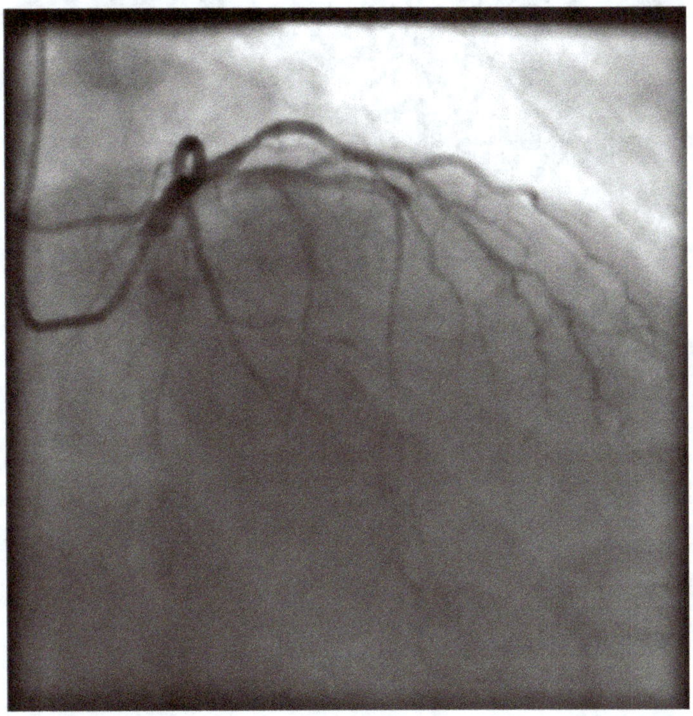

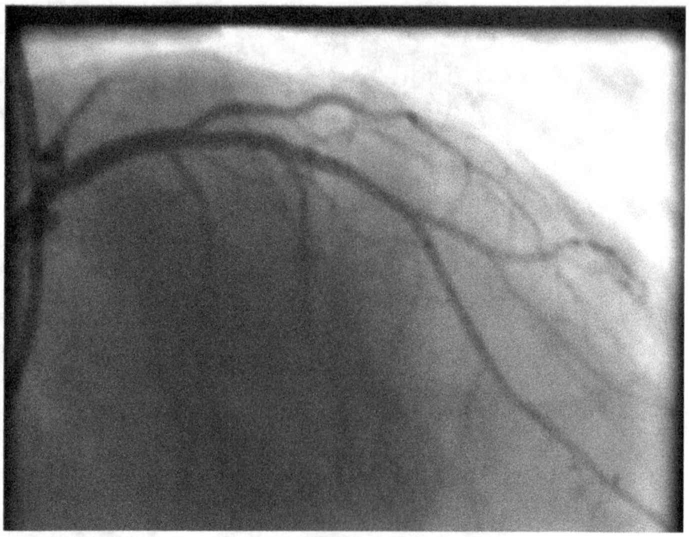

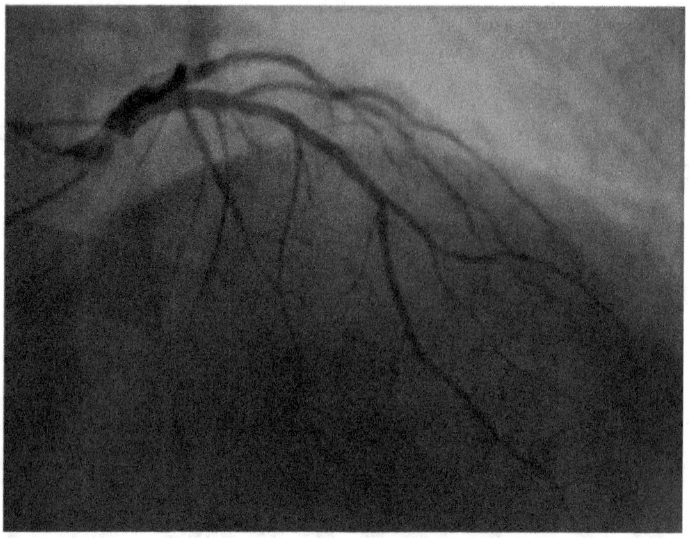

Case illustration 3: A 53-year-old female presenting with a lateral STEMI. Pre-, immediate-, post-DCB-only PCI (showing a type b dissection) and follow-up images at 17 months showing a nicely healed dissection and an excellent result

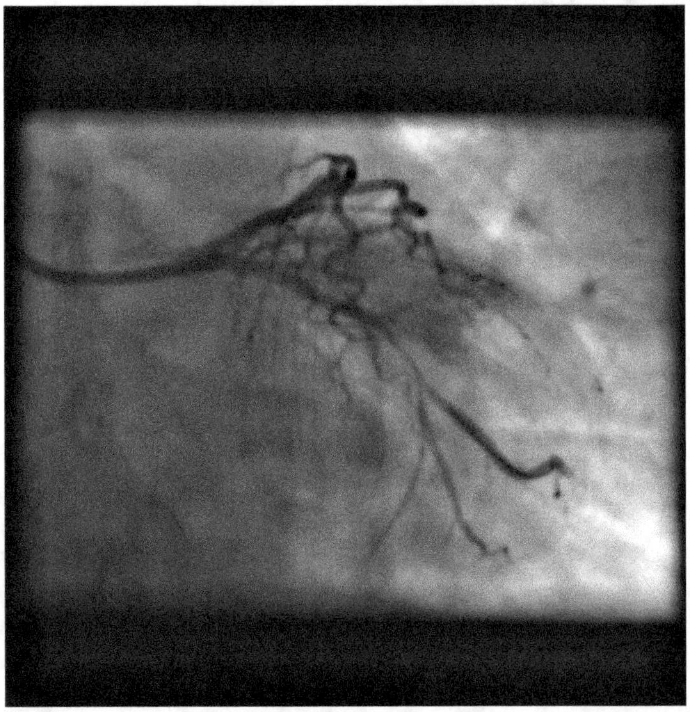

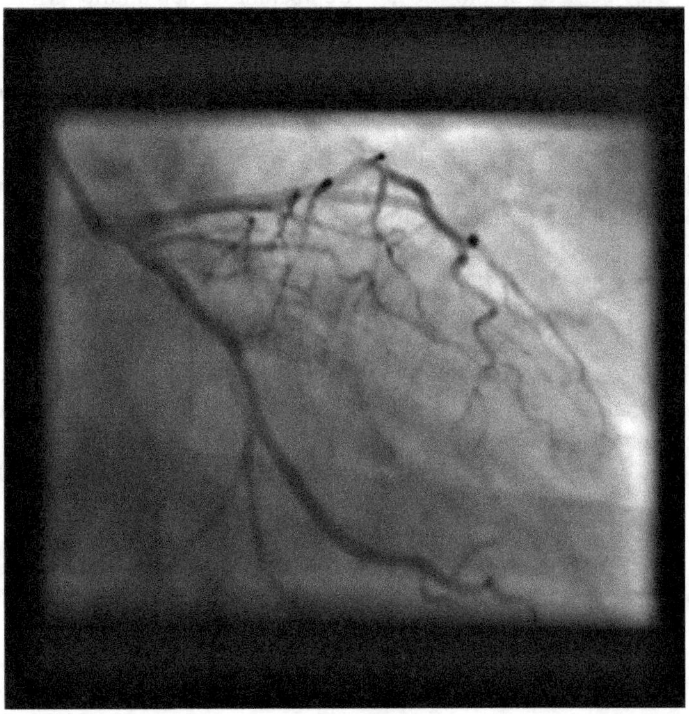

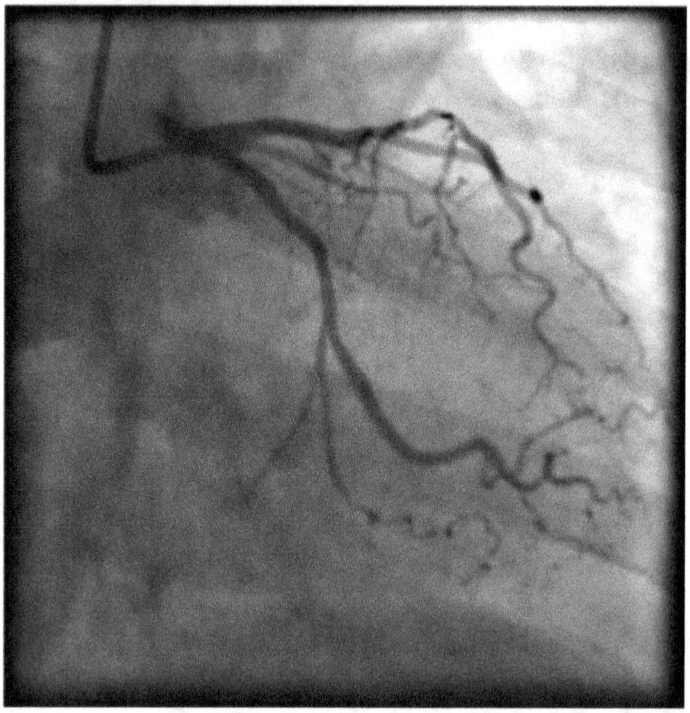

References

1. Gruppo Italiano per lo Studio della Streptochinasi nell'Infarto Miocardico (GISSI). Effectiveness of intravenous thrombolytic treatment in acute myocardial infarction. Lancet. 1986;1:397–402.
2. Randomised trial of intravenous streptokinase, oral aspirin, both, or neither among 17,187 cases of suspected acute myocardial infarction:ISIS-2. ISIS-2 (second international study of infarct survival) collaborative group. Lancet. 1988;2:349–60.
3. Chesebro JH, Knatterud G, Roberts R, et al. Thrombolysis in myocardial infarction (TIMI) trial, phase I: a comparison between intravenous tissue plasminogen activator and intravenous streptokinase. Clinical findings through hospital discharge. Circulation. 1987;76:142–54.
4. GUSTO Angiographic Investigators. The effects of tissue plasminogen activator, streptokinase, or both on coronary-artery patency, ventricular function, and survival after acute myocardial infarction. N Engl J Med. 1993;329(22):1615.
5. Chen ZM, Jiang LX, Chen YP, et al. Addition of clopidogrel to aspirin in 45,852 patients with acute myocardial infarction: randomised placebo-controlled trial. Lancet. 2005;366:1607–21.
6. Sabatine MS, Cannon CP, Gibson CM, et al. Addition of clopidogrel to aspirin and fibrinolytic therapy for myocardial infarction with ST-segment elevation. N Engl J Med. 2005;352:1179–89.
7. Grines CL, Browne KF, Marco J, et al. A comparison of immediate angioplasty with thrombolytic therapy for acute myocardial infarction. The primary angioplasty in myocardial infarction study group. N Engl J Med. 1993;328:673–9.
8. Weaver WD, Simes RJ, Betriu A, et al. Comparison of primary coronary angioplasty and intravenous thrombolytic therapy for acute myocardial infarction: a quantitative review. JAMA. 1997;278:2093–8.
9. Grines CL, Cox DA, Stone GW, et al. Coronary angioplasty with or without stent implantation for acute myocardial infarction. Stent primary angioplasty in myocardial infarction study group. N Engl J Med. 1999;341:1949–56.

10. Stone GW, Grines CL, Cox DA, et al. Comparison of angioplasty with stenting, with or without abciximab, in acute myocardial infarction. N Engl J Med. 2002;346:957–66.
11. Le May MR, Labinaz M, Davies RF, et al. Stenting versus thrombolysis in acute myocardial infarction trial (STAT). J Am Coll Cardiol. 2001;37:985–91.
12. Sabate M, Cequier A, Iniguez A, et al. Everolimus-eluting stent versus bare-metal stent in ST-segment elevation myocardial infarction (EXAMINATION): 1 year results of a randomised controlled trial. Lancet. 2012;380:1482–90.
13. Raber L, Kelbaek H, Ostojic M, et al. Effect of biolimus-eluting stents with biodegradable polymer vs bare-metal stents on cardiovascular events among patients with acute myocardial infarction: the COMFORTABLE AMI randomized trial. JAMA. 2012;308:777–87.
14. Stone GW, Lansky AJ, Pocock SJ, et al. Paclitaxel-eluting stents versus bare-metal stents in acute myocardial infarction. N Engl J Med. 2009;360:1946–59.
15. Kastrati A, Dibra A, Spaulding C, et al. Meta-analysis of randomized trials on drug-eluting stents vs. bare-metal stents in patients with acute myocardial infarction. Eur Heart J. 2007;28:2706–13.
16. Brodie BR, Pokharel Y, Garg A, et al. Very late hazard with stenting versus balloon angioplasty for ST-elevation myocardial infarction: a 16-year single-center experience. J Interv Cardiol. 2014;27:21–8.
17. Scheller B, Speck U, Abramjuk C, et al. Paclitaxel balloon coating, a novel method for prevention and therapy of restenosis. Circulation. 2004;110:810–4.
18. Vos NS, Dirksen MT, Vink MA, et al. Safety and feasibility of a PAclitaxel-eluting balloon angioplasty in primary percutaneous coronary intervention in Amsterdam (PAPPA): one-year clinical outcome of a pilot study. EuroIntervention. 2014;10:584–90.
19. Ho HH, Tan J, Ooi YW, et al. Preliminary experience with drug-coated balloon angioplasty in primary percutaneous coronary intervention. World J Cardiol. 2015;7:311–4.
20. Nijhoff F, Agostoni P, Belkacemi A, et al. Primary percutaneous coronary intervention by drug-eluting balloon angioplasty: the nonrandomized fourth arm of the DEB-AMI (drug-eluting balloon in ST-segment elevation myocardial infarction) trial. Catheter Cardiovasc Interv. 2015;86(Suppl 1):S34–44.
21. Wickramarachchi U, Corballis N, Maart C, et al. Primary PCI with DEB-only angioplasty, first UK experience. EuroPCR, May 2017, Paris, abstract no: Euro17A-POS0364. https://abstract-book.pcronline.com/index/slide/abstract/364/search/deb: PCRonline.com 2017.
22. Kleber FX, Rittger H, Bonaventura K, et al. Drug-coated balloons for treatment of coronary artery disease: updated recommendations from a consensus group. Clin Res Cardiol. 2013;102:785–97.
23. Huber MS, Mooney JF, Madison J, et al. Use of a morphologic classification to predict clinical outcome after dissection from coronary angioplasty. Am J Cardiol. 1991;68:467–71.
24. Mok KH, Wickramarachchi U, Watson T, et al. Safety of bailout stenting after paclitaxel-coated balloon angioplasty. Herz. 2017;42:684–9.
25. Vos NS, van der Schaaf RJ, Amoroso G, et al. REVascularization with paclitaxEL-coated balloon angioplasty versus drug-eluting stenting in acute myocardial infarcTION-A randomized controlled trial: rationale and design of the REVELATION trial. Catheter Cardiovasc Interv. 2016;87:1213–21.

Culprit-Only Artery Versus Multivessel Disease

13

Valeria Paradies and Pieter C. Smits

13.1 Introduction

Primary percutaneous coronary intervention (pPCI) is the treatment of choice in patients presenting with ST-segment elevation myocardial infarction (STEMI). In contemporary practice, among patients who present to the hospital with STEMI, between 40 and 65% have concurrent multi-vessel (MV) coronary artery disease (CAD), a combination of a thrombotic culprit lesion and one or more significant (50% or more diameter stenosis) non-culprit lesions in other coronary artery territories on coronary angiography. Optimal management of these non-culprit lesions in this setting is still a matter of debate. STEMI patients with MV CAD are at higher risk of recurrent cardiovascular events. However, PCI of bystander lesions during pPCI can bring potential complications. The presence of MV CAD in STEMI patients often poses therapeutic dilemma for interventional cardiologists as there are multiple possible strategies and controversial data. Besides clinical relevance, as the burden of cardiovascular disease affects hospital systems around the world, there is growing interest to examine and improve the various treatment strategies involved in the management of STEMI with MV CAD.

13.1.1 Revascularization Strategies for STEMI Patients with MV CAD

Revascularization strategies for non-culprit lesions in haemodynamically stable patients after pPCI currently vary from an aggressive approach with the PCI of all

V. Paradies
National Heart Research Institute Singapore, National Heart Centre, Singapore, Singapore

P. C. Smits (✉)
Department of Interventional Cardiology, Maasstad Hospital, Rotterdam, Netherlands
e-mail: smitsp@maasstadziekenhuis.nl

T. J. Watson et al. (eds.), *Primary Angioplasty*,
https://doi.org/10.1007/978-981-13-1114-7_13

Table 13.1 Factors influencing management of STEMI patients with MV CAD undergoing pPCI

Clinical factors	Procedural factors	Lesion characteristics
Age Comorbidities Haemodynamic stability LV function Renal function Diabetes	Complexity Duration/contrast Final result	Complexity/SYNTAX score Number of vessel disease LM involvement CTO calcifications

significant non-culprit lesions during the index intervention to a very conservative approach with culprit lesion-only treatment and only symptom-driven or ischaemia-driven non-culprit PCI during index hospitalization or after discharge (Table 13.1).

In general three PCI strategies can be identified:

1. Culprit vessel-only pPCI with optimal medical therapy for bystander lesions and PCI of the non-culprit arteries only for spontaneous angina or myocardial ischaemia on stress testing
2. MV PCI at the time of pPCI, guided by angiography or FFR
3. Culprit vessel-only pPCI, followed by angiography or FFR-driven staged PCI of non-culprit arteries during the index hospitalization or after hospital discharge

Incomplete revascularization of STEMI patients presenting with MV CAD has been associated with worse early and late prognosis. The culprit vessel-only PCI strategy may reduce the contrast volume and risk of PCI complications but has been associated with increased risk of repeat revascularization and potential reduction in left ventricle ejection fraction (LVEF) recovery. There are several potential advantages of performing single-stage MV PCI. Firstly, the complete restoration of myocardial blood supply in the acute phase may increase myocardial salvage in hibernating myocardium, therefore improving LVEF. Secondly, this strategy decreases the risk of access site vascular complications associated with repeat vascular punctures. Thirdly, single-stage MV PCI reduces hospitalization with a relevant impact on the healthcare costs. Finally, complete revascularization has been associated with an improved prognosis after PCI: achieving complete revascularization decreases the risk of a future acute coronary syndrome (ACS) or revascularization procedures and improves prognosis. Naturally, there are safety concerns associated with this strategy including prolongation of the interventional procedure, contrast overload and increased radiation exposure. Moreover, the occurrence of procedural complications during non-culprit lesion PCI may further depress LV function which is already compromised from the initial STEMI event. Furthermore, the risk of abrupt vessel closure and stent thrombosis may be increased in this setting due to pro-thrombotic and pro-inflammatory state, while the risk of jeopardizing remote viable myocardium (distal embolization, no reflow, side branch occlusion, loss of collateral circulation) may result in haemodynamic instability.

Despite the additional risks related to PCI access site and additional costs, the staged PCI strategy allows more time to appropriately investigate and weigh on the risks and benefits of non-culprit lesion intervention.

13.1.2 Randomized Trials

There are a number of key clinical trials which provide the wealth of guidance with regard to timing of non-culprit lesion intervention in the setting of STEMI.

13.1.2.1 PRAMI

In the Preventive Angioplasty in Acute Myocardial Infarction (PRAMI) trial, a total of 465 patients were randomly assigned to culprit-only revascularization (n = 231) and complete revascularization during the index procedure (n = 234). The study defined the presence of MV CAD as a non-infarcted-related artery lesion of ≥50% by angiography. Staged revascularization in the asymptomatic patients was discouraged. Patients in cardiogenic shock, unable to provide consent, with previous CABG or non-infarct stenosis of ≥50% in the left main or the ostia of both the left anterior descending and circumflex arteries, or if the only non-culprit stenosis was a chronic total occlusion (CTO), were excluded. After a mean follow-up of 23 months, this study reported a 65% reduction in the primary endpoint (cardiovascular death, new myocardial infarction (MI) and refractory angina defined as angina despite medical therapy supported by evidence of objective ischaemia) in complete revascularization group compared to the culprit-only revascularization group. The study was discontinued early by the data safety monitoring board, due to a significant difference in primary endpoint in favour of complete revascularization which was mainly driven a significant reduction in refractory angina and non-fatal MI; however, no significant reduction in mortality was shown.

Although the study reported convincingly positive study results in favour of single-stage MV PCI, the study had little impact on clinical practice. Several concerns have been raised: the randomization process was not stratified for timing of intervention in relation to symptom onset, nor for site of infarction; the study enrolment included less than 50% of screened patients with possible selection bias; no more information were provided on the non-culprit lesions (i.e. QCA, TIMI flow or lesion characteristics). Moreover, the infarct-related artery (IRA) only revascularization group in this study demonstrated a higher proportion of diabetic patients and anterior MI, which might have influenced the worse prognosis in this group. Finally, this study compared only the most aggressive to the most conservative strategy.

13.1.2.2 CvLPRIT

The Complete versus Lesion-only Primary PCI (CvLPRIT) trial randomized 296 STEMI patients presenting with MV CAD to culprit-only strategy (n = 146) or complete revascularization (n = 150). Patients were excluded in case of age < 18 years, clear contraindication to MV pPCI according to operator judgement, prior MI or CABG, cardiogenic shock, ventricular septal rupture or moderate/severe mitral regurgitation, chronic kidney disease, thrombosis of a previously stented artery and chronic total occlusion of the only non-culprit.

This study reported a 55% reduction of the primary composite endpoint of all-cause mortality, recurrent MI, heart failure and ischaemia-driven revascularization by PCI or CABG within 12 months in the complete revascularization group as compared to the culprit-only group. The investigators found also lower incidence of individual components of the primary endpoint in the complete revascularization group, though not statistically significant. Complete revascularization was performed either at the time of index procedure (64%) or before hospital discharge (36%). The former group showed a trend of greater benefit in terms of MACE incidence as compared to the latter. There was no increase in stroke, major bleeding or contrast-induced nephropathy with complete versus culprit-only revascularization. A pooled analysis of PRAMI and CULPRIT showed a significant reduction in individual endpoints of CV death, recurrent MI and repeat revascularization associated with complete revascularization approach.

13.1.2.3 DANAMI-3 PRIMULTI

In The Third Danish Study of Optimal Acute Treatment of Patients with STEMI: Primary PCI in Multivessel Disease (DANAMI-3 PRIMULTI), 627 patients were randomized to receive culprit lesion-only treatment ($n = 314$) versus fractional flow reserved (FFR)-guided complete revascularization ($n = 312$). Patients with an angiographic diameter stenosis >50% in one or more non-IRA were enrolled and randomized after successful PCI of the culprit lesion. Patients intolerant to contrast media, relevant anticoagulant or antithrombotic drugs, in cardiogenic shock, with stent thrombosis, increased bleeding risk or indication for CABG were excluded from the trial. The FFR-guided staged revascularization was performed 2 days after the index procedure and during the index hospitalization.

One-third of patients within the complete revascularization group had FFR values >0.80 and did not receive PCI. The investigators demonstrated a significant 44% reduction in the composite primary endpoint of death, MI or ischaemia-driven revascularization within 12 months in the FFR-guided complete revascularization group, which was largely driven by a 69% reduction of ischaemia-driven revascularization of the non-IRAs. There were no significant differences in the all-cause mortality or non-fatal MI rates between the two groups. This trial was not powered to evaluate an impact on hard outcomes (such as death and MI).

13.1.2.4 COMPARE-ACUTE Trial

The Comparison Between FFR-Guided Revascularization Versus Conventional Strategy in Acute STEMI Patients with MVD ^^(COMPARE-ACUTE) trial enrolled 885 STEMI patients with MV CAD. After successful revascularization of the culprit artery, patients were randomly assigned in a ratio of 1:2 to FFR-guided complete revascularization ($n = 295$) and culprit-only revascularization ($n = 590$). The most important exclusion criteria were left main CAD, chronic total occlusion, severe stenosis with a Thrombolysis in Myocardial Infarction (TIMI) flow grade of 2 or less in the non-IRA, a suboptimal result or complication after treatment of IRA, severe valve dysfunction and Killip class III or IV. Complete revascularization was performed in lesions with FFR ≤0.80, preferably during the index procedure, but could be delayed within 72 h (complete PCI was performed during index procedure in 83.4% patients). Primary endpoint of the study was the composite of all-cause mortality, non-fatal MI, any revascularization and cerebrovascular events (MACCE) at 12 months. FFR-guided revascularization treatment was associated with lower rate of MACCE compared to culprit-only revascularization, which seems to be driven mainly by the need for repeat revascularization. Similar to previous studies, COMPARE-ACUTE trial was not powered to detect differences in low-frequency events, such as death, re-infarction and stroke. However, in contrast with DANAMI-3PRIMULTI, this study investigated the role of FFR-guided revascularizations during the index procedure, supporting this strategy as safe and cost-saving, from both a patient and economic perspective.

One main criticism of the trial was potential operator bias concerning the decision process about staging the revascularization of non-IRAs beyond the 45 days. In the IRA-only group, urgent revascularizations performed within this time window but after the index procedure or further revascularizations performed thereafter were indeed counted as events. Moreover, in the same treatment group, the indication to treat the non-culprit lesions was heterogeneous and based on detection of ischaemia, symptoms or clinical judgement. However, the rate of MACCE at 1 year remained significantly lower with the complete revascularization strategy even extending the treatment window from 45 to 60 or 90 days and excluding nonurgent revascularizations.

13.1.3 Safety of Complete Revascularization

The recommendation against PCI of non-culprit lesions was largely driven by results of non-randomized observational studies with conflicting results. These recommendations arose from historical safety concerns that included an increased potential risk for procedural complications. However, more complete acute revascularization in patients with STEMI may be safer in the current era due to advances in stent technology and antiplatelet therapy. Recent evidences suggest that potential longer procedural time or increased use of contrast in complete revascularization does not translate into an increased risk of adverse events. A pooled analysis of PRAMI, CULPRIT and the trial by Politi et al. found no increase in cerebrovascular (CVA) events, bleeding or contrast-induced nephropathy associated with PCI of non-culprit lesions performed at the time of index procedure. DANAMI3-PRIMULTI study demonstrated similar rates of peri-procedural MI, stroke, contrast-induced nephropathy or bleeding between IRA-only and complete revascularization treatment. In a similar way, the recent COMPARE-ACUTE found no differences in terms of peri-procedural MI and bleeding between the two strategies.

13.1.4 Timing of Revascularization

The optimal timing for revascularization of the non-culprit lesions remains extremely debated. Potential options include performing complete revascularization during index procedure or as planned elective procedure during index hospitalization or after discharge. To date there are no RCTs investigating both staged and immediate complete revascularization and analysing them separately. PRAMI specifically compared single-stage MV PCI to culprit-only strategy, while DANAMI3- PRIMULTI analysed only staged versus culprit-only revascularization. The two RCTs CvLPRIT and COMPARE-ACUTE were designed to perform complete revascularization in the acute phase, but allowed staged revascularization, which happened in a minority of the cases. Although all RCT trials show an advantage of immediate or early staged complete revascularization guided by angiography or FFR in comparison to culprit-only treatment, still uncertainties exist about when the complete revascularization should be performed. Looking at the time to event curves in all the above-mentioned trials, we can observe that the event curves start to diverge from the outset, presumably indicating that an immediate or very early revascularization strategy is likely to be beneficial. This assumption is complemented by a meta-analysis by Wang et al. comparing complete revascularization during the index procedure with staged revascularization that found a significantly lower incidence of MACE, all-cause death and/or MI, non-fatal MI and repeat revascularization associated with the former strategy.

Interestingly, the benefit of the immediate complete revascularization strategy has not been confirmed in other meta-analyses and in the various published observational studies. In the post hoc analysis of HORIZONS-AMI trial, MV PCI during index procedure was associated with an increased all-cause and cardiovascular mortality compared to the staged MV PCI in a total of 668 STEMI patients. Similarly, a recent meta-analysis by Tarantini et al. demonstrated that a staged MV revascularization strategy may improve both early and late survival. Moreover, a propensity-matched analysis of 3984 patients presenting with STEMI and MV disease suggested an improved survival and improved MACE with culprit-only PCI during the index procedure. The confusion is compounded by a paired and network meta-analysis of 14 studies including 40,280 patients and compared three timing strategies in STEMI patients with MV disease: staged PCI (defined as separate procedure during index admission or within 1 month of the primary PCI), immediate complete revascularization during index pPCI procedure and culprit-only PCI. This analysis found lowest short- and long-term mortality rates in patients undergoing staged complete revascularization.

Overall, the above studies suggest staged revascularization as the best option. Nevertheless, these data are from prior observational studies and meta-analyses of revascularization strategies derived from an extremely heterogeneous set of inclusion criteria, study protocols, PCI techniques, timing of MV PCI and comparator groups. Also with divergent analytical methods and variable endpoints, definite conclusions are difficult to draw.

13.1.5 Trials on the Horizon

The large ongoing randomized, Complete versus Culprit-only Revascularization to Treat Multivessel Disease After Primary PCI for STEMI (COMPLETE) trial will enrol a total of 3900 STEMI patients with MV disease and is estimated to be completed in December 2018. Patients are randomized to receive either staged revascularization or culprit-only revascularization, on top of optimal medical therapy (including low-dose aspirin and ticagrelor in both arms and FFR guidance in intermediate lesions (50–70% diameter stenosis)) in the complete revascularization arm. The FULL REVASC trial from Sweden is another large-scale trial randomizing 4052 MV-STEMI or high-risk MV-NSTEMI patients between FFR-guided complete revascularization in the acute or staged phase and angiography-guided. The primary endpoint of both trials are the combination of recurrent myocardial infarction and all death (FULL REVASC) or cardiovascular death (COMPLETE) and will provide final answers with hard endpoints as to whether staged revascularization is better than culprit-only revascularization or FFR guidance is better compared to angiography in acute MI patients with MV disease.

13.2 State of the Art: Current Recommendations

Both the 2014 European Society of Cardiology guidelines and 2013 American College of Cardiology/American Heart Association guidelines did not recommend revascularization of non-culprit lesions in the setting of STEMI unless complicated by cardiogenic shock. These recommendations were influenced strongly by safety concerns based on observational studies. The publication of larger scale RCTs has prompted ACC/AHA to change the recommendation for complete revascularization to class IIb in the recent 2015 ACC/AHA/SCAI Focused Update on Primary Percutaneous Intervention for Patients with ST-Elevation Myocardial Infarction. These guidelines specifically allow consideration of single-stage MV PCI in selected patients, either at the time of pPCI or as a delayed, staged procedure. Similarly, 2017 ESC guidelines for the management of acute myocardial infarction in patients presenting with STEMI recommend that revascularization of non-IRA should be considered in STEMI patients with MV CAD at index or before hospital discharge (class IIa). The optimal timing of revascularization (immediate vs. staged) has not been adequately investigated; therefore, no recommendation is provided in these guidelines.

13.3 Role of Fractional Flow Reserve

Most of the observational and randomized studies have so far used angiographic diameter stenosis severity to determine non-culprit lesions requiring PCI. Fractional flow reserve (FFR) has historically not been utilized in ACS due to concern that acute microvascular dysfunction might influence these results. It has been suggested that non-IRA stenosis severity may be acutely exaggerated as the result of circulating catecholamine-mediated vasoconstriction. Moreover, virtual histology intravascular ultrasound (VH-IVUS) analysis of non-culprit lesions in ACS patients has shown a greater prevalence of vulnerable plaques, with greater necrotic core and thin-cap fibroatheroma as compared with stable coronary lesions.

Nevertheless, reliability of FFR of non-culprit lesions in the acute phase of STEMI has been extensively demonstrated. Ntalianis et al. reported the reproducibility of FFR measurements in 75 STEMI patients undergoing PCI when repeated at a mean of 35 ± 4 days post initial procedure. The same was observed by a similar study performed by Musto et al. when similar FFR and instantaneous wave-free ratio (iFR) values were obtained in the acute phase and 7 days later in 60 MV-STEMI patients undergoing pPCI. Moreover, the COMPARE-ACUTE trial demonstrated a discrepancy between angiographic and haemodynamically significant lesions in STEMI patients; approximately half of non-culprit lesions that were considered to be critical on coronary angiography were found to have an FFR value >0.80 and therefore not physiologically relevant.

Both DANAMI3-PRIMULTI and COMPARE-ACUTE trial showed that FFR-guided PCI decreased acute and repeat revascularization rates, though did not impact mortality or re-infarction rates. However, performing FFR during index procedure, as investigated in COMPARE-ACUTE trial, was found to be safe and to reduce cost and risk associated with a delayed procedure, justifies a selective anatomically incomplete revascularization, expedites post-STEMI care and discharge, facilitates decision-making in the heart team and may offer reassurance to the patient.

13.4 Prognostic Value of Complete Revascularization

Although recent RCTs showed a benefit of composite MACE endpoints associated with complete revascularization as compared to culprit-only strategy, this was mainly driven by a reduction in ischaemia-driven revascularization. Of note, none of these trials was powered to evaluate prognostic clinical endpoints such as death and myocardial infarction. Interestingly, a meta-analysis of four RCTs including CvLPRIT, PRAMI, Politi and HELP-AMI for a total of 1044 patients that compared complete revascularization and culprit-only demonstrated significant reduction in long-term (≥1 year) all-cause mortality, cardiovascular death and MI associated with the former treatment. A low degree of heterogeneity between the studies was reported for this meta-analysis. Despite all the limits related to differences of individual studies, these findings suggest a trend towards improved death and MI with complete revascularization. Further clarification is expected from the COMPLETE trial which will investigate the benefit of complete revascularization in terms of composite of cardiovascular death and MI as primary endpoint.

13.5 STEMI with Multivessel Coronary Artery Disease Complicated by Cardiogenic Shock

Cardiogenic shock is present in 6–12% of cases with acute myocardial infarction, varying according to the population analysed and definition of cardiogenic shock. The presence of MV CAD has been reported in up to 60–70% of STEMI patients complicated by cardiogenic shock. In the Should We Emergently Revascularize

Occluded Coronaries for Cardiogenic Shock (SHOCK) trial, three-vessel CAD was found in 60% of patients undergoing PCI. MV CAD in STEMI patients complicated by cardiogenic shock has been found to be an independent predictor of in-hospital mortality.

Most of the current available data regarding the management of MV CAD in the context of cardiogenic shock are based on retrospective analysis of registries, therefore producing heterogeneous and conflicting results.

In the milestone SHOCK trial, 352 patients with acute myocardial infarction complicated by cardiogenic shock were randomized to receive either emergency revascularization with either PCI or CABG (n = 152) or initial medical stabilization (n = 150). Despite the high rate of intra-aortic balloon pump used in both groups, the investigators found no differences in terms of 30-day mortality and lower 6-month mortality rates in the complete revascularization group as compared to culprit-only treatment. This study showed that a strategy of early revascularization resulted in 6-year higher survival rates compared with initial medical stabilization. Retrospective sub-analysis of KAMIR registry evaluating 510 STEMI patients with cardiogenic shock and evidence of MV CAD at angiography revealed reduction of early mortality with complete revascularization. Similarly, a prospective observational study of 266 STEMI patients with cardiogenic shock showed improved 6-month survival associated with single-stage MV PCI strategy.

Results of the CULPRIT-SHOCK (Culprit Lesion-Only PCI Versus MV PCI in Cardiogenic Shock) trial have been recently published. This multicentre, open-label trial randomized 706 patients with cardiogenic shock and evidence of MV CAD at index angiography to receive either culprit vessel revascularization (during index procedure with possible staged revascularization) or single-stage MV PCI. The use of intra-aortic balloon pump and mechanical support device use was left at operator's discretion. The 30-day risk of a composite of death or severe renal failure leading to renal replacement therapy was lower among those who initially underwent PCI of the culprit lesion-only than among those who underwent immediate MV PCI. One potential limitation of this study is advocating attempts at CTO revascularization in the acute setting, which is usually performed only with evidence of ischaemia and viability demonstrated in the CTO territory.

Current ESC guidelines recommend that non-IRA PCI during the index procedure should be considered in STEMI patients with cardiogenic shock (Class IIA, Level of evidence C). The ACC/AHA/SCAI guidelines recommend emergency revascularization with either PCI or CABG irrespective of the time delay from myocardial infarction onset in STEMI patients complicated by cardiogenic shock (Class I, Level of evidence B). The rationale behind complete revascularization is to improve perfusion to non-IRA territories in order to reverse the spiral of decline that characterizes this status. In the context of myocardial ischaemia, a pan-myocardial inflammatory process as well as systemic hypotension might impact on the entire coronary circulation and exacerbate ischaemia in non-IRA lesions, leading to further coronary hypoperfusion and impaired myocardial function. However, despite current recommendations, multiple registries have shown that only one-fourth to one-third of STEMI patients with cardiogenic shock and evidence of MV CAD undergo immediate MV PCI.

13.6 Clinical Practice

The recently reported RCTs have shown potential benefit of complete revascularization strategy which have led to guideline updates. These studies reflect more contemporary clinical practice where the use of DES, radial access and more effective P2Y12 inhibitors has improved clinical outcomes and reduced procedure-related complications. These findings have shed new light on the potential management of such patients. The use of FFR in this context has been proposed as a safe tool able to guide a functionally complete revascularization.

However, there are still unsolved issues with regard to the optimal timing of intervention as the current data present conflicting evidence. Moreover, the recent RCTs have shown improved MACE outcomes with complete revascularization mostly driven by need for repeat revascularization but are underpowered to determine hard clinical endpoints of death and MI. Furthermore, whether the goal of complete revascularization should be the treatment of ischaemia-related lesions or vulnerable plaques prone to thrombosis has yet to be determined.

Despite the available evidence and ongoing trials, defining a common strategy for all STEMI patients with MVD remains challenging. These patients are extremely heterogeneous, and any revascularization strategy should be individualized based on patient and lesion characteristics. Physiological evaluation of non-culprit lesions should be encouraged in order to define appropriate revascularization strategy.

13.7 Case Report

Valeria Paradies and Peter C. Smits

A 58-year-old man, without cardiac history, was admitted to our hospital for acute onset of chest pain and diagnosis of inferior STEMI. The ECG showed clear ST elevation in inferior leads, and the coronary angiography confirmed occlusion of RCA (Fig. 13.1a). However, a clear image of thrombus was detected in the mid-LAD involving the ostium of a diagonal branch (Fig. 13.1b). Our strategy began with PCI of RCA with a drug-eluting stent (DES) 4.0 × 12 mm (Fig. 13.2a). Due to plaque shift, a second 4.0 × 18 mm DES was implanted proximal to the previous one (Fig. 13.2b). No reflow occurred but rapidly improved with i.c. verapamil injection. Despite the culprit lesion having been identified and successfully treated, a clear image of thrombus that was evident in the mid-LAD was concerning, although not immediately compromising flow or generating apparent rest ischaemia. As the culprit lesion was successfully treated in a relatively short time and the patient remained haemodynamically stable despite transient no reflow, we considered the option to proceed with immediate PCI of LAD and diagonal branch, both of which were non-culprit lesions (despite the presence of obvious but non-occlusive thrombus)

A provisional approach was taken, and predilatation of the LAD with a 2.5 × 10 mm balloon followed by DES 3.5 × 23 mm implantation in mid-LAD was performed (Fig. 13.3a). After LAD stenting, plaque shift occurred towards the ostium of the diagonal (Fig. 13.3b). At this point, our decision-making process considered the

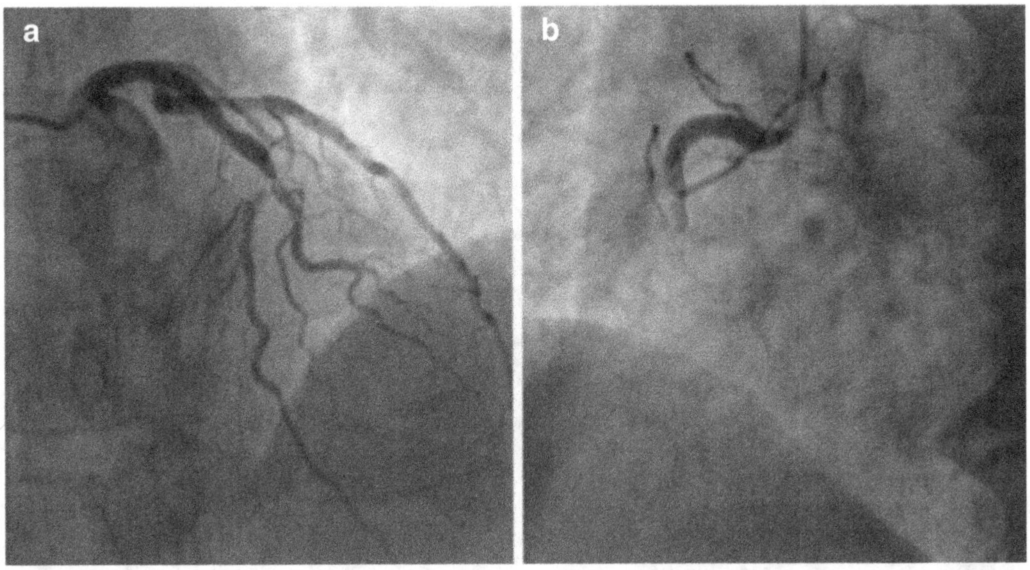

Fig. 13.1 (**a**) Left coronary angiography showed images of non-occlusive thrombus in the mid-LAD involving the origin of a relevant diagonal branch. (**b**) Right coronary angiography showed complete thrombotic occlusion of the right coronary artery in line with ECG findings of inferior STEMI

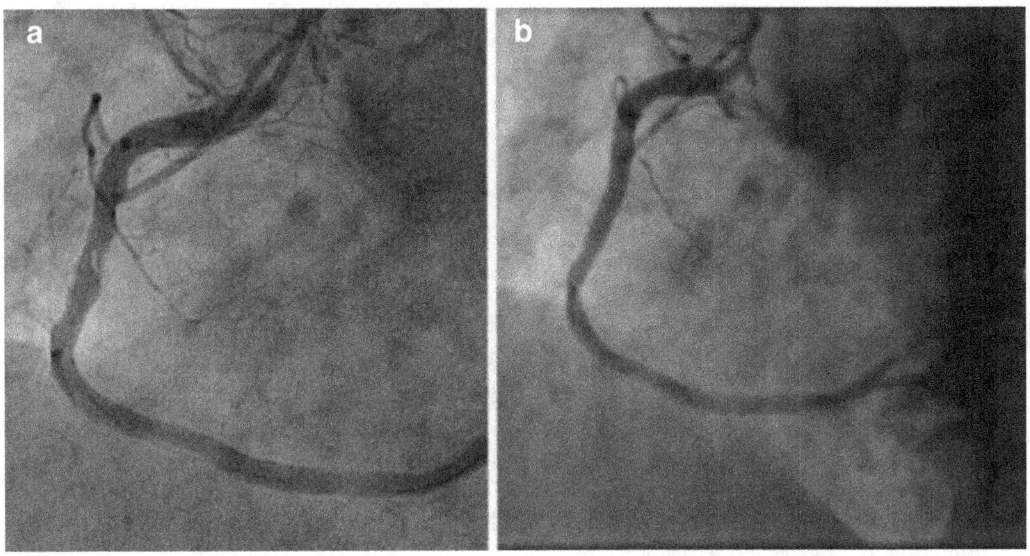

Fig. 13.2 (**a**) Proximal plaque shift after DES 4.0 × 12 implantation on mid-RCA. (**b**) Final result after second stent implantation, i.c. verapamil administration and postdilatation of RCA lesion

potentially complicated issue of leading to a two-stent bifurcation PCI of a non-culprit vessel in a STEMI setting. However, given the degree of stenosis at ostium of the diagonal and calibre of this vessel, we decided to complete the procedure with a TAP stenting technique. A DES 2.75 × 8 mm was implanted in the diagonal branch and final kissing balloon dilatation performed using oversized NC balloons (Fig. 13.3c). The patient remained haemodynamically stable and was discharged home a few days later. Although there is currently a vivid debate on complete revascularization during

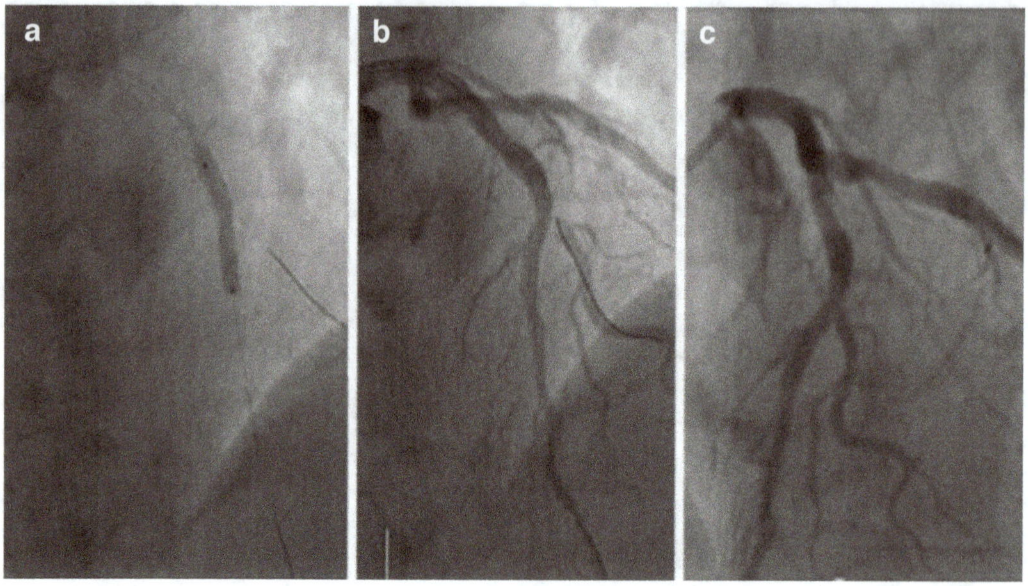

Fig. 13.3 (**a**) DES 3.5 × 23 mm implantation on mid-LAD. (**b**) Result after LAD stenting. (**c**) Final result after D1 stenting with TAP technique and final kissing balloon

pPCI, this case highlights how the risk/safety balance of non-culprit PCI was steered by the angiographic findings of high thrombus burden in mid-LAD, which if left untreated may have had severe consequences.

Further Readings

Engstrøm T, Kelbæk H, Helqvist S, et al. Complete revascularisation versus treatment of the culprit lesion only in patients with ST-segment elevation myocardial infarction and multivessel disease (DANAMI-3—PRIMULTI): an open-label, randomised controlled trial. Lancet. 2015;386:665–71.

Gershlick AH, Khan JN, Kelly DJ, et al. Randomized trial of complete versus lesion-only revascularization in patients undergoing primary percutaneous coronary intervention for STEMI and multivessel disease: the CvLPRIT trial. J Am Coll Cardiol. 2015;65:963–72.

Smits PC, Abdel-Wahab M, Neumann FJ, et al. Fractional flow reserve-guided multivessel angioplasty in myocardial infarction. N Engl J Med. 2017;376:1234–44.

Wald DS, Morris JK, Wald NJ, et al. Randomized trial of preventive angioplasty in myocardial infarction. N Engl J Med. 2013;369:1115–23.

14 Role of Intravascular Imaging in Primary PCI

William K. T. Hau and Bryan P. Y. Yan

14.1 Introduction

Acute ST-segment elevation myocardial infarction (STEMI) usually results from acute thrombotic occlusion of a major epicardial coronary artery. Primary percutaneous coronary intervention (PPCI) is the reperfusion strategy of choice if it can be done in a timely manner, its aim being to rapidly achieve complete myocardial reperfusion. Overwhelming evidence has shown that prompt reperfusion reduces infarct size, preserves left ventricular function, and improves survival [1, 2].

Studies have demonstrated the benefits of drug-eluting stents (DESs) in patients with acute myocardial infarction (MI) undergoing primary stent implantation. The HORIZONS-AMI (*Harmonizing Outcomes with Revascularization and Stents in Acute Myocardial Infarction*) trial demonstrated that the use of DESs in patients with STEMI is safe and effective compared with bare metal stents (BMSs) at 1-year follow-up. The use of DESs definitively reduces the need for repeat revascularization without additional risk of death or MI [3]. Besides, a meta-analysis of 13 randomized trials, which compared the outcomes of DES and BMS in 7352 randomized patients, suggested that DES use significantly decreases restenosis compared with BMS use in patients with STEMI. DES use yields a relative and absolute reduction in target vessel revascularization (TVR) of 56% and −7%, respectively ($p < 0.001$). The meta-analysis also suggested that this benefit does not come at the expense of stent thrombosis, reinfarction, or increased death within 2 years of the PCI [4].

Even though DES use has proven to be safe in the setting of primary PCI, stent thrombosis remains a serious complication associated with increased morbidity and mortality [5, 6]. Thus, careful attention must be paid to ensure complete stent

B. P. Y. Yan · W. K. T. Hau (✉)
Division of Cardiology, Department of Medicine and Therapeutics, The Chinese University of Hong Kong, Prince of Wales Hospital, Hong Kong, SAR, China
e-mail: william.hau@cuhk.edu.hk

T. J. Watson et al. (eds.), *Primary Angioplasty*,
https://doi.org/10.1007/978-981-13-1114-7_14

coverage of the culprit lesion in terms of diameter and stenosis. In STEMI patients, rapid reperfusion is the most crucial issue, so primary PCI is always targeted on the angiographically identified culprit lesion. However, the actual culprit lesion may not be lumen-compromising and could be located proximally or distally to the angiographic target lesion. As a result, the risk of incomplete lesion coverage could be high when the primary PCI is guided solely by angiography. Furthermore, stent implantation must be optimized, as incomplete apposition and/or edge dissection may result in in-stent restenosis or thrombosis. Thus, invasive coronary imaging (Fig. 14.1) using intravascular ultrasound (IVUS) or optical coherence tomography (OCT) is useful for guiding the PCI procedure in the primary setting by locating the true culprit lesion and may lead to better stent coverage of the lesion. Besides, invasive imaging also helps to resolve diagnostic uncertainty and to identify the mechanism underlying the acute event. Thin-cap

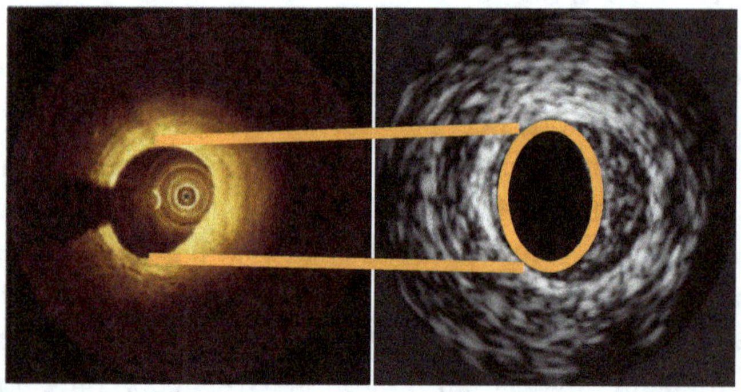

	OCT	IVUS
Resolution	15 µm	150 µm
Penetration	2 mm	10 mm
Field of View	10 mm	10 mm
Frame Rate	100 FPS	15-30 FPS
Pullback Speed	75 mm/sec	0.5/1.0 mm/sec
Catheter Size	Sub 3F	3.2 F

Fig. 14.1 A comparison table of OCT and IVUS

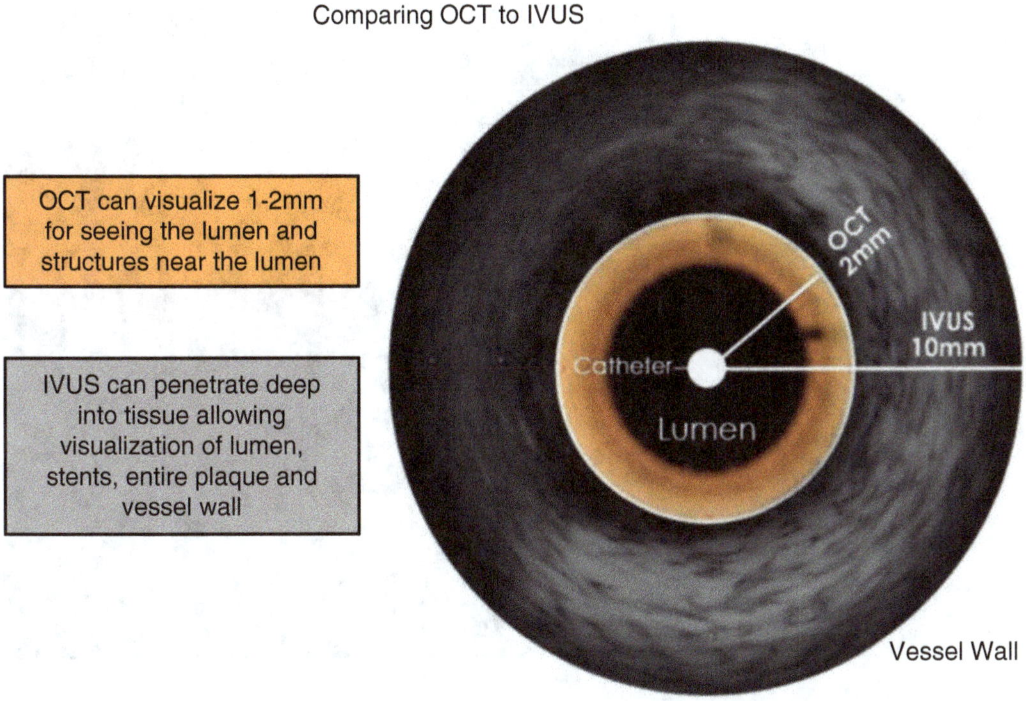

Fig. 14.2 IVUS can penetrate deep into tissue allowing visualization of the lumen, entire plaque, and vessel wall. However, the high resolution of OCT provides superior delineation of the superficial structures

fibroatheroma (TCFA) is the most common type of vulnerable plaque and is defined as a lesion with a fibrous cap thickness ≤ 65 μm containing a large lipid pool with a necrotic core and infiltrated by macrophages. It is believed to be the precursor of thrombotic plaque rupture [7]. Autopsy studies have shown that TCFA is more commonly found in coronary segments with positive remodeling [8], and due to its better penetration power than OCT (Fig. 14.2), IVUS is very useful in identifying coronary vessels with positive remodeling [9]. However, the high resolution of OCT is able to provide accurate quantification of fibrous cap thicknesses ≤65 μm (Fig. 14.3). Other than coronary plaque rupture, plaque erosion and calcified nodules are frequent pathophysiological mechanisms responsible for acute coronary syndrome (ACS) [7], and OCT enables differentiation of all three features in vivo [10]. Other rare causes of acute coronary symptoms such as spontaneous coronary artery dissection [11], myocardial bridging [12], or mechanical problems due to stent underexpansion [13] and/or stent fracture [14] can also be identified by invasive imaging. However, the impact of intravascular imaging in terms of clinical outcomes in the setting of acute MI remains a matter of controversy.

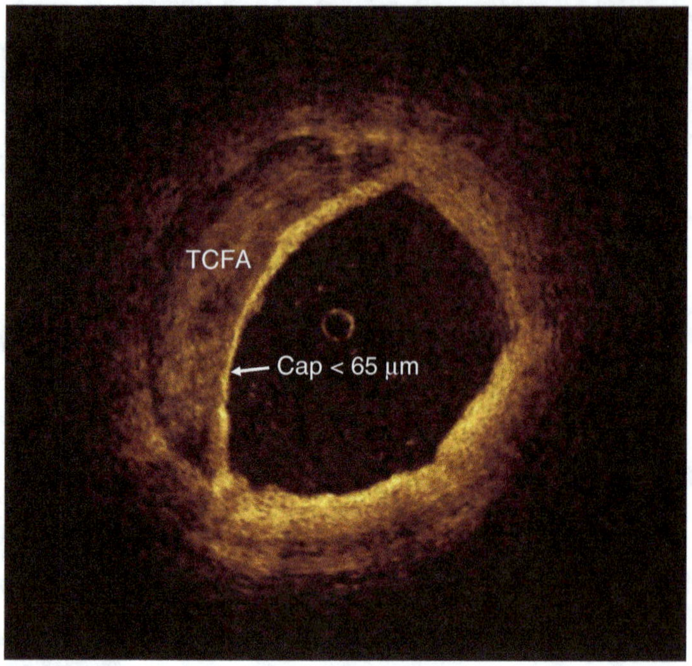

Fig. 14.3 Thin-cap fibroatheroma (TCFA) is the most common type of vulnerable plaque and is defined as a lesion with a fibrous cap thickness ≤65 μm containing a large lipid pool with a necrotic core and infiltrated by macrophages. The high resolution of OCT is able to provide accurate quantification of fibrous cap thicknesses ≤65 μm

14.2 Role of Invasive Imaging in the Management of STEMI and Non-STEMI

14.2.1 Intravascular Ultrasound

IVUS uses reflected high-frequency (10–60 MHz) sound waves to visualize the arterial wall in a two-dimensional tomographic format. IVUS permits not only a greater understanding of the characteristics of the coronary plaque and its response to interventional coronary procedures but also allows more precise quantification of the coronary luminal dimensions and atherosclerotic plaque burden [15–17]. In the setting of elective PCI, randomized trials and meta-analyses indicate that IVUS-guided PCI is associated with a lower incidence of TVR and fewer major adverse cardiac events (MACEs), MI, and stent thromboses than angiography-guided PCI [18, 19]. IVUS provides useful information about the morphology of the coronary lesion, as well as helping stent size selection, optimization of stent expansion, and detection of incomplete apposition and/or edge dissection, resulting in reduced restenosis or stent thrombosis. IVUS- measured minimal stent cross-sectional area (CSA) is the best IVUS predictor of DES failure. The results from the IVUS substudy of the HORIZONS-AMI trial showed that mechanical problems such as a smaller final stent CSA (<5 mm^2) and inflow/outflow disease (residual stenosis or dissection) but not acute mal-apposition were associated with early stent thrombosis after intervention for acute MI. The minimal stent CSA measured by IVUS and the degree of stent expansion were significantly smaller in patients with early stent thrombosis than in the control group. The finding that the minimal stent CSA was significantly smaller in acute MI patients with early stent thrombosis could be either because of tissue protrusion (plaque and/or thrombus) or stent underexpansion or both, as the culprit lesions in acute MI patients are presumed to be thrombus-containing, and thus tissue protrusion into the lumen through stent struts is common [20]. Besides, another IVUS sub-study of the HORIZONS-AMI trial also suggested that the final post-procedure minimal stent CSA in patients with STEMI after primary stent implantation was the only independent IVUS predictor of angiographic binary restenosis, similar to patients with stable coronary disease as previously reported. Angiographic restenosis rates were 26.7% in lesions with a CSA <4 mm^2, 22.2% in lesions with a CSA <5 mm^2, and 20.5% in lesions with a CSA <6 mm^2 [21]. Therefore, a well-expanded stent with a final minimal stent CSA ≥5 mm^2 by IVUS is needed in patients undergoing primary PCI to prevent stent thrombosis as well as restenosis at follow-up.

However, it is still controversial whether routine IVUS guidance improves outcomes in patients receiving primary PCI treatment. The Assessment of Dual Antiplatelet Therapy with Drug-Eluting Stents (ADAPT-DES) trial reported that IVUS-guided PCI with DESs was associated with significantly lower rates of stent thrombosis, MI, and MACEs. In this particular trial, 813 STEMI patients were enrolled, and it was found that IVUS use was associated with substantially improved outcomes in these patients [22]. Besides, studies by Singh et al. have shown that the use of IVUS in patients with acute MI was associated with reduced in-hospital mortality but at the expense of increased cost of care and vascular complications, compared with angiography-guided PCI [23]. On the contrary, a few other studies did not support the routine use of IVUS for patients who present with an acute MI and undergoing primary PCI. A study by Maluenda et al. showed no clear clinical benefit of routine use of IVUS-guided stenting in 905 patients with acute MI undergoing primary PCI. The overall rates of the composite primary outcome were similar, as were the rates of stent thrombosis in the IVUS-guided and the non-IVUS-guided groups. However, the number of treated lesions and the number of stents used were higher in the IVUS-guided group, with a longer procedural time as well [24]. Consistently, two studies from Korea reported similar findings; IVUS guidance during primary PCI did not provide a better clinical outcome and prevent stent thrombotic events. Although the stent size and the final minimal stented CSA were larger in the IVUS-guided group, the use of IVUS was also associated with a longer stent length and higher number of stents used [25, 26]. Traditionally, longer and more stents used are associated with much worse clinical outcomes and thus may minimize the potential benefits of IVUS use in acute MI patients undergoing primary PCI. Supporting this notion, a recent study from Japan, the CREDO (Coronary Revascularization Demonstrating Outcome)-Kyoto AMI registry sub-analysis, evaluated the outcomes of 932 patients undergoing IVUS-guided PCI among the 3028 STEMI patients enrolled in the registry and also found no apparent benefit of IVUS for reducing TVR and stent thrombosis as well as mortality in STEMI patients undergoing primary PCI [27]. Despite the fact that, in the setting of elective PCI, IVUS use has been demonstrated to reduce the MACE rate and improve clinical outcomes, in the setting of primary PCI, it seems that IVUS use can be a two-edged sword; it may help in stent implantation guidance—and in terms of proper stent size selection and

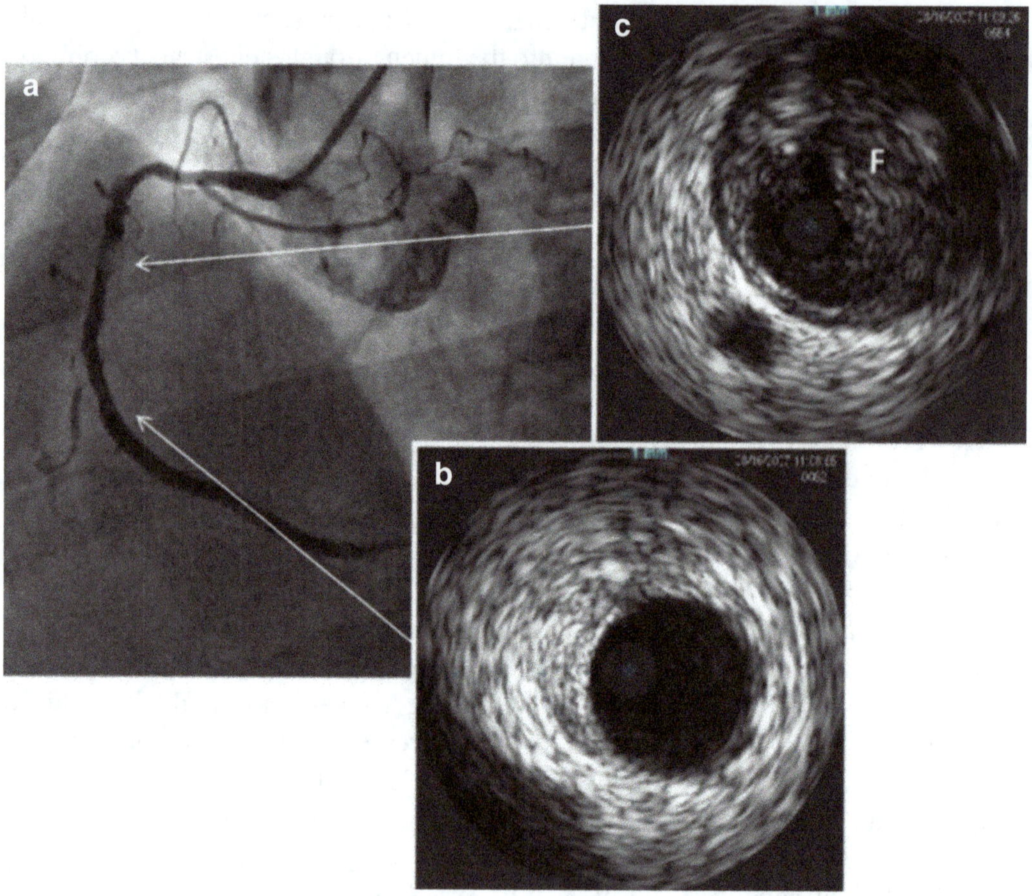

Fig. 14.4 (**a**) Coronary angiography suggestive of thrombus formation at the mid-right coronary artery. (**b**) IVUS image of the normal reference distal to the culprit site. (**c**) IVUS image at the culprit site with positive remodeling contains a large thrombus (F) burden

postimplantation stent optimization, it may result in reduction of restenosis or stent thrombosis. On the other hand though, it may also be associated with a higher rate of coronary complications, and this could be because of poor IVUS interpretation due to a large thrombus burden in the culprit lesions of STEMI patients (Fig. 14.4), making it rather difficult to determine proper stent sizing and optimization of stent deployment, resulting in under- or oversize stent selection, and this may lead to disastrous consequences like perforation and stent thrombosis. In addition, the underlying pathological process in acute settings is very different from that in elective settings. The culprit lesions responsible for causing the acute events are very soft with less calcification and naturally contain a large thrombus burden; thus post-dilatation to optimize stent deployment with high-pressure ballooning in acute MI patients may potentially cause thrombus protrusion or tissue prolapse through the stent strut and increase the likelihood of distal embolization. Besides, acute MI patients might have a higher chance of late-acquired stent mal-apposition due to the thrombus resolving over time, and that may lead to thrombotic events as well. It has been shown on IVUS that at the time of acute MI, IVUS use is not able to predict the occurrence of late-acquired incomplete stent apposition, as this could result from either thrombus dissolution and/or positive vessel wall remodeling [28]. Thus, it is possible that IVUS use in the setting of primary PCI may increase the overall procedural time and cost without providing additional clinical outcome benefits.

14.2.2 Optical Coherence Tomography

OCT generates real-time high-resolution cross-sectional images of the vascular wall from backscattered reflections of infrared light. The greatest advantage of this infrared light-based imaging technology is its significantly higher resolution (tenfold higher) than that of the sound-based technology, but at the cost of having to inject contrast medium to flush blood from the vessel, as the OCT signal is attenuated by the presence of red blood cells. Current commercially available intravascular OCT technologies have an axial resolution of 10–20 μm and a lateral resolution of 20–25 μm. The higher resolution of OCT provides superior delineation of the superficial structures and is able to visualize calcium (Fig. 14.5) without acoustic shadowing [29], as seen with IVUS. However, signal penetration through the diseased vessel is more limited due to its lower penetration power, making it difficult to quantify the plaque burden or to investigate large vessels. Besides, since OCT requires the injection of a contrast medium during image acquisition in order to create a blood-free environment, OCT cannot be performed in scenarios such as totally occluded vessels or coronary arteries with massive dissection. The results from the CLI-OPCI (Centro per la Lotta contro l'Infarto-Optimisation of Percutaneous Coronary Intervention) registry suggested that the use of OCT in patients undergoing PCI could improve clinical outcomes. A significant reduction in the primary end

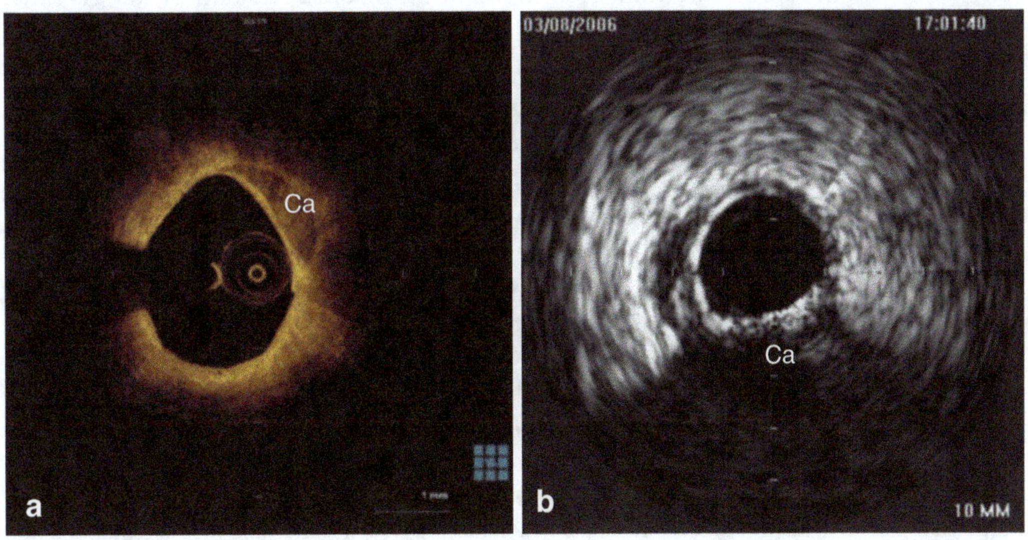

Fig. 14.5 (**a**) The higher resolution of OCT is able to visualize calcium (Ca) without acoustic shadowing. (**b**) The IVUS image shows superficial calcium (Ca) from 4 o'clock to 8 o'clock with acoustic shadowing

point of cardiac death or MI was found in patients undergoing OCT-guided PCI compared with patients treated with angiographic guidance alone [30]. Suboptimal stent deployment was associated with an increased risk of MACEs during follow-up. More recently, a randomized controlled trial reported that OCT-guided PCI procedures using a specific reference segment external elastic lamina-based stent optimization strategy resulted in clinical outcomes equivalent to those with IVUS-guided PCI [31]. Due to the ultra-high resolution, OCT is more sensitive in detecting mal-apposition, tissue prolapse, small edge dissection, and intra-stent thrombus than IVUS. However, studies have also shown that small dissections and tissue protrusion detected by OCT tend to resolve over a 6-month follow-up period [32], so all these small details detected by OCT may be clinically irrelevant and could potentially lead to unnecessary interventions and might eventually cause more complications.

Most acute coronary events, including MI, occur in relation to subsequent coronary thrombus formation. Due to its high resolution, OCT can identify a thrombus better than IVUS and is able to discriminate two types of thrombi (Fig. 14.6): red thrombus (red blood cell-rich), which has high backscatter and high attenuation, and white thrombus (platelet-rich) characterized by signal-rich low backscatter and low attenuation [33]. However, the impact of characterization of these two types of thrombi in clinical decision-making is still unclear, and further studies are needed. Furthermore, in the ACS setting, OCT has been shown to identify plaque morphologies associated with a worse prognosis. Plaque erosion and plaque rupture (Fig. 14.7) are the two most frequent pathophysiological mechanisms responsible for ACS and contribute to almost 95% of the acute coronary events; OCT enables the differentiation of these two plaque features in vivo. At OCT, plaque erosion appears as a plaque covered by thrombus (typically a white, platelet-rich thrombus) without signs of fibrous cap disruption. This occurs at sites with impaired endothelium, rich in smooth muscle cells and proteoglycans. In contrast, plaque rupture is identified by the presence of a fibrous cap

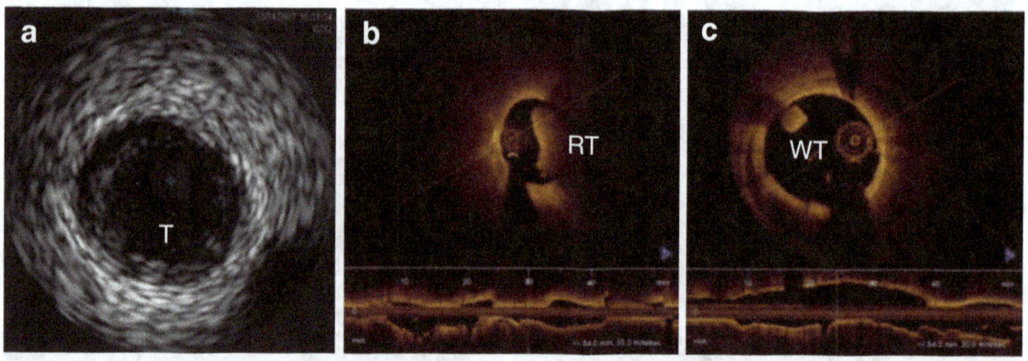

Fig. 14.6 (**a**) IVUS image of a vessel contains a large thrombus burden. OCT is able to discriminate two types of thrombi: (**b**) red thrombus, which has high backscatter and high attenuation, and (**c**) white thrombus characterized by signal-rich low backscatter and low attenuation. *T* thrombus, *RT* red thrombus, *WT* white thrombus

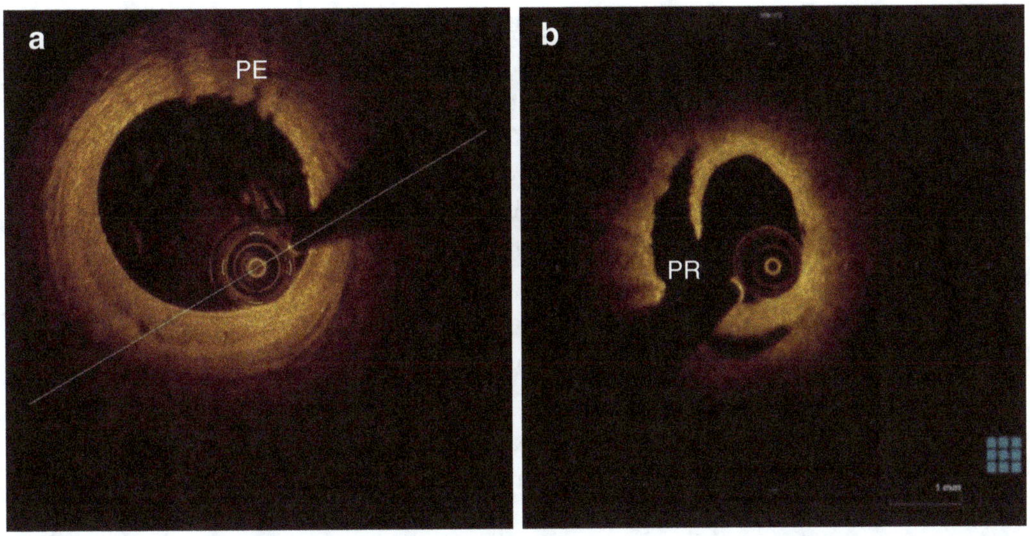

Fig. 14.7 OCT enables the differentiation of plaque erosion (PE) and plaque rupture (PR) in vivo. (**a**) PE appears as a plaque covered by thrombus (typically a white, platelet-rich thrombus) without signs of fibrous cap disruption. (**b**) PR is identified by the presence of a fibrous cap discontinuity, creating communication between a cavity within the plaque and the arterial lumen

discontinuity, creating communication between a cavity within the plaque and the arterial lumen. Calcified nodules contribute to ≤5% of acute coronary events, and these are characterized by fibrous cap disruption due to protrusion of calcium [34, 35]. Differentiation of these three plaque features can be useful in the choice of therapeutic strategy. The recent EROSION (Effective Antithrombotic Therapy Without Stenting: Intravascular OCT-Based Management in Plaque Erosion) trial suggested that patients with ACS caused by plaque erosion may be stabilized by antithrombotic therapy alone, without stenting, and thereby potentially have fewer stent-related early and late complications [36].

The high resolution of OCT clearly enables a better understanding of the atherosclerotic plaque and helps to identify the mechanism underlying the acute event. Studies aiming to investigate an association between OCT and improvement in clinical outcomes may further strengthen the evidence in favor of using OCT to guide PCI in ACS patients. The DOCTORS (Does Optical Coherence Tomography Optimize Results of Stenting) trial is the first randomized, prospective, multicenter trial to investigate the use of OCT in optimizing the results of PCI for non-ST-segment elevation ACS. The results showed that OCT findings led to a change in procedural strategy in 50% of the patients in the OCT-guided group, mainly driven by the optimization of stent expansion, and were associated with higher fractional flow reserve values at the end of the procedure than angiography-guided PCI alone. However, this benefit was obtained at the cost of longer fluoroscopy and procedural times, as well as a greater volume of contrast medium and a higher dose of radiation, but without an increase in periprocedural complications, MI, or kidney dysfunction [37].

14.3 Role of Invasive Imaging in the Management of Spontaneous Coronary Artery Dissection

14.3.1 Pathogenesis of Spontaneous Coronary Artery Dissection

The usual pathogenesis of acute MI involves unstable plaque rupture or plaque erosion that is distinct from spontaneous coronary artery dissection (SCAD). SCAD is a rare cause of acute MI, and is due to hemorrhage within the arterial wall, resulting in separation of the intimal-medial layers rather than atherosclerotic plaque rupture or erosion. The presence of true arterial lumen compression by the hematoma in the intimal-medial layers can subsequently result in myocardial ischemia or acute MI. Early recognition and precise diagnosis of SCAD is very important in order to implement the appropriate medical treatment; otherwise it will lead to disastrous consequences. Two potential mechanisms for the cause of SCAD have been proposed. The first is that an intimal tear creates an entry point that promotes intramural bleeding inside the false lumen, leading to separation of the intimal-medial layers. The second is that rupture of the vasa vasorum leads to an intramural hematoma, which increases the pressure and potentially causes an intimal rupture into the true lumen. Thus SCAD caused by the latter mechanism can occur with or without a distinct intimal rupture [38]. SCAD is not uncommon in young females presenting with acute MI in the absence of traditional cardiovascular risk factors [39] and is the most frequent cause of acute MI among pregnant women [40].

The symptoms of SCAD usually do not differ from those of ACS, as SCAD impairs myocardial perfusion by reducing the vessel lumen in a manner very similar to atherosclerotic stenosis, and thus accurate recognition and management of SCAD may improve both short- and long-term outcomes. However, SCAD is mainly caused by spontaneous dissection of the coronary artery wall. As a matter of fact, it is very difficult to correctly diagnose based on angiography alone as angiography is only a two-dimensional luminogram and is not able to visualize the vessel wall, explaining why SCAD is frequently underdiagnosed. The angiographic appearance of SCAD consists of extraluminal contrast staining, spiral dissection, an intraluminal filling defect, and smooth narrowing of varying length and severity which depends on the amount of blood accumulation within the false lumen. Based on the angiographic appearance, Saw proposed a classification of SCAD (Fig. 14.8) to aid its diagnosis [41]. Type 1 angiographic SCAD describes the pathognomonic appearance of arterial wall contrast staining with multiple radiolucent lumens. Type 2 angiographic SCAD describes long diffuse stenosis of varying severity (typically >20 mm), but often subtle, abrupt changes in arterial caliber from the normal diameter to diffuse smooth narrowing, and often extends to the distal ends of the arteries. Type 3 angiographic SCAD describes focal tubular (typically <20 mm) stenosis that mimics atherosclerotic lesions. Invasive coronary imaging techniques like IVUS and OCT that can image the arterial wall improve SCAD diagnosis and are also very useful in guiding coronary intervention when revascularization is needed. However, they are not available in some catheterization laboratories and are also associated with additional risks and cost. Thus, angiography remains the frontline imaging

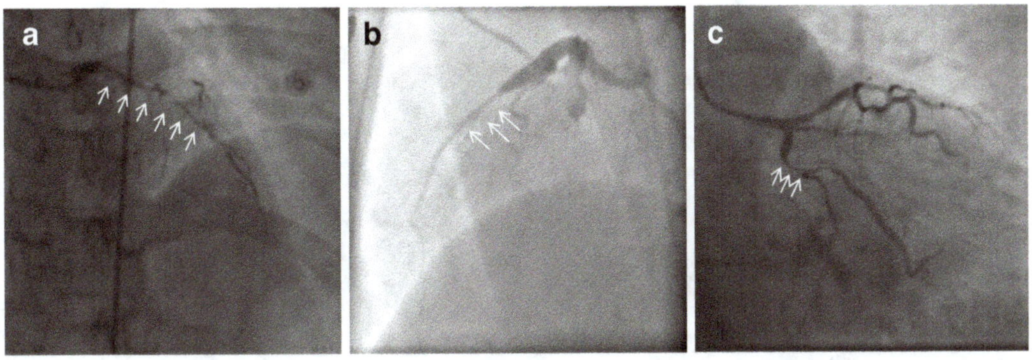

Fig. 14.8 Saw proposed an angiographic classification of SCAD to aid its diagnosis. (**a**) Type 1 angiographic SCAD describes the pathognomonic appearance of arterial wall contrast staining with multiple radiolucent lumens. (**b**) Type 2 angiographic SCAD describes long diffuse stenosis of varying severity (typically >20 mm), but often subtle, abrupt changes in arterial caliber from the normal diameter to diffuse smooth narrowing, and often extends to the distal ends of the arteries. (**c**) Type 3 angiographic SCAD describes focal tubular (typically <20 mm) stenosis that mimics atherosclerotic lesions

technology for the diagnosis of SCAD. However, when it comes to SCAD patient management, coronary revascularization is only indicated for those with ongoing or recurrent ischemia with favorable anatomy but is associated with high complication rates [42]. On the other hand, patients without evidence of ongoing ischemia can be treated medically, and most have an uneventful clinical course [43]. Medical management consists of blood pressure control with dual antiplatelet and beta-blockers.

14.3.2 Intravascular Ultrasound

As noted above, in both elective and acute settings, IVUS is very useful in the determination of the severity and characteristics of atherosclerotic plaques and has played a vital role in PCI guidance in terms of vessel sizing and the optimization of stent implantation. In patients suspected of having SCAD, the diagnosis of SCAD requires visualization of the intramural hematoma and separation of the intimal-medial layers creating double true and false lumens. Thus, due to its better tissue penetration power, IVUS allows a more complete and deeper vessel visualization of the extent of the intramural hematoma, as well as the dissected layers, while the true and false lumens can be clearly identified. Also, the distribution of the false lumen and the compromise of the true lumen can also be clearly visualized on IVUS [44]. An intramural hematoma on IVUS appears homogeneous and hyperechoic, with a crescent-shaped area of blood accumulation (Fig. 14.9). However, due to its relatively poor image resolution, IVUS is not able to identify the intimal rupture site. On the other hand, IVUS is able to confirm the guide-wire position within the true lumen (Fig. 14.10), and IVUS findings have also been used to optimize the results of stent implantation in patients with SCAD requiring coronary intervention [45].

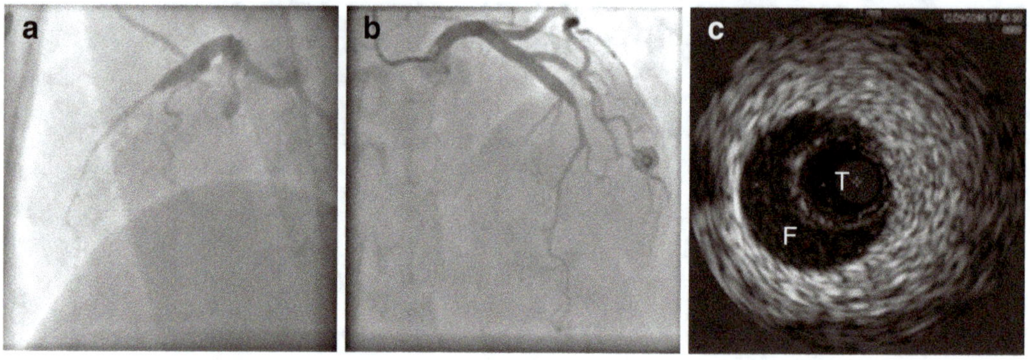

Fig. 14.9 (**a**) and (**b**) Coronary angiography suggesting a type 2 SCAD. (c) IVUS revealing the presence of a dissection; both the true (T) and false (F) lumens can be clearly identified

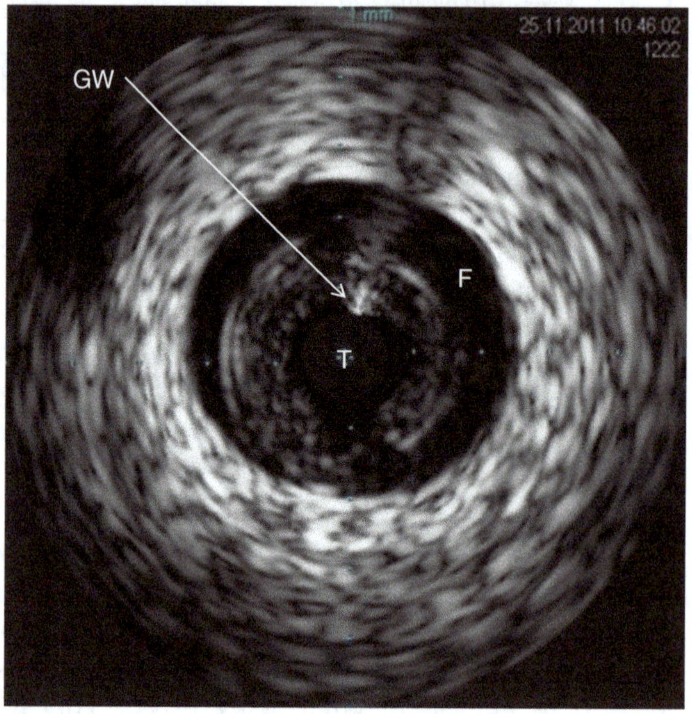

Fig. 14.10 IVUS confirms the guide-wire (GW) is in the true (T) lumen, not the false (F) lumen

14.3.3 Optical Coherence Tomography

Coronary angiography is unable to establish a definitive diagnosis of SCAD. Conversely, OCT allows accurate visualization of the coronary artery wall with unprecedented resolution and thus is very useful to rule out this diagnosis in patients with images mimicking SCAD. OCT provides unique insights by visualizing most of the morphological features of the condition including intimal tears, intraluminal thrombi, double-lumen morphology, and intramural hematoma. However, inadequate optical penetration may impede full visualization of the circumferential extent of an intramural hematoma. Like IVUS, the distribution of the false lumen and the compromise of the true lumen can also be very clearly visualized on OCT. An intramural hematoma, on the other hand, has a dark appearance on OCT (Fig. 14.11).

In addition, due to its superb near-field resolution compared with IVUS, OCT is superior in identifying the precise location of the intimal rupture tear and readily depicts the length of the dissecting membrane [46]. However, IVUS provides deeper penetration of the vessel wall and is therefore able to fully visualize large hematomas (Fig. 14.12). On the other hand, caution must be exercised when performing OCT imaging on SCAD patients, as OCT requires flush injection of contrast medium to

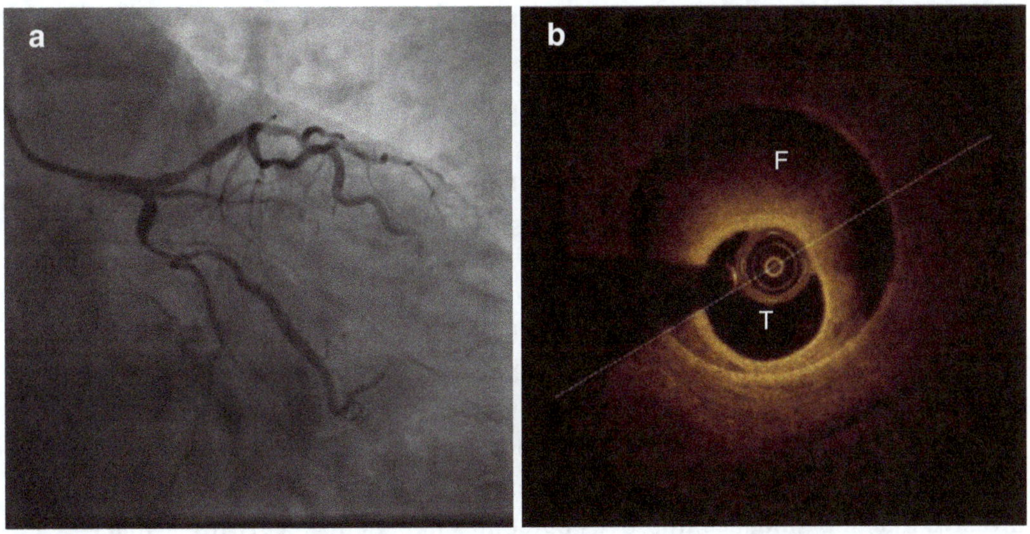

Fig. 14.11 (**a**) Coronary angiography suggesting a type 3 SCAD. (**b**) OCT revealing the presence of a dissection; both the true (T) and false (F) lumens can be clearly identified

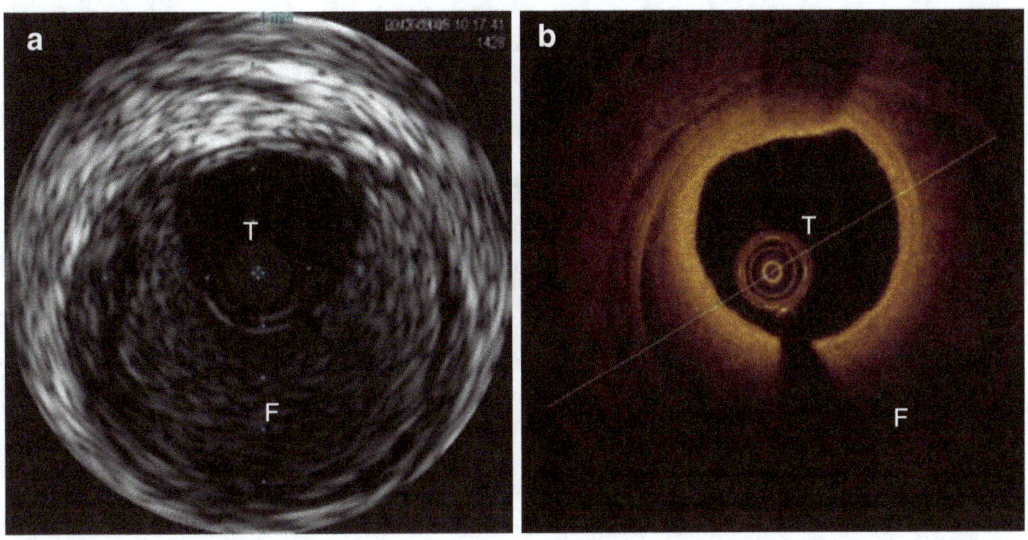

Fig. 14.12 (**a**) Intramural hematoma on IVUS appears homogeneous and hyperechoic, with a crescent-shaped area of blood accumulation. The distribution of the false lumen (F) and the compromise of the true lumen (T) are clearly visualized. (**b**) Intramural hematoma has a dark appearance on OCT. The distribution of the false lumen (F) and the compromise of the true lumen (T) can also be very clearly visualized on OCT. However, IVUS provides deeper penetration of the vessel wall and is therefore able to fully visualize large hematomas

create a blood-free environment during image acquisition in order to obtain good images. This may cause the hematoma to extend distally. Also, abnormalities such as an extramural vessel hematoma or perivascular hematoma can be detected on IVUS, but not on OCT. Finally, for patients undergoing coronary intervention, OCT imaging is also able to help to confirm the guide-wire position within the true lumen, as well as helping in vessel sizing and stent optimization [47].

14.4 Summary

Even though angiography is the gold standard to guide procedural decision-making during primary PCI, it has various well-known limitations. Angiography is only a luminology without providing any information on the vessel wall and atherosclerotic plaque characteristics. Besides, it is suboptimal in detecting stent underexpansion, stent edge dissection, plaque protrusion, or thrombi. Invasive imaging techniques like IVUS and OCT provide complementary details to help primary PCI guidance, such as to ensure stent coverage of the culprit lesion and optimization of stent implantation. OCT is superior in the visualization of superficial structures, such as stent edge dissection, intimal tear, tissue protrusion, and intraluminal thrombi, whereas IVUS is better for deep vessel imaging, vessel sizing, and identifying positive remodeling. However, it remains controversial as to whether routine invasive imaging guidance improves outcomes in patients receiving primary PCI.

References

1. Keeley EC, Boura JA, Grines CL. Primary angioplasty versus intravenous thrombolytic therapy for acute myocardial infarction: a quantitative review of 23 randomized trials. Lancet. 2003;361:13–20.
2. Mauri L, Silbaugh TS, Garg P, et al. Drug-eluting or bare-metal stents for acute myocardial infarction. N Engl J Med. 2008;359:1330–42.
3. Stone GW, Lansky AJ, Pocock SJ, et al. Paclitaxel-eluting stents versus bare-metal stents in acute myocardial infarction. N Engl J Med. 2009;360:1946–59.
4. Brar SS, Leon MB, Stone GW, et al. Use of drug-eluting stents in acute myocardial infarction. A systematic review and meta-analysis. J Am Coll Cardiol. 2009;53:1677–89.
5. Sianos G, Papafaklis MI, Darmen J, et al. Angiographic stent thrombosis after routine use of drug-eluting stents in ST-segment elevation myocardial infarction: the importance of thrombus burden. J Am Coll Cardiol. 2007;50:573–83.
6. Iakovou I, Schmidt T, Bonizzoni E, et al. Incidence, predictors, and outcome of thrombosis after successful implantation of drug-eluting stents. JAMA. 2005;293:2126–30.
7. Virmani R, Kolodgie FD, Burke AP, et al. Lessons from sudden coronary death: a comprehensive morphological classification scheme for atherosclerotic lesions. Arterioscler Thromb Vasc Biol. 2000;20:1262–75.
8. Burke AP, Farb A, Malcolm GT, et al. Coronary risk factors and plaque morphology in men with coronary disease who died suddenly. N Engl J Med. 1997;336:1276–82.
9. Nakamura M, Nishikawa H, Mukai S, et al. Impact of coronary artery remodeling on clinical presentation of coronary artery disease: an intravascular ultrasound study. J Am Coll Cardiol. 2001;37:63–9.

10. Niccoli G, Montone RA, DiVito L, et al. Plaque rupture ad intact fibrous cap assessed by optical coherence tomography portend different outcomes in patients with acute coronary syndrome. Eur Heart J. 2015;36:1377–84.
11. Tweet MY, Hayes SN, Pitta SR, et al. Clinical features, management, and prognosis of spontaneous coronary artery dissection. Circulation. 2012;126:579–88.
12. Ishikawa Y, Akasaka Y, Akishima-Fukasawa Y, et al. Histopathologic profiles of coronary atherosclerosis by myocardial bridge underlying myocardial infarction. Atherosclerosis. 2013;226:118–23.
13. Fujii K, Carlier SG, Mintz GS, et al. Stent underexpansion and residual reference segment stenosis are related to stent thrombosis after sirolimus-eluting stent implantation. J Am Coll Cardiol. 2005;45:995–8.
14. Makaryus AN, Lefkowitz L, Lee AD. Coronary artery stent fracture. Int J Cardiovasc Imaging. 2007;23:305–9.
15. Mintz GS, Painter JA, Pichard AD, et al. Atherosclerosis in angiographically "normal" coronary artery reference segments: an intravascular ultrasound study with clinical correlations. J Am Coll Cardiol. 1995;25:1479–85.
16. Mintz GS. Intravascular ultrasound and outcome after drug-eluting stent implantation. Coron Artery Dis. 2017;28:346–52.
17. Mintz GS, Nissen SE, Anderson WD, et al. American college of cardiology clinical expert consensus document on standards for acquisition, measurement and reporting of intravascular ultrasound studies (IVUS): a report of the American college of cardiology task force on clinical expert consensus documents. J Am Coll Cardiol. 2001;37:1478–92.
18. Steinvil A, Zhang YJ, Lee SY, et al. Intravascular ultrasound-guided drug eluting stent implantation: an updated meta-analysis of randomized control trials and observational studies. Int J Cardiol. 2016;216:133–9.
19. Bavishi C, Sardar P, Chatterjee S, et al. Intravascular ultrasound-guided vs angiography-guided drug-eluting stent implantation in complex coronary lesions: meta-analysis of randomized trials. Am Heart J. 2017;185:26–34.
20. Choi SY, Witzenbichler B, Maehara A, et al. Intravascular ultrasound findings of early stent thrombosis after primary percutaneous intervention in acute myocardial infarction. A harmonizing outcomes with revascularization and stents in acute myocardial infarction (HORIZONS-AMI) substudy. Circ Cardiovasc Interv. 2001;4:239–47.
21. Choi SY, Maehara A, Cristea E, et al. Usefulness of minimum stent cross sectional area as a predictor of angiographic restenosis after primary percutaneous coronary intervention in acute myocardial infarction (from the HORIZONS-AMI trial IVUS substudy). Am J Cardiol. 2012;109:455–60.
22. Witzenbichler B, Maehara A, Weisz G, et al. Relationship between intravascular ultrasound guidance and clinical outcomes after drug-eluting stents: the assessment of dual antiplatelet therapy with drug-eluting stents (ADAPT-DES) study. Circulation. 2014;129:463–70.
23. Singh V, Badheka AO, Arora S, et al. Comparison of inhospital mortality, length of hospitalization, costs, and vascular complications of percutaneous coronary interventions guided by ultrasound versus angiography. Am J Cardiol. 2015;115:1357–66.
24. Maluenda G, Lemesle G, Ben-Dor I, et al. Impact of intravascular ultrasound guidance in patients with acute myocardial infarction undergoing percutaneous coronary intervention. Catheter Cardiovasc Interv. 2010;75:86–92.
25. Ahmed K, Jeong MH, Chakraborty R, et al. Role of intravascular ultrasound in patients with acute myocardial infarction undergoing percutaneous coronary intervention. Am J Cardiol. 2011;108:8–14.
26. Youn YJ, Yoon JH, Lee JW, et al. Intravascular ultrasound-guided primary percutaneous coronary intervention with drug-eluting stent implantation in patients with ST-segment elevation myocardial infarction. Clin Cardiol. 2011;34:706–13.
27. Nakatsuma K, Shiomi H, Morimoto T, et al. Intravascular ultrasound guidance vs. angiographic guidance in primary percutaneous coronary intervention for ST-segment elevation

myocardial infarction – long term clinical outcomes from the CREDO-Kyoto AMI registry. Circ J. 2006;80:477–84.
28. Cheneau E, Leborgne L, Mintz GS, et al. Predictors of subacute stent thrombosis results of a systematic intravascular ultrasound study. Circulation. 2003;108:43–7.
29. Kume T, Okura H, Kawamoto T, et al. Assessment of the coronary calcification by optical coherence tomography. EuroIntervention. 2011;6:768–72.
30. Prati F, Di Vito L, Biondi-Zoccai G, et al. Angiography alone versus angiography plus optical coherence tomography to guide decision-making during percutaneous coronary intervention: the Centro per la Lotta contro I'Infarto-Optimisation of Percutaneous Coronary Intervention (CLI-OPCI) study. EuroIntervention. 2012;8:823–9.
31. Ali ZA, Maehara A, Genereux P, et al. Optical coherence tomography compared with intravascular ultrasound with angiography to guide coronary stent implantation (ILUMIEN III: OPTIMIZE PCI): a randomized controlled trial. Lancet. 2016;388:2618–28.
32. Kawamori H, Shite J, Shinke T, et al. Natural consequence of post-intervention stent malapposition, thrombus, tissue prolapse, and dissection assessed by optical coherence tomography at mid-term follow-up. Eur Heart J Cardiovasc Imaging. 2013;14:865–75.
33. Kume T, Akasaka T, Kawamoto T, et al. Assessment of coronary arterial thrombus by optical coherence tomography. Am J Cardiol. 2006;97:1713–7.
34. Kubo T, Imanishi T, Takarada S, et al. Assessment of culprit lesion morphology in acute myocardial infarction: ability of optical coherence tomography compared with intravascular ultrasound and coronary angioscopy. J Am Coll Cardiol. 2007;50:933–9.
35. Jia H, Abtahian F, Aguirre AD, et al. In vivo diagnosis of plaque erosion and calcified nodule in patients with acute coronary syndrome by intravascular optical coherence tomography. J Am Coll Cardiol. 2013;62:1748–58.
36. Jia H, Dai J, Hou J, et al. Effective anti-thrombotic therapy without stenting: intravascular optical coherence tomography-based management in plaque erosion (the EROSION study). Eur Heart J. 2017;38:792–800.
37. Meneveau N, Souteyrand G, Motreff P, et al. Optical coherence tomography to optimize results of percutaneous coronary intervention in patients with non-ST-elevation acute coronary syndrome – results of multicenter randomized DOCTORS study (does optical coherence tomography optimize results of stenting). Circulation. 2016;134:906–17.
38. Maehara A, Mintz GS, Castagna MT, et al. Intravascular ultrasound assessment of spontaneous coronary artery dissection. Am J Cardiol. 2002;89:466–8.
39. Tweet MS, Best P, Hayes SN. Unique presentations and etiologies of myocardial infarction in women. Curr Treat Options Cardiovasc Med. 2017;19:66.
40. Tweet MS, Hayes SN, Codsi E, et al. Spontaneous coronary artery dissection associated with pregnancy. J Am Coll Cardiol. 2017;70:426–35.
41. Saw J. Coronary angiogram classification of spontaneous coronary artery dissection. Catheter Cardiovasc Interv. 2014;84:1115–22.
42. Tweet MS, Eleid MF, Best PJM, et al. Spontaneous coronary artery dissection revascularization versus conservative therapy. Circ Cardiovasc Interv. 2014;7:777–86.
43. Alfonso F, Paulo M, Lennie V, et al. Spontaneous coronary artery dissection: long-term follow-up of a large series of patients prospectively managed with a "conservative" therapeutic strategy. J Am Coll Cardiol Intv. 2012;5:1061–70.
44. Maehara A, Mintz GS, Bui AB, et al. Incidence, morphology, angiographic findings, and outcomes of intramural hematomas after percutaneous coronary interventions: an intravascular ultrasound study. Circulation. 2002;105:2037–3042.
45. Arnold JR, West NEJ, Gaal WJV, et al. The role of intravascular ultrasound in the management of spontaneous coronary artery dissection. Cardiovasc Ultrasound. 2008;6:24.
46. Alfonso F, Paulo M, Gonzalo N, et al. Diagnosis of spontaneous coronary artery dissection by optical coherence tomography. J Am Coll Cardiol. 2012;59:1073–9.
47. Nakagawa M, Shite J, Shinke T, et al. Ability of optical coherence tomography to visualize the entry port of spontaneous coronary artery dissection. Circ J. 2011;75:2505–7.

Physiological Lesion Assessment in STEMI and Other Acute Coronary Syndromes

15

Katherine M. Yu and Morton J. Kern

15.1 Introduction

Although coronary artery disease (CAD), the most common cause of morbidity and mortality in the USA, is identified principally by coronary angiography, the relationship between the degrees of angiographic narrowing (% stenosis) is poorly correlated to its functional response (e.g., stress testing or intracoronary physiology). Over the past two decades, the use of in-lab coronary physiology has demonstrated that angiography alone is not accurate in determining ischemia for intermediate lesions. Compared with angiographically guided percutaneous coronary intervention (PCI), physiology-guided PCI is associated with improved clinical outcomes and cost-effectiveness. The most commonly used invasive physiologic indices include fractional flow reserve (FFR), coronary flow reserve (CFR), and instantaneous wave-free ratio (iFR). Understanding applied coronary physiology and the tools for measuring it in the cath lab is paramount to best clinical decision-making in interventional cardiology.

While FFR has been well validated in patients with chronic stable coronary artery disease, in ACS, physiological assessment of the culprit coronary artery is not performed because reduced flow to the myocardial bed can lead to false negatives. However, FFR can be measured in the non-culprit vessels because theoretically it is presumed that flow is not reduced to myocardial regions remote for the culprit

K. M. Yu
Department of Cardiology, Veterans Administration Long Beach Health Care System, Long Beach, CA, USA

University of California, Irvine, CA, USA

M. J. Kern (✉)
University of California, Irvine, CA, USA

Division of Medicine, Veterans Administration Long Beach Health Care System, Long Beach, CA, USA

T. J. Watson et al. (eds.), *Primary Angioplasty*,
https://doi.org/10.1007/978-981-13-1114-7_15

infarct vessel territory. This chapter will be to review the different methods of invasive physiological assessment of coronary stenoses and their outcomes with a focus on their practical applications in patients with ST-elevation myocardial infarction (STEMI) and other ACS.

15.2 ACS and FFR Case

A 58-year-old man presented with 1 day of intermittent chest pain. His medical history was significant for hypertension and hyperlipidemia. The ECG showed anterior T wave inversions and his troponin was 4. Urgent cardiac catheterization revealed a 95% stenosis in the proximal left circumflex (LCX) artery and a 60% stenosis in the proximal left anterior descending (LAD) artery (Figs. 15.1 and 15.2). The presumed culprit vessel, the left circumflex artery, was stented (Fig. 15.3). Turning to the LAD, should we proceed to stent, defer and treat medically, or measure FFR and treat based on the ischemic potential of the lesion? Based on the evidence (see below), FFR of the non-infarct LAD artery is not only reasonable but favored to reduce operator uncertainty and shorten the current and future hospitalizations. As the lesion was fairly remote from the injured lateral wall myocardial zone, FFR should be valid (especially if positive). FFR of the proximal LAD lesion was 0.78 (Fig. 15.4) and stented (Fig. 15.5) in the same procedure. The patient was discharged uneventfully.

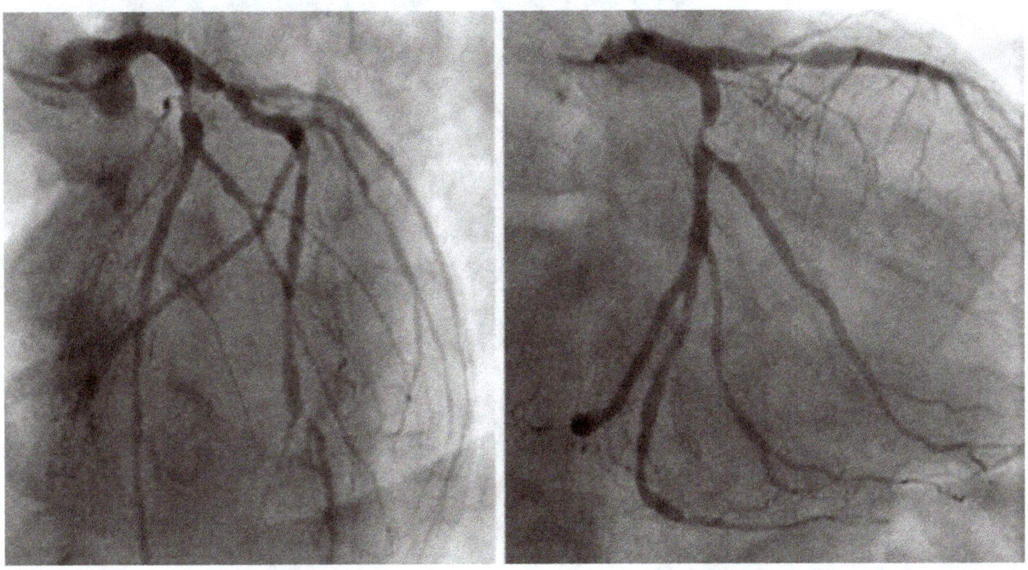

Fig. 15.1 Cineangiogram from ACS and FFR case (LAO cranial and RAO projections) showing 95% circumflex and 60% LAD lesions

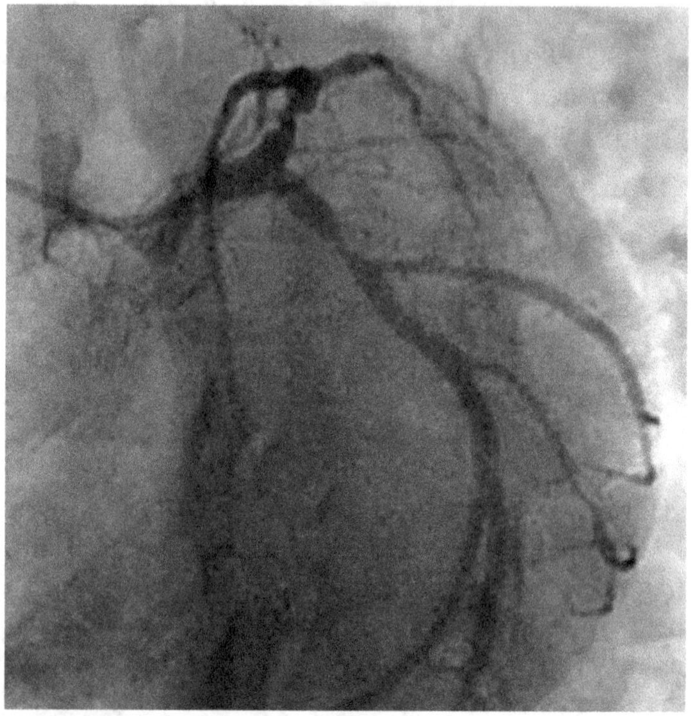

Fig. 15.2 Cineangiogram from ACS and FFR case (LAO Caudal) showing 95% circumflex and 60% LAD lesions

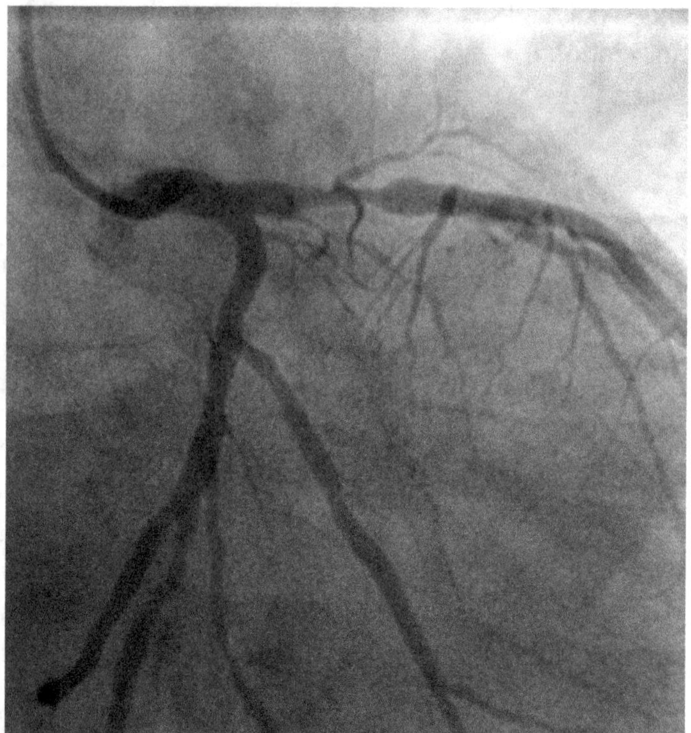

Fig. 15.3 Cineangiogram frame after circumflex stenting

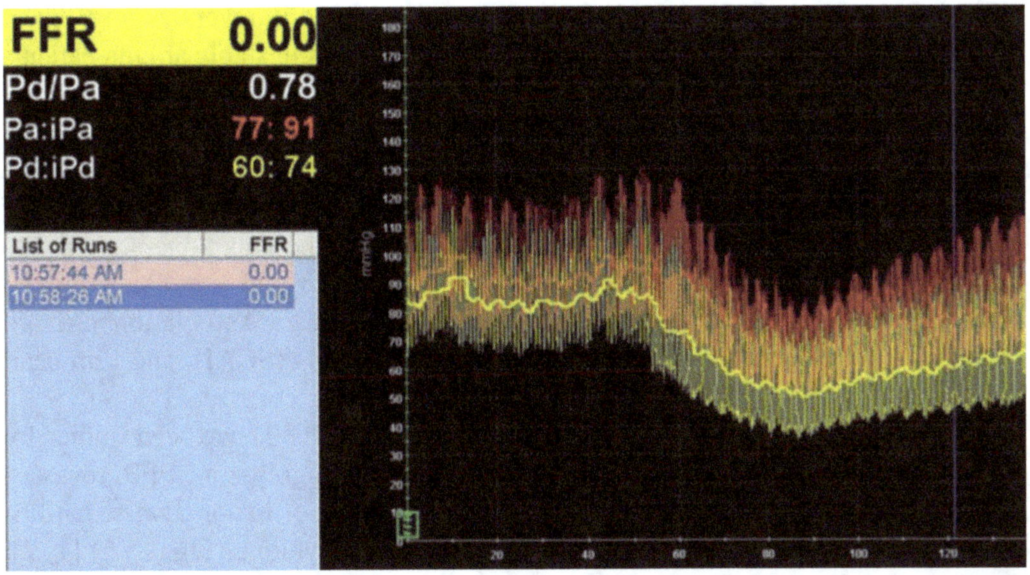

Fig. 15.4 LAD FFR (Pd/Pa) is 0.78

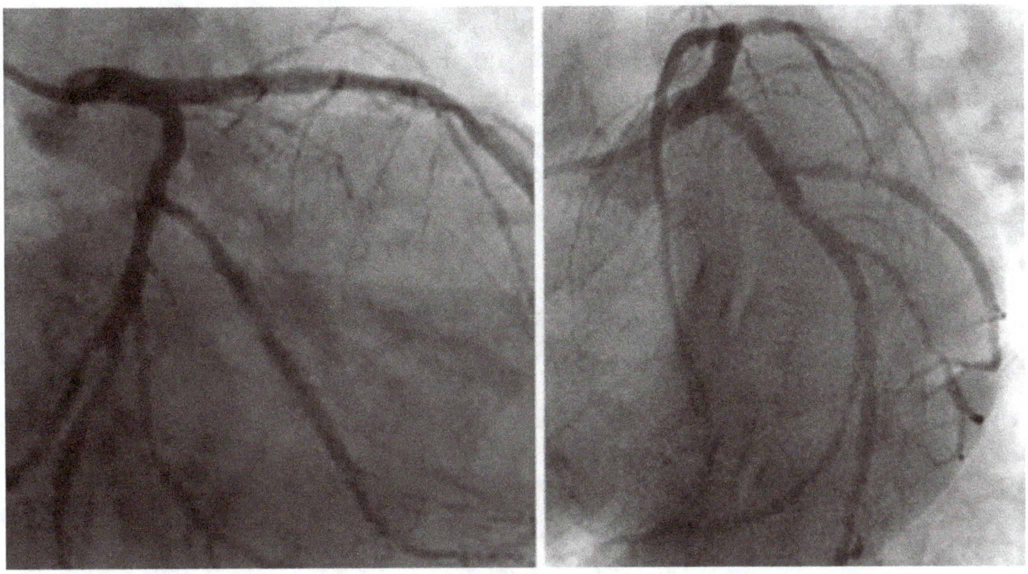

Fig. 15.5 Cineangiogram frame after LAD stenting

15.3 Fractional Flow Reserve Foundations

FFR is the ratio of the mean coronary pressure distal (Pd) to a stenosis to the mean aortic pressure (Pa) at maximal hyperemia when myocardial resistance is at its presumed absolute minimum. This condition permits pressure and flow to be linearly related, and thus the ratio represents the fraction of normal coronary blood flow across a stenosis with a normal value being 1 (i.e., Pd = Pa). FFR requires the induction of maximal hyperemia, most commonly with an intravenous infusion or intracoronary bolus of adenosine. Initial validation studies in stable angina patients have shown that an FFR <0.75, a reduction in coronary perfusion pressure by 25% of normal, was indicative of ischemia on stress testing. Additional investigations comparing FFR to different types of stress tests found that nearly all were negative when FFR > 0.80 and positive with FFR < 0.75, thereby establishing a gray zone of uncertainty. Clinical trials opted to use the upper end of the gray zone, 0.80 as the clinical threshold for outcome decision-making. This threshold is endorsed by the American College of Cardiology (ACC), American Heart Association (AHA), Society for Cardiovascular Angiography and Interventions (SCAI), and European Society of Cardiology (ESC) in their guidelines for PCI.

The outcomes of patients within the gray zone of 0.75–0.80 have been studied by Adjedj J et al. [1] who found that among 238 patients with gray-zone FFR, revascularization was associated with a significantly reduced risk of major adverse cardiovascular events (MACE) compared with medical therapy alone (Fig. 15.6) [1, 2]. On the other hand, the risk of MACE was not significantly different between deferred and revascularized lesions for FFR ≥0.76 (including the gray zone) in the large, prospective, multicenter Interventional Cardiology Research Incooperation Society Fractional Flow Reserve (IRIS-FFR) registry [3]. For patients with an FFR between 0.75 and 0.8, the decision to revascularize requires the operators' synthesis of findings based on the clinical context of the patient.

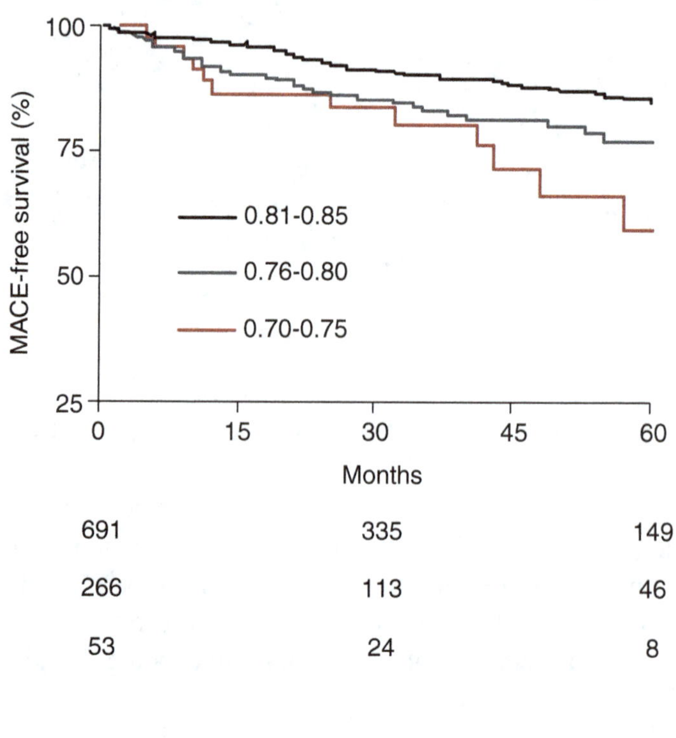

Fig. 15.6 MACE-free survival (%) in patients of the medical therapy group stratified by FFR strata (log-rank, 15; $P < 0.001$). *FFR* fractional flow reserve, *MACE* major adverse cardiovascular event. Source: Adjedj J, et al. Circulation. 2016;133:502–508 [1]

15.4 Fundamentals of Fractional Flow Reserve in STEMI and Other ACS

The utility of FFR to guide revascularization of intermediate lesions in patients with chronic stable multivessel coronary artery disease has been validated in several landmark clinical trials including the Fractional Flow Reserve to Determine the Appropriateness of Angioplasty in Moderate Coronary Stenosis (DEFER), FFR Versus Angiography for Multivessel Evaluation (FAME 1), and FFR-Guided Percutaneous Coronary Intervention Plus Medical Treatment Versus Medical Treatment Alone in Patients with Stable Coronary Artery Disease (FAME 2) trials [4–6]. The utility of FFR in acute coronary syndrome (ACS) has been controversial.

During a STEMI, the degree of damage to the infarct-related or culprit myocardial bed in the first hours of the injury makes the accuracy of FFR in the culprit artery highly questionable when >0.80. Since microcirculatory injury reduces flow, a low flow across a stenosis can produce a high FFR. Depending on the severity of the infarct, flow may recover in the days following the infarct, and hence the prior negative FFR may become positive, i.e., <0.80. To recap, a sub-hyperemic response to adenosine would result in an underestimation of stenosis severity so that an FFR >0.80 at the time of STEMI may initially be considered nonsignificant, but it may decrease several days later as the injured myocardial bed recovers and flow increases to the area. In other words, it may create a false negative. However, an FFR of <0.80 is truly functionally significant (Fig. 15.7).

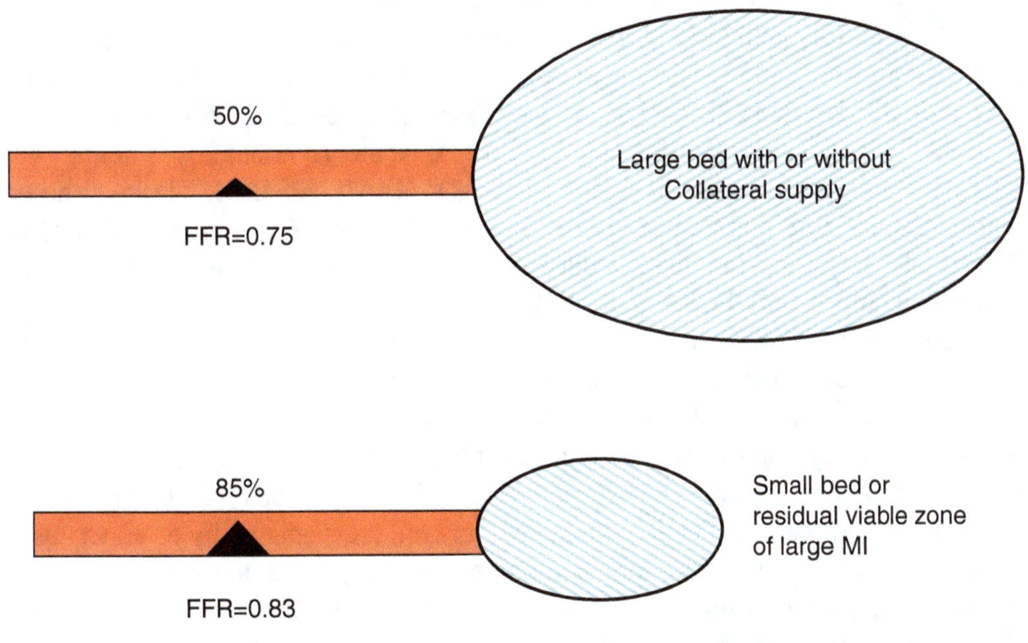

Fig. 15.7 STEMI and FFR cartoon on influence of myocardial bed size. The upper image shows a 50% stenosis supplying a large myocardial bed. Because flow to the bed is large, the FFR is 0.75. After a myocardial infarction of this bed, the injured myocardium has lower flow, and despite a more severe stenosis of 85%, the FFR is now higher 0.83

In the case of the non-culprit ACS artery, the flow to the myocardium supplied by non-infarct-related arteries should not be as affected as the culprit artery. The microcirculation should be normal, and FFR should accurately reflect the functional significance of a lesion in a non-culprit artery. All studies investigating the utility of FFR in STEMI or other ACS have assessed the non-culprit arteries. There are several studies that have found the microcirculation of the remote region can be abnormal [7], and the closer the non-culprit vessel is to the STEMI territory, the higher the potential for a false negative (due to impaired border zone microcirculatory function and less inducible hyperemia).

15.5 Fractional Flow Reserve and STEMI Revascularization Guidance

Traditionally, treating only the culprit vessel during STEMI has been considered superior to treating all lesions supported in part by several meta-analyses, and non-randomized registry studies showed that treating all vessels at the same time as the STEMI culprit was associated with more adverse events. Even the 2015 update of the 2013 ACC/AHA/SCAI STEMI guidelines gave a class III (do not do) recommendation to intervening on a non-infarct-related artery at the time of primary PCI in patients who are hemodynamically stable [8].

However, several recent studies have shown FFR is accurate in ACS, including the Fractional Flow Reserve Versus Angiography in Guiding Management to Optimize Outcomes in Non-ST-Elevation Myocardial Infarction Cardiac Magnetic Resonance (FAMOUS NSTEMI CMR) substudy that showed an excellent accuracy of FFR <0.80 for predicting perfusion defects on cardiac magnetic resonance [9]. Furthermore, multiple trials including the Preventive Angioplasty in Acute Myocardial Infarction (PRAMI), Complete Versus Lesion-Only Primary PCI Trial (CvLPRIT), and Third Danish Study of Optimal Acute Treatment of Patients With STEMI: Primary PCI in Multivessel Disease (DANAMI3-PRIMULTI) have shown that revascularizing non-culprit arteries in a STEMI, either at the time of primary PCI or later in a staged manner, reduce risk of MACE by a relative 44–65% compared with culprit-only PCI (Fig. 15.8) [10–12].

The PRAMI trial looked at 435 patients with acute STEMI and multivessel coronary artery disease. Patients were randomized to receive immediate preventive PCI in non-infarct arteries with stenosis >50% or no further PCI procedures. Recruitment was stopped early due to a highly significant between-group difference in the incidence of primary outcome favoring preventive PCI. Preventive PCI reduced the combined rate of cardiac death, nonfatal MI, or refractory angina by 65%, an absolute risk reduction of 14% over 23 months. Of note, revascularization was not included as a primary outcome. In this study, the severity of disease in non-infarct arteries was determined by angiographic assessment alone [10]. The effect of using FFR to determine the significance of disease in non-infarct arteries in STEMI patients was subsequently studied in DANAMI3-PRIMULTI and COMPARE-ACUTE trials.

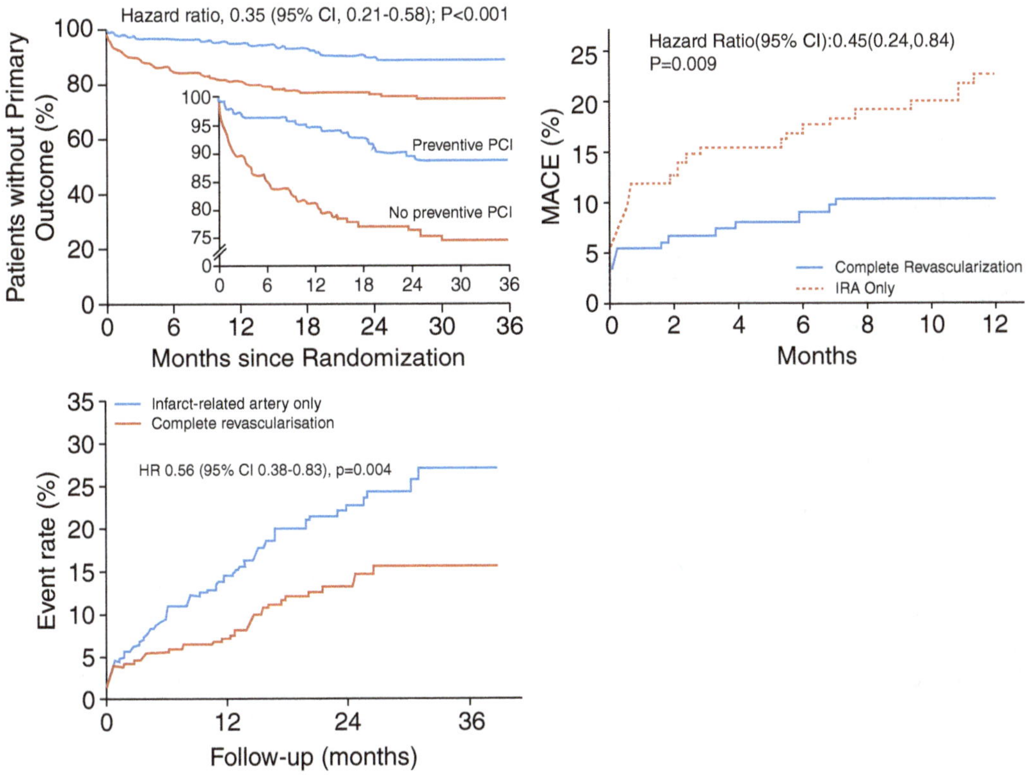

Fig. 15.8 Kaplan-Meier curves of PRAMI, CvLPRIT, and DANAMI3-PRIMULTI. Source: Wald, et al., 2013; Gershlick, et al., 2015; Engstrom, et al., 2015 [10–12]

DANAMI3-PRIMULTI was an open-label, randomized controlled trial that enrolled 627 patients with STEMI who had ≥1 clinically significant coronary stenosis in addition to the culprit lesion. After successful PCI to the culprit lesion, patients were randomized into no further invasive treatment or complete FFR-guided revascularization before discharge. A threshold of FFR <0.80 was used, and FFR was performed 2 days after primary PCI to avoid the risk of invalid FFR measurements inferred from acute changes in macrovascular tone or microvascular flow obstruction. The primary endpoint of a composite of all-cause mortality, nonfatal reinfarction, and ischemia-driven revascularization of lesions in non-infarct-related arteries was significantly lower in the complete revascularization group (13%) compared with the infarct-related-only group (22%). The favorable effect was driven by significantly fewer revascularizations. A substudy of the DANAMI3-PRIMULTI trial found that the benefit of staged FFR-guided complete revascularization was observed primarily in patients with three-vessel disease and at least one non-infarct-related stenosis with a ≥ 90% diameter (Fig. 15.9) [13].

In the Fractional Flow Reserve-Guided Multivessel Angioplasty in Myocardial Infarction, COMPARE-ACUTE trial, 885 patients with STEMI and multivessel disease who had undergone primary PCI of the infarct-related artery were randomized to undergo FFR-guided complete revascularization of non-infarct-related coronary arteries or no revascularization of non-infarct-related arteries. Unlike DANAMI3-PRIMULTI, FFR of the non-infarct-related artery was done in the acute STEMI

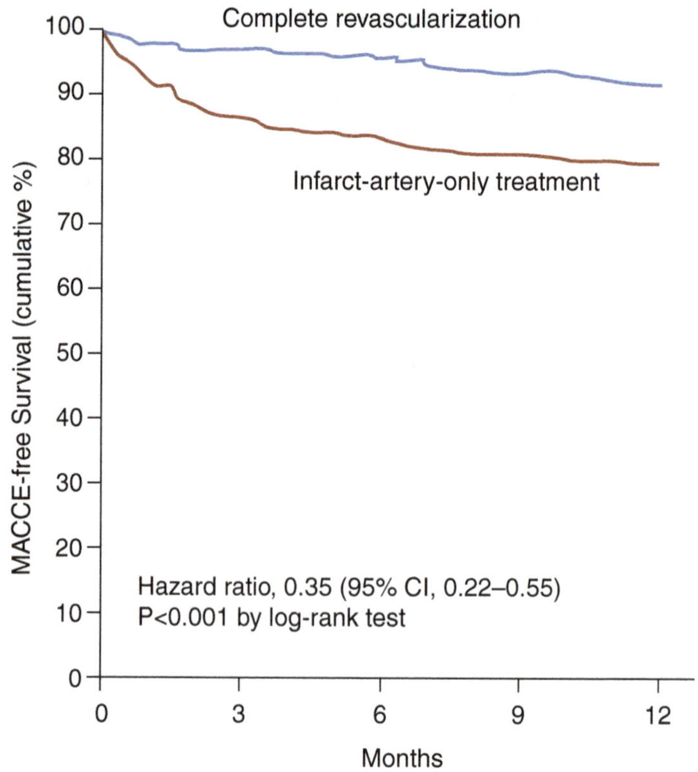

Fig. 15.9 Results from the DANAMI3-PRIMULTI study. In STEMI patients, the primary composite endpoint of all cause death, reinfarction, and ischemia-driven revascularization was lower in those who received FFR-guided complete revascularization compared to infarct-related PCI alone. The primary endpoint was further reduced in patients with at least one non-infarct-related stenosis ≥90% compared to those with <90%. *FFR* fractional flow reserve, *STEMI* ST-elevation myocardial infarction. Source: Lønborg, et al., 2017 [13]

setting, during the time of primary PCI. At 1 year those who underwent FFR-guided complete revascularization of non-infarct-related arteries had a lower risk of death (1.4 vs. 1.7%), MI (2.4 vs. 4.7%), revascularization (6.1 vs. 17.5%), and cerebrovascular events (0.0 vs. 0.7%) compared with those who were treated for the infarct-related artery only [14]. Approximately half of the non-infarct-related artery lesions that were angiographically significant were not physiologically significant by FFR (≥0.80).

15.6 FFR in Other Acute Coronary Syndrome

FFR also plays a role in patients with non-STEMI ACS. This population may be more difficult to study than patients with STEMI because the culprit vessel is not always clear in NSTEMI or unstable angina (USA) group. The Impact of Routine Fractional Flow Reserve on Management Decision and 1-Year Clinical Outcome of Patients with Acute Coronary Syndrome (PRIME-FFR) pooled the results of the French FFR Registry (R3F) and the Portuguese Study on the Evaluation of FFR-Guided Treatment of Coronary Disease (POST-IT). A total of 1983 patients with NSTEMI or unstable angina (USA) were included in the large, international prospective study. They found that the use of FFR was associated with a high rate of reclassification of treatment. The percent of patients with ACS who were reclassified by FFR was similar to those with non-ACS (38 vs. 39%, P = NS). There was no significant difference in MACE (8.0 vs. 11.6%,

$p = 0.2$) or symptoms (92.3 vs. 94.8%, $p = 0.25$) in patients reclassified based on FFR compared to those who were not reclassified. Fewer patients with ACS were reclassified from revascularization to medical treatment compared with those with non-ACS (P = 0.01). Furthermore, deferral to medical treatment based on FFR was as safe in ACS as it was in non-ACS patients. Patients with disregarded FFR had higher rates of MACE [15].

The ideal threshold for FFR in the ACS population has been debated. The FFR threshold of 0.80, which is used to determine functional significance in the stable ischemic heart disease (SIHD) population, was applied to the ACS population in the above studies. The accuracy of this threshold for ACS patients has been challenged. Hakeem et al. found that using the standard FFR threshold of 0.80 for clinical decision-making in ACS patients was associated with a threefold increase in the risk of subsequent MI and target vessel failure compared with SIHD patients and advised caution in using FFR-derived values for clinical decision-making in patients with ACS. They found that ACS patients had a higher FFR threshold of functional significance, and those with an FFR <0.85 had significantly higher event rates than those with FFR >0.85 [16].

Lee et al. found that regardless of the FFR value (FFR = 0.8–1.0), non-culprit lesions of ACS had a more than twofold higher rate of MACE that that of SIHD. The clinical outcomes of 449 non-culprit lesions in 301 patients with ACS were compared with the outcomes of lesions in patients with SIHD. The primary outcome of MACE (a composite of cardiac death, target vessel-related MI, and ischemia-driven revascularization) was higher in the ACS population (3.8 vs. 1.6%, HR_{adj} 2.97, 95%

Table 15.1 Table of key trials in FFR and ACS

	PRAMI	CvLPRIT	DANAMI3-PRIMULTI	COMPARE-ACUTE	PRIME-FFR
Study design	Single-blind randomized	RCT	RCT	Prospective randomized trial	Prospective study
N	465	296	627	885	1983
Follow-up period	23 months	296 months	627	36 months	12 months
Long-term mortality	Complete revascularization better	Complete revascularization better	Complete revascularization better	Complete revascularization better	Deferral based on FFR is safe in ACS
Assessment of non-culprit lesion	Angiography	Angiography	FFR	FFR	FFR
Timing	Immediate complete revascularization	Immediate complete revascularization or staged PCI	Staged PCI	Immediate complete revascularization or staged PCI	--

Source: Wald, et al., 2013; Gershlick, et al., 2015; Engstrom, et al., 2015; Smits, et al. 2017; Van Belle, et al. 2017 [10–12, 14]

CI: 1.23–7.17, $p = 0.016$) after 2 years and was mainly driven by a higher rate of ischemia-driven revascularization [17]. Table 15.1 summarizes the key trials of FFR in STEMI and other ACS.

15.7 Coronary Flow Reserve and the Index of Microvascular Resistance

Coronary flow reserve measures flow through both the epicardial resistance conduit and the microcirculation. It represents the vasodilator capacity of the coronary vascular bed during hyperemia and is another validated index of the functional significance of a coronary stenosis. Since most resistance occurs in the microcirculation, it is a primary method to measure microvascular flow. It is well-established that the failure to achieve myocardial reperfusion in a STEMI results in myocardial hemorrhage and infarct. Despite timely reperfusion therapy with PPCI, microvascular obstruction still occurs in up to 25–50% of STEMI patients who go on to have a higher degree of MACE. Therefore, measuring microvascular function may be a useful way to risk stratify STEMI patients.

In a STEMI, the microvasculature of the myocardium supplied by the non-infarct coronary arteries, in addition to the infarct-related artery, is abnormal. Cheng et al. evaluated 18 patients with acute MI and found that the CFR in the remote region (i.e., the region supplied by the non-infarct artery) was linked to CFR in the infarcted region and correlated with infarct size and severity. Even after successful PCI, the CFR in the myocardium supplied by the infarct-related artery was lower than normal [18]. A CFR > 2.0 is generally considered normal.

The index of microvascular resistance (IMR) is a direct invasive measure of microvascular resistance. It is defined as the distal coronary pressure multiplied by the mean transit time of a 3 mL bolus of saline at room temperature during maximal coronary hyperemia. It has been less well studied compared to FFR, but it may be a useful tool in evaluating the microcirculation during primary PCI. An IMR > 40 is considered abnormal and has been found to be associated with microvascular pathology, changes in LV function and EDV, and all-cause death and heart failure [19]. In a meta-analysis of six studies, a median IMR > 40 was an independent predictor of death [20]. In some studies, the combination of a high IMR and reduced CFR enhances the detection of microvascular obstruction, but in other studies, the combination did not have any prognostic value [21, 22].

An invasive measurement of the coronary microcirculation at the end of primary PCI may be a more sensitive measure of successful reperfusion compared with standard tests such as angiography or ECG. This could help identify high-risk patients who may benefit from continued treatment such as with glycoprotein IIb/IIIa inhibitors or intracoronary thrombolysis.

15.8 Instant Wave-Free Ratio

iFR is a resting index used to assess the severity of an intracoronary stenosis. It measures the ratio of the Pd to the Pa during an isolated period of diastole (i.e., the "wave-free period"). It is an attractive alternative to FFR because it does not require hyperemia and therefore has a lower incidence of patient discomfort, side effects, and a shorter procedural time. iFR has been shown to be non-inferior compared to FFR in two large, multicenter, randomized controlled trials: the Instantaneous Wave-Free Ratio Versus Fractional Flow Reserve in Patients with Stable Angina Pectoris or Acute Coronary Syndrome (iFR-SWEDEHEART) trial and the Functional Lesion Assessment of Intermediate Stenosis to Guide Revascularization (DEFINE-FLAIR) trial. Both included patients with NSTEMI ACS, while DEFINE-FLAIR also included STEMI patients. The iFR-SWEDEHEART trial included 2037 patients with stable angina, unstable angina, or NSTEMI and randomly assigned them to undergo either iFR- or FFR-guided revascularization. For patients with unstable angina or NSTEMI, only non-culprit lesions were evaluated, and the culprit lesions were managed as clinically indicated. The rate of primary endpoint (composite of death from any cause, nonfatal MI, or unplanned revascularization within 12 months after the procedure) was not significantly different between the iFR and FFR groups [23].

In the DEFINE-FLAIR trial, 2492 patients with CAD were randomized to have iFR-guided or FFR-guided coronary revascularization. Patients with ACS were included but only non-culprit vessels and outside of primary intervention during acute STEMI. The primary endpoint of a composite of death from any cause, non-fatal MI, or unplanned revascularization did not differ significantly between groups. Additionally, the number of patients in the iFR group had lower rates of adverse side effects from the procedure (3.1 vs. 30.8%) and a shorter median procedural time (40.5 vs. 45.0 min) compared with the FFR group [24].

Conclusion

The physiological assessment of coronary stenoses is an integral part of the decision-making process for interventional cardiologists. Functional assessment in the STEMI and other ACS situation should consider the altered milieu of the microvasculature in an infarcted territory. While FFR is not valid in the infarct-related artery until recovery of the injured myocardium, the microcirculation in the non-infarct-related artery is not generally affected to reduce the accuracy of FFR and iFR. Future applications of translesional physiologic indices will expand the use of these methods into unique clinical scenarios to improve outcomes and prognosis.

Disclosures MJK is a consultant and speaker for Abbott/St. Jude, Philips/Volcano, Acist Medical Inc., Opsens Inc., and HeartFlow Inc.

KMY has no conflict of interest to declare.

References

1. Adjedj J, De Bruyne B, Floré V, et al. Significance of intermediate values of fractional flow reserve in patients with coronary artery disease. Circulation. 2016;133:502–8. https://doi.org/10.1161/CIRCULATIONAHA.115.018747.
2. Agarwal SK, Kasula S, Edupuganti MM, et al. Clinical decision-making for the hemodynamic "gray zone" (FFR 0.75–0.80) and long-term outcomes. J Invasive Cardiol. 2017;29(11):371–6.
3. Ahn JM, Park DW, Shin ES, et al. Fractional flow reserve and cardiac events in coronary artery disease: data from a prospective IRIS-FFR registry (interventional cardiology research Incooperation society fractional flow reserve). Circulation. 2017;135:2241–51. https://doi.org/10.1161/CIRCULATIONAHA.116.024433.
4. Zimmermann FM, Ferrara A, Johnson NP, et al. Deferral vs performance of percutaneous coronary intervention of functionally non-significant coronary stenosis: 15-year follow-up of the DEFER trial. Eur Heart J. 2015;36:3182–8. https://doi.org/10.1093/eurheartj/ehv452.
5. Tonino PA, De Bruyne B, Pijls NH, et al. Fractional flow reserve versus angiography for guiding percutaneous coronary intervention. N Engl J Med. 2009;360:213–24. https://doi.org/10.1056/NEJMoa0807611.
6. De Bruyne B, Pijls NHJ, Kalesan B, et al. Fractional flow reserve-guided PCI versus medical therapy in stable coronary disease. N Engl J Med. 2012;367:991–1001. https://doi.org/10.1056/NEJMoa1205361.
7. Bodí V, Sanchis J, Núñez J, López-Lereu MP, Mainar L, Bosch MJ, et al. Abnormal myocardial perfusion after infarction in patients with persistent TIMI grade-3 flow. Only an acute phenomenon? Rev Esp Cardiol. 2007;60:486–92.
8. O'Gara PT, Kushner FG, Ascheim DD, et al. ACCF/AHA guideline for the management of ST-elevation myocardial infarction: a report of the American College of Cardiology Foundation/American Heart Association task force on practice guidelines. J Am Coll Cardiol. 2013;61:e78–e140. https://doi.org/10.1016/j.jacc.2012.11.019.
9. Layland J, Rauhalammi S, Watkins S, et al. Assessment of fractional flow reserve in patients with recent non-ST-segment-elevation myocardial infarction: comparative study with 3-T stress perfusion cardiac magnetic resonance imaging. Circ Cardiovasc Interv. 2015;8:e002207. https://doi.org/10.1161/CIRCINTERVENTIONS.114.002207.
10. Wald DS, Morris JK, Wald NJ, et al. Randomized trial of preventive angioplasty in myocardial infarction. N Engl J Med. 2013;369:1115–23. https://doi.org/10.1056/NEJMoa1305520.
11. Gershlick AH, Khan JN, Kelly DJ, et al. Randomized trial of complete versus lesion-only revascularization in patients undergoing primary percutaneous coronary intervention for STEMI and multivessel disease: the CvLPRIT trial. J Am Coll Cardiol. 2015;65:963–72. https://doi.org/10.1016/j.jacc.2014.12.038.
12. Engstrøm T. The third Danish study of optimal acute treatment of patients with ST-segment elevation myocardial infarction: Primary PCI in Multivessel disease. Presented at American College of Cardiology/i2 Scientific Session, San Diego, California, 16 March 2015.
13. Lønborg J, Engstrøm T, Kelbæk H, et al. Fractional flow reserve-guided complete revascularization improves the prognosis in patients with ST-segment-elevation myocardial infarction and severe nonculprit disease: a DANAMI 3-PRIMULTI substudy (primary PCI in patients with ST-elevation myocardial infarction and multivessel Disease: treatment of culprit lesion only or complete revascularization). Circ Cardiovasc Interv. 2017;10:e004460. https://doi.org/10.1161/CIRCINTERVENTIONS.116.004460.
14. Smits PC, Abdel-Wahab M, Neumann FJ, et al. Fractional flow reserve-guided multivessel angioplasty in myocardial infarction. N Engl J Med. 2017;376:1234–44. https://doi.org/10.1056/NEJMoa1701067.
15. Van Belle E, et al. Impact of routine fractional flow reserve on management decision and 1-year clinical outcome of patients with acute coronary syndromes. Circ Cardiovasc Interv. 2017;10(6):e004296. https://doi.org/10.1161/CIRCINTERVENTIONS.116.004296.

16. Hakeem A, Edupuganti MM, Almomani A, et al. Long-term prognosis of deferred acute coronary syndrome lesions based on nonischemic fractional flow reserve. J Am Coll Cardiol. 2016;68:1181–91. https://doi.org/10.1016/j.jacc.2016.06.035.
17. Lee JM, Choi KH, Koo BK, et al. Prognosis of deferred non-culprit lesions according to fractional flow reserve in patients with acute coronary syndrome. EuroIntervention. 2017;13(9):e1112–9.
18. Cheng R, et al. Coronary flow reserve in the remote myocardium predicts left ventricular remodeling following acute myocardial infarction. Yonsei Med J. 2014;55(4):904–11.
19. Carrick D, et al. Comparative prognostic utility of indices of microvascular function alone or in combination in patients with an acute ST-segment elevation myocardial infarction. Circulation. 2016;134(23):1833–47. https://doi.org/10.1161/CIRCULATIONAHA.116.022603.
20. Bulluck H, et al. Index of microvascular resistance and microvascular obstruction in patients with acute myocardial infarction. JACC. 2016;9:2172–3.
21. Park SD, Baek YS, Lee MJ, Kwon SW, Shin SH, Woo SI, Kim DH, Kwan J, Park KS. Comprehensive assessment of microcirculation after primary percutaneous intervention in ST segment elevation myocardial infarction: insight from thermodilution-derived index ofmicrocirculatory resistance and coronary flow reserve. Coron Artery Dis. 2016;27:34–9.
22. Ahn SG, Hung OY, Lee JW, Lee JH, Youn YJ, Ahn MS, Kim JY, Yoo BS, Lee SH, Yoon J, Kwon W, Samady H. Combination of the thermodilution-derived index of microcirculatory resistance and coronary flow reserve is highly predictive of microvascular obstruction on cardiac magnetic resonance imaging after ST-segment elevation myocardial infarction. JACC Cardiovasc Interv. 2016;9:793–801.
23. Götberg M, Christiansen EH, Gudmundsdottir IJ, et al. Instantaneous wave-free ratio versus fractional flow reserve to guide PCI. N Engl J Med. 2017;376:1813–23. https://doi.org/10.1056/NEJMoa1616540.
24. Davies JE, Sen S, Dehbi HM, et al. Use of the instantaneous wave-free ratio or fractional flow reserve in PCI. N Engl J Med. 2017;376:1824–34. https://doi.org/10.1056/NEJMoa1700445.

16 Role of Coronary Artery Bypass Surgery in Acute Myocardial Infarction

William Y. Shi and Julian A. Smith

16.1 Introduction

Coronary artery bypass grafting (CABG) is one of the most commonly performed procedures worldwide. Its place in the treatment of coronary artery disease has been established for decades with the benefits of CABG versus percutaneous coronary intervention (PCI) in various scenarios being extensively investigated. Recent major landmark randomised clinical trials such as SYNTAX,[1] EXCEL[2] and NOBLE[3] have helped to define the patients in which each approach is likely to be most successful. Indeed, the last decade has seen most centres embrace the "Heart Team" concept, whereby a collaborative approach helps to optimise patients' outcomes.

The benefit of timely revascularisation in acute myocardial infarction (MI) is well established. The role of PCI and thrombolysis is discussed elsewhere; however, the former has now become the preferred strategy worldwide and is associated with

[1] Mohr FW et al., Lancet 2013.

[2] Stone GW et al., N Eng J Med 2016

[3] Makikallio T et al., Lancet 2016

W. Y. Shi
Department of Cardiothoracic Surgery, Monash Health, Melbourne, VIC, Australia

Faculty of Medicine, Melbourne Medical School, University of Melbourne, Melbourne, VIC, Australia

J. A. Smith (✉)
Department of Cardiothoracic Surgery, Monash Health, Melbourne, VIC, Australia

Department of Surgery, School of Clinical Sciences at Monash Health, Monash University, Melbourne, VIC, Australia
e-mail: julian.smith@monash.edu

T. J. Watson et al. (eds.), *Primary Angioplasty*,
https://doi.org/10.1007/978-981-13-1114-7_16

good outcomes. In general, PCI and thrombolysis can restore blood flow to the myocardium in the timeliest manner, whereas CABG is generally associated with a time delay and as such, is utilised in only around 5% of acute MI cases in today's practice.

Historically, large multicentre randomised trials were designed to assess the efficacy of thrombolysis and PCI. CABG was never investigated as a primary treatment modality for STEMI in major randomised trials. Thus, high-level evidence for its place in the management of acute MI has never been firmly established. Practical, logistic and economic restraints mean that surgery remains, in most cases, a third option behind PCI and thrombolysis in the management acute MI. Nevertheless—as this chapter will discuss—CABG serves an important role in a select subgroup of patients.

16.2 Indications for CABG in Acute MI

16.2.1 Unsuccessful PCI and Incomplete Revascularisation

Patients with unsuccessful PCI, or those in which a less than satisfactory result has been achieved with PCI, should be referred for surgery if the coronary anatomy and patient factors are suitable. A substantial portion of patients with acute MI have multi-vessel coronary disease which may be long-standing and difficult to manage percutaneously.

Despite effective management of the culprit lesion via PCI, CABG may be required once the patient is stabilised in order to complete revascularisation of diseased territories not amenable to PCI. Studies have suggested reasonable early and late outcomes for those undergoing emergent CABG after failed angioplasty. Even in patients with cardiogenic shock post PCI, CABG may be associated with improved survival compared to post-PCI medical therapy alone.

Although uncommon, complications encountered during PCI for STEMI may necessitate emergency CABG. These include failed stent deployment, stent fracture, coronary artery dissection, coronary artery perforation or recurrent acute thrombosis. In these scenarios, patients with ongoing ischaemia will benefit from CABG so as to minimise further myocardial damage.

In general, restoration of blood flow should be a priority, and patients who continue to have clinical evidence of ongoing ischaemia post-PCI should be offered CABG if no further percutaneous options are available. The appropriateness of surgery differs on a case-by-case basis, and co-operation between cardiologists and cardiac surgeons is crucial.

16.2.2 Mechanical Complications of Acute Myocardial Infarction

Common mechanical complications of myocardial infarction are acute mitral regurgitation, rupture of the interventricular septum and rupture of the left ventricular (LV) free wall. These patients almost always require emergency surgery to repair the defect.

While a culprit lesion may be addressed via PCI, the restoration of blood flow will not reduce the haemodynamic burden of the mechanical defect. In select cases, it may be appropriate to perform PCI to the culprit lesion—if it can be done so in a timely manner—and then subsequently transfer the patient to the operating theatre for repair of the mechanical defect and grafting of other diseased vessels not addressed via PCI. In general, this approach is unsuitable in patients with rupture of the LV or ventricular septal defect as in these cases, the infarcted area cannot be salvaged with PCI and repair of the defect and restoration of normal haemodynamics is of higher priority. In the operating theatre, grafting of the culprit vessel in those with LV rupture or ventricular septal defect (VSD) is generally not performed due to absence of viable myocardium.

Surgery for mechanical complications of myocardial infarction is associated with a high early mortality risk, ranging between 30 and 50%. Predictors of death are older age, worsening renal function, emergency surgery and higher filling pressures. Infero-posterior ventricular septal rupture is associated with the worst prognosis, owing to a more technically challenging repair and a higher rate of right ventricular dysfunction. Five-year survival ranges between 40 and 60%.

16.2.3 CABG as the Primary Revascularisation Strategy in STEMI

There are no randomised trials directly comparing CABG with PCI in the setting of acute MI. In the acute setting, PCI is most often the appropriate approach if there is a clear culprit lesion, the distal flow is poor, and a stent can be deployed safely and more rapidly than performing CABG. However, approximately 50% of patients presenting with acute MI will have multivessel disease, and in stabe patients with complex coronary anatomy and higher SYNTAX scores, CABG may be preferable to PCI given its superior long-term clinical results, as demonstrated from observational and randomised studies.

There are cases in acute MI where CABG may be preferable. Patients who no longer have signs of active ischaemia but exhibit complex coronary anatomy may be better suited for CABG. Clinical factors such as diabetes and poor ventricular function also represent indications for CABG over PCI, even in the acute setting. The decision on which modality to pursue should be individualised and may also relate to whether surgical facilities are available in the local setting.

The advantage of CABG—even in the acute scenario—is that complete revascularisation can be achieved, rather than only targeting the culprit lesion. Complete revascularisation restores myocardial perfusion and provides the best opportunity for myocardial salvage. The importance of complete revascularisation is even more pronounced in patients with multivessel disease, as myocardium may continue to be compromised even after a culprit lesion is addressed via PCI.

16.3 Timing of CABG After Acute Myocardial Infarction

The optimal timing of CABG after acute MI is controversial. In many cases, there are clear indications for emergency surgery. In situations of ongoing ischaemia, mechanical complications or severe cardiogenic shock, patients should be transferred directly to the operating theatre. However, in the absence of these, the ideal timing of surgery is less well established.

While early surgical revascularisation may limit the size of the infarct and reduce the potential for mechanical sequelae, there is the risk of reperfusion injury associated with early restoration of blood flow. This may lead to haemorrhagic infarction, extension of the infarct and greater scar development. It has been postulated that early CABG—either with or without cardiopulmonary bypass—after MI may augment the systemic inflammatory response seen after STEMI.

In a multicentre study of 32,099 cases, Lee and colleagues[4] showed that for transmural myocardial infarction, in-hospital mortality decreased with increasing time interval between myocardial infarct and surgery. Mortality was 14.2% for those undergoing surgery within 6 h, and 2.7% for those having surgery beyond 15 days after presentation. Revascularisation within 3 days of MI was an independent predictor of in-hospital mortality on multivariable regression analyses.

Similarly, Thielmann et al.[5] reported their results of 138 cases of CABG in acute MI and found an overall mortality rate of 8.7%. The mortality rate however varied between 23.8% for those operated on between 7 and 24 h after presentation and 2.4% for those receiving surgery at 8–14 days post-presentation.

At our centre, we generally avoid CABG on patients presenting with an acute STEMI and prefer to wait a period of 3–5 days until surgery in the absence of absolute indications for emergent CABG. Indeed, in cases where early surgery is an absolute necessity, we are usually prepared to offer post-operative mechanical circulatory support if the patient had reasonable premorbid function, as mortality is likely to result from pump failure.

In addition to timing of surgery, risk factors for mortality in surgery for MI are increasing age, renal impairment, number of previous MIs, hypertension, re-operative surgery, cardiogenic shock, reduced left ventricular ejection fraction, the need for cardiopulmonary resuscitation, left main stem coronary disease and the need for intra-aortic counterpulsation. On the other hand, preserved left ventricular function, younger age, male gender and non-transmural MI are associated with more favourable outcomes.

Some have advocated the use of mechanical circulatory support to stabilise patients presenting with MI and shock. Dang and colleagues,[6] in an analysis of 74 patients undergoing left ventricular assist device implantation for post-MI shock, showed that 1-year survival was higher in patients undergoing direct left ventricular assist device (LVAD) placement rather than revascularisation followed by LVAD implantation.

16.4 CABG in Cardiogenic Shock

In patients with acute MI complicated by cardiogenic shock, CABG has been shown to result in a reasonable survival rate. Earlier reports from the 1980s and 1990s suggested in-hospital mortality of approximately 10–30% for those with cardiogenic shock undergoing CABG.

[4] Lee DC et al., J Thorac Cardiovasc Surg 2003.

[5] Thielmann et al., Ann Thorac Surg 2007.

[6] Dang NC et al., J Thorac Cardiovasc Surg 2005

More recently, the SHOCK trial[7] randomised 302 patients with acute MI and cardiogenic shock to medical therapy versus early revascularisation. Of the early revascularisation group, 38% underwent CABG and 55% PCI. One-year survival was improved for those receiving early revascularisation compared to medical therapy. However, the design of the trial meant that patients could receive PCI or CABG up to 54 h after symptom onset and still be considered to have received early revascularisation. Nevertheless, for patients with cardiogenic shock, CABG represents a reasonable strategy, despite the higher risk of post-operative low cardiac output and end-organ dysfunction.

16.5 Peri-operative and Operative Considerations

Compared to elective CABG, surgery in the context of AMI presents unique challenges for cardiac surgeons. The heightened risk of mortality and morbidity of emergency surgery compared to more conventional elective surgery must be carefully considered by surgeons and cardiologists when deciding upon the best mode of therapy.

16.5.1 Antiplatelet Therapy

Antiplatelet agents such as clopidogrel and ticagrelor are now commonly administered to patients in combination with aspirin as dual antiplatelet therapy (DAPT) at presentation with an acute coronary syndrome, or around the time of angiography and stent implantation to reduce the risk of stent thrombosis.

In urgent scenarios, or those in whom a stent has been placed to treat a culprit lesion, patients often require surgery while on dual antiplatelet therapy. The risk of peri-operative bleeding after CABG in patients receiving DAPT is substantially increased, with the risk of reoperation for ongoing bleeding being reported as being up to 6 times higher. A meta-analysis investigating timing of surgery in patients on clopidogrel found that patients on DAPT were more likely to have ongoing bleeding, require reoperation and experience adverse outcomes compared to those in whom a washout period of >5 days was observed. However, patients in whom a washout period of >5 days was observed, use of clopidogrel was associated with lower rates of mortality and myocardial infarction compared to those not on clopidogrel, suggesting a valuable role for DAPT in those presenting with an acute MI.

The American Heart Association/American College of Cardiology (AHA/ACC) and European Society of Cardiology/European Association of Cardiothoracic Surgery (ESC/EACTS) guidelines suggest cessation of clopidogrel or ticagrelor for at least 5 days prior to nonurgent CABG (Table 16.1). For urgent cases, clopidogrel or ticagrelor should be discontinued for at least 24 h. At our centre, we generally cease clopidogrel or ticagrelor 3–5 days prior to CABG.

---

[7] Hochman et al., N Eng J Med 1999

Table 16.1 Summary of AHA and ESC recommendations

Recommendation	2013 AHA[a]	2017 ESC[b]
Urgent CABG is indicated in patients with STEMI and coronary anatomy not amenable to PCI who have ongoing or recurrent ischaemia, cardiogenic shock, severe HF or other high-risk features	Class I	
Immediate PCI is indicated for patients with cardiogenic shock if coronary anatomy is suitable. If coronary anatomy is not suitable for PCI, or PCI has failed, emergency CABG is recommended		Class I
CABG should be considered in patients with ongoing ischaemia and large areas of jeopardised myocardium if PCI of the ischaemia-related artery cannot be performed		Class IIa
CABG is recommended in patients with STEMI at time of operative repair of mechanical defects	Class I	
The use of mechanical circulatory support is reasonable in patients with STEMI who are haemodynamically unstable and require urgent CABG	Class IIa	Class IIb
Emergency CABG within 6 h of symptom onset may be considered in patients with STEMI who do not have cardiogenic shock and are not candidates for PCI or fibrinolytic therapy	Class IIa	
For nonurgent CABG, discontinue clopidogrel and ticagrelor for at least 5 days before surgery and prasugrel for at least 7 days	Class I	Class I (2014)[c]
Clopidogrel or ticagrelor should be discontinued at least 24 h before urgent on-pump CABG, if possible	Class I	Class I (2014)
The use of intra-aortic balloon pump (IABP) counter-pulsation can be useful for patients with cardiogenic shock after STEMI	Class IIa	Class IIa

[a]O'Gara P et al., Circulation 2013
[b]Ibanez et al., Eur Heart J 2017
[c]Windecker S, Eur Heart J 2014

16.6 Intra-aortic Balloon Pump (IABP)

For patients who are haemodynamically unstable, the IABP is a useful adjunct when performing CABG in the context of acute MI. The IABP has been shown to decrease myocardial oxygen requirements. Earlier studies suggested a reduction in early mortality associated with IABP use. However, the IABP-SHOCK II trial,[8] which randomised 600 patients with cardiogenic shock complicating acute MI to IABP or no IABP, showed that IABP therapy did not significantly reduce early mortality. The ACC/AHA guidelines have also changed the recommendation for IABP use in cardiogenic shock from a class I down to a class IIa recommendation.

At our centre, we generally insert an IABP for acute MI in patients with cardiogenic shock in preparation for transfer to the operating theatre so as to provide temporary stabilisation until cardiopulmonary bypass can be established.

[8]Thiele H et al., Lancet 2013.

16.7 Intra-operative Considerations

In the last decade, observational and randomised studies have suggested a benefit in using additional arterial conduits (radial artery, right internal thoracic artery) to revascularise the myocardium in addition to the standard left internal thoracic artery to left anterior descending artery configuration. Indeed, the ACC/AHA guidelines give class II indications to the use of additional arterial conduits.

In general, the selection of conduits is similar to that of elective CABG cases. Unless patients are haemodynamically unstable, a LITA should still be harvested for revascularising the LAD territory, with additional supplemental conduits such as the long saphenous vein or radial artery.

Where patients are unstable with cardiogenic shock, it may be more prudent to cannulate the heart and establish cardiopulmonary bypass immediately following sternotomy, thus avoiding the 20–30 min delay associated with LITA harvest. Cardiopulmonary bypass with decompression of the heart substantially reduces wall tension and metabolic requirements. The LITA can then be harvested while on cardiopulmonary bypass. With unstable cases, we will generally harvest a LITA on cardiopulmonary bypass in younger patients with few comorbidities, while in older patients, we will use only peripheral conduits (radial artery, saphenous vein).

Both on-pump and off-pump CABG are acceptable techniques for surgery in acute MI. Fattouch et al. randomised 128 patients with STEMI to either on- or off-pump CABG and found off-pump surgery to be associated with low mortality (1.6%). Off-pump CABG was associated with lower rates of low cardiac output syndrome, mechanical ventilation, inotrope use and reoperation for bleeding. In our centre, on-pump CABG is our preferred technique; as such off-pump CABG in the acute setting is reserved for those cases where significant aortic calcification renders aortic cannulation and cross-clamping unsafe.

Some surgeons prefer to perform on-pump surgery without cardioplegic arrest (on-pump beating heart CABG) in the acute setting, as this has the potential to reduce the impact of ischaemic-reperfusion injury associated with aortic cross-clamping. The beating heart technique has been shown to achieve similar results compared to conventional CABG with comparable rates of early mortality and morbidity.[9]

16.8 Results of CABG in Acute MI

Earlier reports of CABG in acute MI showed mortality rates of 5–10%. As thrombolysis and PCI have evolved to become first-line the therapies, the spectrum of patients presenting for surgery has changed significantly compared to patients included in those earlier reports. Contemporary reports of surgery in acute MI show early mortality rates of 5–20%, with cardiogenic shock being a major predictor of early mortality. Long-term survival after emergency CABG is influenced chiefly by patient comorbidities and ventricular function.

[9] Chaudhry UA et al., Ann Thorac Surg 2015

16.9 Conclusions

Bypass surgery, despite not being first-line, remains an important modality in the management of patients unsuccessful acute MI. It is reserved for cases where PCI is not feasible, or has been unsuccessful, and in those where revascularisation cannot be completed with PCI alone. The optimal time to operate on patients can be difficult to determine. In those with ongoing ischaemia, emergency surgery is indicated. However, in stable patients, delayed surgery is associated with improved outcomes. For cardiac surgeons, surgery for acute MI presents additional challenges including bleeding risk, conduit selection and the decision to utilise mechanical support. A collaborative "Heart Team" approach ensures the management approach is tailored specifically to the patient.

16.10 Coronary Artery Bypass Surgery for STEMI

William Y. Shi and Julian A. Smith

16.11 Illustrative Cases

When managing patients with acute MI, cardiologists and cardiac surgeons may be faced with a number of difficult clinical decisions. The two cases below represent "real-life" clinical cases from our institution and illustrate the key themes discussed in this chapter.

16.11.1 Case 1: Delayed Surgery After PCI for Acute MI

A 54-year-old man presented with an acute STEMI. He had experienced intermittent chest pain for several months. ECG revealed ST elevation in the inferior leads with ST depression in the anterolateral leads. He was loaded with 300 mg aspirin and 180 mg ticagrelor. He had no other past medical history. Coronary angiography revealed chronic total occlusion of the left anterior descending and left circumflex systems. The right coronary system was dominant. There was occlusion of the proximal segment with TIMI I flow due to acute plaque rupture. The right coronary artery was providing retrograde collateral blood supply to the left coronary system. The right coronary occlusion was deemed to be the culprit lesion, and this was stented using a drug-eluting stent (Fig. 16.1).

The patient was subsequently referred for consideration of surgery given the left coronary system was not suitable for PCI. Subsequent transthoracic echocardiogram demonstrated severe left ventricular dysfunction (LV ejection fraction 30%). Troponin I peaked at 7500ng/L.

The patient experienced short episodes of chest pain upon return to the ward; as such he was commenced on heparin and glyceryl trinitrate infusion and thereafter

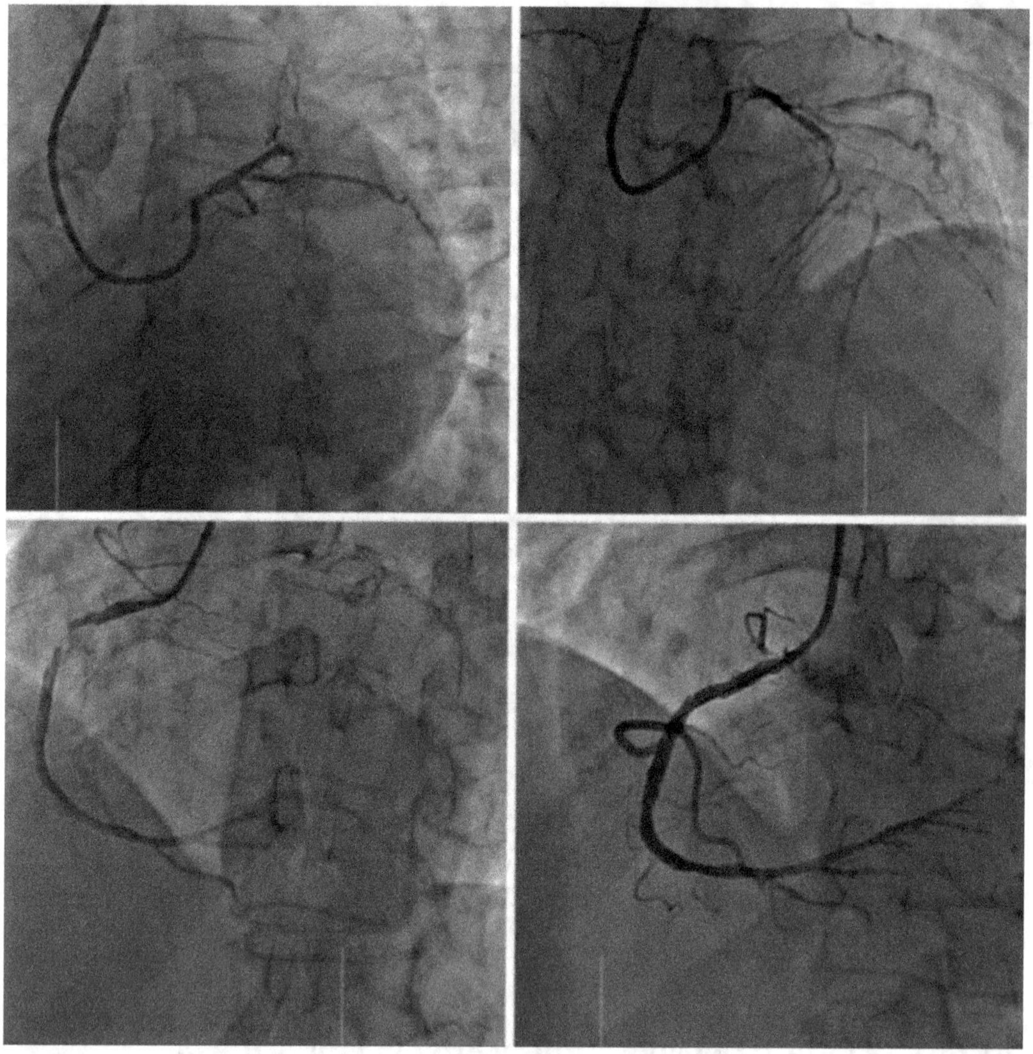

Fig. 16.1 Coronary angiogram demonstrating chronic occlusions of the LAD and circumflex vessels and acute occlusion of the proximal right coronary artery. Post-PCI result is demonstrated on the bottom right

remained pain-free. Given his haemodynamically stable state, poor ventricular function and substantial infarct size, the decision was made to delay surgery due to the high mortality risk associated with early surgery for acute MI. Due to recent PCI, dual antiplatelet therapy could not be ceased prior to surgery, and as such aspirin 100 mg daily and ticagrelor 90 mg twice daily were administered up until the day of surgery.

The patient subsequently underwent surgery for CABG 7 days later and received a left internal thoracic artery to his left anterior descending artery and a radial artery to an obtuse marginal branch of the circumflex. An epicardial left ventricular lead was placed to facilitate cardiac resynchronisation therapy should the patient require it in the future. An intra-aortic balloon pump was considered but ultimately not used as the patient was weaned off cardiopulmonary bypass on low-dose inotropes. Thromboelastography demonstrated abnormal platelet function, and platelet transfusion was required to obtain satisfactory haemostasis prior to surgical closure.

The patient was extubated on day 1 post-surgery. Aspirin was commenced on post-operative day 1, and ticagrelor was recommenced on post-operative day 2. Recovery was complicated by post-operative atrial fibrillation for which he received amiodarone. The patient was ultimately discharged home on post-operative day 11.

16.11.2 Case 2: Emergency CABG for Ongoing Ischaemia

A 72-year-old man presented with an inferior ST-elevation myocardial infarction. He had a past history of type 2 diabetes mellitus, hypercholesterolaemia, chronic obstructive pulmonary disease, obesity and chronic renal impairment. He presented with several hours of chest pain with inferior ST elevation. He developed cardiogenic shock and acute pulmonary oedema requiring an adrenaline infusion and mechanical ventilation before transfer to the cardiac catheterisation laboratory.

Coronary angiography demonstrated an occluded distal right coronary artery with evidence of thrombus. His left anterior descending artery also showed severe disease with mid-segment occlusion (Fig. 16.2). Attempted PCI to the right coronary lesion was unsuccessful due to inability to pass the guidewire beyond the lesion. There was ongoing inferior ST elevation and hypotension. The patient was referred for emergency CABG. Given the patient's haemodynamic instability, an IABP was inserted in the catheterisation laboratory prior to transfer to the operating theatre. Transthoracic echocardiography demonstrated severe left ventricular impairment (EF 15%).

In the operating theatre, after sternotomy, cardiopulmonary bypass was immediately established. Simultaneously, the long saphenous vein was harvested. The LITA was not harvested. Saphenous vein was used to revascularise the LAD and the PDA. The patient was weaned off cardiopulmonary bypass using the IABP as an adjunct.

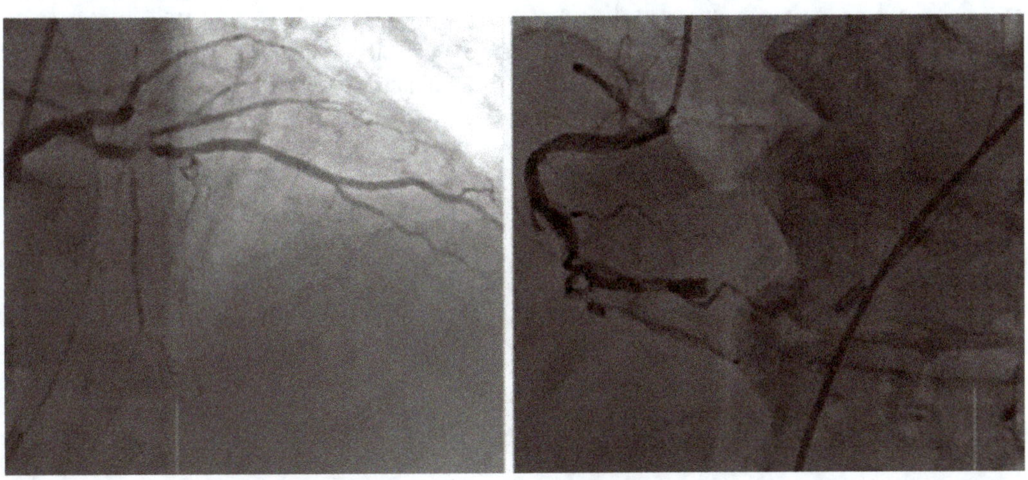

Fig. 16.2 Coronary angiogram of case 2, demonstrating occluded LAD and RCA. The RCA had evidence of thrombus formation, suggesting its role as the culprit lesion

Post-operatively, the patient was supported on adrenaline infusion. The IABP was weaned and removed on post-operative day 2. The patient's recovery was complicated by prolonged ventilation, requiring tracheostomy and renal failure, requiring temporary dialysis. The patient was discharged after 1 month to a rehabilitation facility and then subsequently discharged home.

Further Readings

Ibanez B, James S, Agewall S, et al. 2017 ESC Guidelines for the management of acute myocardial infarction in patients presenting with ST-segment elevation: The Task Force for the management of acute myocardial infarction in patients presenting with ST-segment elevation of the European Society of Cardiology (ESC). Eur Heart J. 2017;39(2):119–77. https://doi.org/10.1093/eurheartj/ehx393.

Lee DC, Oz MC, Weinberg AD, Ting W. Appropriate timing of surgical intervention after transmural acute myocardial infarction. J Thorac Cardiovasc Surg. 2003;125:115–9.

Mohr FW, Morice MC, Kappetein AP, et al. Coronary artery bypass graft surgery versus percutaneous coronary intervention in patients with three-vessel disease and left main coronary disease: 5-year follow-up of the randomised, clinical SYNTAX trial. Lancet. 2013;381:629–38.

O'Gara PT, Kushner FG, Ascheim DD, et al. 2013 ACCF/AHA guideline for the management of ST-elevation myocardial infarction: a report of the American College of Cardiology Foundation/American Heart Association Task Force on Practice Guidelines. Circulation. 2013;127:e362–425.

Thiele H, Zeymer U, Neumann FJ, et al. Intra-aortic balloon counterpulsation in acute myocardial infarction complicated by cardiogenic shock (IABP-SHOCK II): final 12 month results of a randomised, open-label trial. Lancet. 2013;382:1638–45.

A Handbook of Primary PCI: No-Reflow Management

17

Julien Adjedj, Olivier Muller, and Eric Eeckhout

17.1 Introduction

Although substantial progress has been made in recent decades in reducing mortality and performing optimal revascularization in patients with acute coronary syndrome (ACS) and stable coronary artery disease (CAD), one of the remaining challenges is to better prevent and treat extended myocardial damage despite "apparent" angiographic optimal percutaneous coronary intervention (PCI). The presence of no-reflow is related to higher risk of major adverse cardiac events (MACE) due to the poor healing of the infarct, adverse left ventricular remodelling, congestive heart failure occurrence and death. Despite optimal epicardial coronary artery reperfusion performed by PCI, distal microembolization into the coronary microcirculation limits myocardial salvage especially during ACS. No-reflow represents the ultimate stage of extended myocardial damage after PCI with absence of contrast medium progression in the coronary artery. This complication occurs mainly during ACS or during PCI of rotational atherectomy and venous graft in stable patients. The objective of this chapter is to describe how to manage a no-reflow phenomenon from the pathophysiology to the management in order to help physician to prevent this complication and if no-reflow occurs adapt therapeutics to limit myocardial damage and reduce poor outcomes.

17.2 Definition

The no-reflow phenomenon is defined as inadequate myocardial perfusion through a given segment of the coronary circulation without angiographic evidence of mechanical obstruction [1].

J. Adjedj · O. Muller · E. Eeckhout (✉)
CHUV, Cardiology Department, Lausanne University Hospital, Lausanne, Switzerland
e-mail: eric.eeckhout@chuv.ch

T. J. Watson et al. (eds.), *Primary Angioplasty*,
https://doi.org/10.1007/978-981-13-1114-7_17

17.3 Pathophysiology

Understanding the pathophysiology of the no-reflow phenomenon is the key to manage this phenomenon and prevent poor outcome. After prolonged coronary occlusion and restoration of coronary blood flow, structural damage to the microvasculature reduces the amount of blood flow to the cardiac myocytes. This may lead to inadequate healing of the cardiac scar.

17.4 Aetiology

No-reflow phenomenon is commonly the consequence of distal embolization and reperfusion injury such as:

- Thrombus containing lesions (ACS)
- Oxygen free radical or cellular-mediated endothelial injury (ACS)
- Loss of microvascular compartment due to completed myocardial infarction
- Cellular and interstitial oedema
- Atherosclerotic debris (venous bypass graft or rotational atherectomy)
- Microvascular constriction of vasospasm (drugs, choc)

No-reflow generally occurs immediately after PCI between 1 and 3% of PCI and can arise in different clinical settings [2–8]:

- Late presentation ACS
- Large thrombus burden
- Venous bypass graft PCI
- Rotational atherectomy
- Cardiogenic shock

17.5 Diagnosis

17.5.1 Clinical Presentation

Generally during ACS, revascularization is associated with relief of symptoms such as chest pain and regression of the ST-segment elevation in the electrocardiogram (ECG) in absence of no-reflow. In the presence of no-reflow, in the catheterization laboratory, the clinical presentation of no-reflow is often sudden and tragic. Control of coronary angiography confirms contrast medium staining in the coronary artery; the patient might complain of chest pain and symptoms persistence with a residual or increase elevation of the ST segment generally followed by haemodynamic instability.

17.5.2 Coronary Angiography

Contrast medium progression speed into the coronary artery is preserved in the absence of sub occlusive coronary stenosis (<90%) and in the absence of microcirculation damage. Therefore, after successful revascularization of an epicardial coronary stenosis, contrast medium progression impairment could reflect microcirculation damage. From the Thrombolysis in Myocardial Infarction (TIMI) study group, two indices were described: TIMI flow grade 0–3 is a semi-quantitative variable that ranges from no contrast medium progression (0) to normal progression (3); TIMI frame count is a quantitative index calculating the number of frames between two landmarks proximal and distal to the interrogated coronary artery [9]. In patients with ACS and preserved TIMI grade flow after revascularization, microcirculation can also be evaluated with myocardial blush, which corresponds to a densitometric method, assessing maximum intensity of contrast medium in the microcirculation. In practice, coronary microvascular obstruction is defined as TIMI grade flow ≤3 with myocardial blush stagnation (grade 0 or 1) [10] and no-reflow as the absence of contrast progression in the coronary vessel of interest in his most evident form. However, this may be subtle with preserved TIMI flow and absence of myocardial blush.

17.6 Management of No-Reflow

17.6.1 No-Reflow Prevention: Before the Procedure

No-reflow phenomenon is rare among overall PCI (1–3%) although some situations are associated with higher rate of no-reflow; therefore, management of some factors could help to prevent its occurrence according to the aetiology. Traditional cardiovascular risk factors are associated with poor outcome and no-reflow increase rate. In patients with diabetes, optimal blood sugar control before the procedure could reduce the occurrence of no-reflow [11, 12]. An animal study suggests that hypertension might be associated with increased risk of no-reflow [13]. Meta-analysis showed that pre-procedural use of statins was associated with significant reduction rate of no-reflow by 4.2% in all PCI patients (risk ratio (RR) 0.56, 95% confidence interval (CI) 0.35–0.90, $P = 0.016$) and attenuated by 5.0% in non-STEMI patients (RR 0.41, 95% CI 0.18–0.94, $P = 0.035$). This benefit was mainly observed in the early or acute intensive statin therapy populations (RR 0.43, 95% CI 0.26–0.71, $P = 0.001$) [14]. Active double antiplatelet therapy will prevent PCI complications such as acute stent thrombosis, periprocedural myocardial infarction (MI) and no-reflow (Fig. 17.1).

17.6.2 No-Reflow Prevention: During the Procedure

General good practice of PCI could limit the no-reflow occurrence. Anticoagulation should be performed at the early phase of the procedure with unfractionated heparin

(70–100 UI/Kg) and monitored with the activated clotting time (ACT) (200–250). Intracoronary nitrates should be administered (100–200 mcg) as well at the early phase, i.e. second angiographic view of diagnostic procedure. Optimal catheter selection is key to avoid damping intracoronary pressures, which can reduce coronary flow due to catheter induced obstruction and thereby lead to thrombus formation. Regular and systematic flushing of catheters can avoid thrombus and air emboli. Because new microthrombus composed of platelet and fibrin is an important contributor to the pathogenesis of the no-reflow phenomenon, glycoprotein IIb/IIIa platelet receptor inhibitor (anti-GPIIb/IIIa) may be beneficial in prevention during PCI. Studies suggest that anti-GPIIb/IIIa is beneficial in reducing rates of death, reinfarction and urgent revascularization when used in conjunction with PCI particularly as a rescue strategy [15] (Fig. 17.1).

17.6.2.1 Rotational Atherectomy

Balloon angioplasty exerts beneficial effects by enlarging the weakest part of coronary artery wall thereby producing intimal splits and medial dissections in calcified lesions. In contrast, rotational atherectomy aims to weaken calcified lesions, erode calcium spicule protrusion and thereby obtains a relatively smooth luminal surface. Rotational atherectomy use a burr rotation with high speed which generate friction (microembolization) and heat (platelet activation) between the burr and calcify plaque.

In experimental modelling, heat varies with technique from 2.6 °C using intermittent ablation and permitting minimal decelerations (5000 rpm) to 13.9 °C using continuous ablation allowing excessive decelerations (16,000 rpm) [16]. Along with microembolization of debris associated with thrombi, thermal injury may contribute to microvascular obstruction and no-reflow. To prevent these phenomena, medical therapy includes effective dual antiplatelet therapy, vasodilators and proper use of rotablational atherectomy. The benefit of antiplatelet therapy was established with the use of anti-GPIIb/IIIa reducing procedural morbidity and CK-MB elevation [17]. Preventive vasodilators are used for the purpose of reducing slow-flow and no-reflow, combining nitrates with calcium inhibitors and sometimes adenosine in the flush solution associated with heparin. Nicardipine may be effective when administered in a flush solution with other drugs during rotational atherectomy [18]. Recommended manipulation of the rotational atherectomy to reduce the risk of

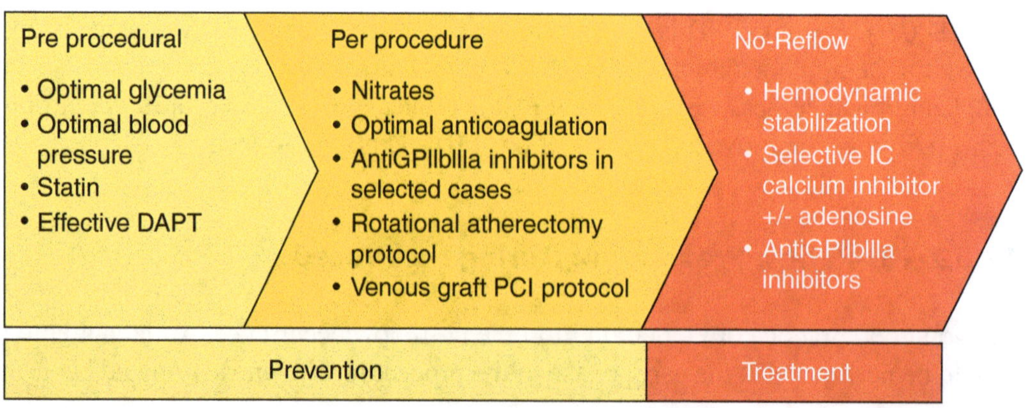

Fig. 17.1 No-reflow prevention and treatment

complications is to perform short runs (15 s) with a pecking motion to preserve flow at a speed rate of 140,000 rpm and avoid deceleration >5000 rpm with maintained patient haemodynamics [19].

17.6.2.2 Venous Graft PCI

Venous graft intervention is associated with higher rates of periprocedural MI and in-hospital mortality compared with PCI of native coronary arteries due to highly friable atherothrombotic debris of venous graft lesion. Therefore, distal embolization may result in slow or no-reflow phenomenon in more than 10% of cases. To prevent this distal embolization, it is recommended (IA) [20] to use distal protection device during stent implantation. In practice an American national registry showed that this protection device was used only in less than 25% of venous graft PCI, but still, the use of protection device was independently associated with a lower incidence of no-reflow but not in-hospital mortality [21]. It is interesting to notice this study evaluated the use of intragraft infusion of adenosine during peri procedure venous graft PCI. The study showed a significant reduction of no-reflow rate and increase average peak velocity compared to control group [22]. Nicardipine may be effective when administered before PCI in vein grafts to prevent no-reflow with minimal systemic depressant effect [18].

17.6.3 No-Reflow Confirmation

Priority is to exclude other mechanical aetiology which could occur after PCI and limit the contrast progression (Fig. 17.2). After PCI other causes such as coronary spasm, diffusion of coronary haematoma, coronary dissection, intracoronary occlusive thrombus or distal coronary stenosis could have similar angiographic and clinical presentation. Therefore, the easiest way to confirm this diagnosis is to perform,

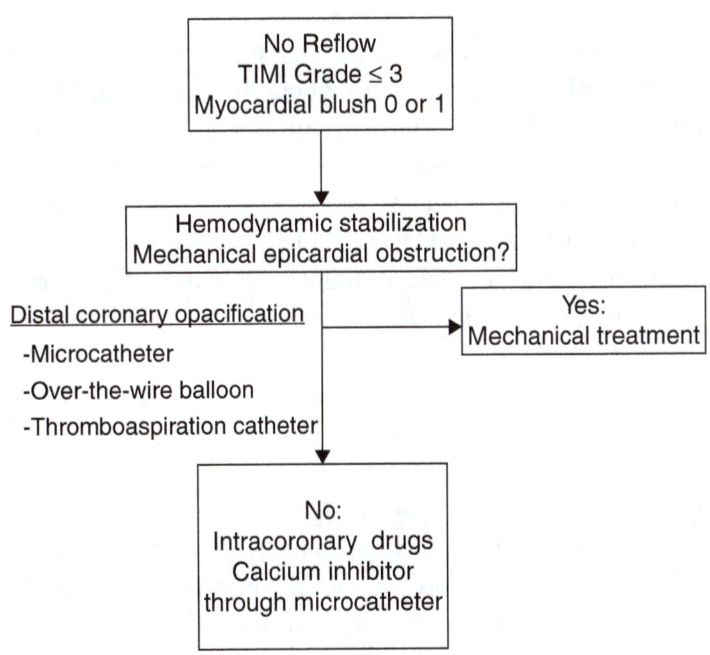

Fig. 17.2 No-reflow diagnosis and management

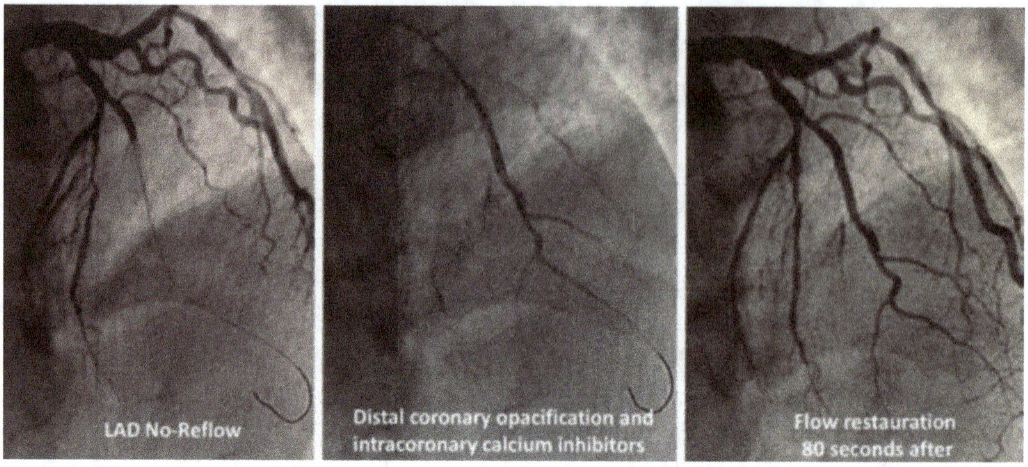

Fig. 17.3 Example of no-reflow management in a 72-year-old patient with anterior MI and no-reflow after DES implantation in the mid-left anterior descending artery

after nitrates administration, distal coronary opacification using extension of guiding catheter, intracoronary microcatheter, thromboaspiration catheter or over-the-wire angioplasty balloon. Careful and gentle distal contrast injection should be performed after aspirating some blood to confirm the true lumen position and the absence of obstruction due to thrombus or coronary wall at the exit of the catheter. Visualization of the distal part of the coronary artery is precious to exclude other causes of epicardial obstruction and confirm the no-reflow. Furthermore, microcatheters allow distal administration of drugs such as calcium inhibitors or adenosine which, by definition, could not reach the microvasculature in the no-reflow area from a guiding administration. An example is provided in Fig. 17.3.

17.6.4 No-Reflow Treatment

In no-reflow, microvascular damage is usually confined in the related coronary artery territory which constitutes a myocardial necrosis area. Therefore, treating no-reflow may not necessarily reduce the infarcted size but might improve blood flow to the necrotic area to improve area healing, infarction expansion and prevent left ventricular remodelling. Furthermore, restauration of flow will salvage the small vessels which may help promote collateral circulation and ensure drug delivery to the necrotic zone. To decrease the incidence of this phenomenon, short-term intracoronary and systemic drugs were studied to restore coronary flow within the no-reflow area (Table 17.1).

17.6.5 Haemodynamic Stabilization

Before starting dedicated therapeutics to treat no-reflow, it is essential to evaluate the patient haemodynamic to maintain optimal aortic blood pressure. Of note, no-reflow of the right coronary artery is prone to reflex hypotension or bradycardia which needs atropine administration. General supportive measures are usually used to maintain stable haemodynamic such as fluid administration and if necessary

Table 17.1 No-reflow aetiology, prevention and treatment

	Aetiology	Prevention	Treatment
Myocardial infarction	Thrombotic	Optimal anticoagulation Consider thrombectomy or balloon inflation to restore TIMI III flow with minimal invasive strategy	Anti-GPIIb/IIIa Intracoronary calcium inhibitors Adenosine
	Microvascular vasospasm	Nitrates	
Rotablator	Atherothrombotic embolization Platelet activation Vasospasm	Optimal anticoagulation Nitrates Maintained stable haemodynamic (temporary pacemaker/atropine in case of severe bradycardia) Flush infusion with nitrates and or calcium inhibitors	Intracoronary calcium inhibitors Adenosine
Venous graft	Atherothrombotic	Distal protection Adenosine intra graft Nicardipine	Intragraft calcium inhibitors Adenosine
Iatrogenic	Thrombotic	Optimal anticoagulation with ACT monitoring	Heparin anti-GPIIb/IIIa Consider balloon inflation or thrombectomy

inotrope support such as epinephrine. In rare refractory cases intra-aortic balloon pump might be an option to maintain overall coronary perfusion.

17.6.6 Thromboaspiration

One must realize that manipulating the occluded thrombotic vessel with balloons and stents often results in distal embolization of the thrombus, which might contribute to no-reflow occurrence. To prevent distal embolization, thromboaspiration might help to reduce the thrombus burden and therefore the degree of no-reflow. Thromboaspiration was widely used in the past years in STEMI patients, but recent study results and meta-analyses failed to show benefit with an increased risk of stroke. Therefore, actual guidelines do not recommend to perform systematic thromboaspiration [23].

17.6.7 Pharmacological Therapeutics

17.6.7.1 Adenosine

Adenosine used in myocardial infarction might have some benefit in terms of preventing extensive microcirculation injury. Intravenous adenosine, given before reperfusion therapy, was suggested to reduce infarct size compared with placebo in the AMISTAD randomized clinical trial [24]. Similarly, the larger AMISTAD II trial demonstrated infarct size reduction in the adenosine group compared with the placebo group, but without significant benefit in terms of clinical outcome [25].

When looking at the post hoc analysis of the AMISTAD II trial, in the subgroup with successful reperfusion within 3 h, the adjunct of adenosine infusion enhanced early and late survival and reduced the composite clinical endpoint of death or congestive heart failure at 6 months [26]. In addition, during reperfusion, the addition of intracoronary adenosine after thromboaspiration, through the thrombectomy catheter, showed a significant improvement in STR, with better 1-year left ventricular remodelling and reduction in clinical events compared with saline and nitroprusside [27, 28].

17.6.7.2 Statins

Based on STR, TIMI frame count and myocardial blush, Kim et al. showed that a high dose of atorvastatin may produce an optimal result in patients with STEMI undergoing PCI by improving microvascular myocardial perfusion, without significant clinical improvement [29].

17.6.7.3 Calcium Inhibitors and Other Drugs

Finally, intracoronary calcium inhibitors (verapamil, diltiazem and nicardipine) are probably the most evaluated and effective drugs available for the prevention and treatment of no-reflow phenomenon. In a meta-analysis by Su et al., including 7 trials involving 539 patients with intracoronary verapamil administration at a dosage of 200 µg to 2 mg, the authors showed a significant decrease in no-reflow incidence, a better TIMI grade and frame count and a reduction in major adverse cardiac events (MACE), 2 months after PCI (relative risk 0.56, 95% confidence interval 0.33–0.95) [30]. Another Meta-analysis of 8 randomized controlled trials involving 494 patients evaluated the efficacy of the combination of verapamil and diltiazem or verapamil alone to treat no-reflow which suggested significant clinical benefit over standard of care with respect to no-reflow [31].

Nitroprusside is an effective intracoronary drug in the treatment of no-reflow. Two meta-analyses showed that intracoronary nitroprusside is beneficial in preventing no-reflow in reducing TIMI frame count and in improving left ventricular ejection fraction. It is also likely to reduce MACE [32, 33].

17.7 Outcome

After the procedure, non-invasive indexes are of importance to evaluate the myocardial damage and assess potential poor outcome.

17.7.1 ECG

Among several indices to assess microvascular obstruction with ECG, only the residual ST-segment elevation was an independent predictor of microvascular injury (odds ratio 19.1, 95% confidence interval 2.4–154; $P = 0.005$) in multivariable analysis in a study evaluating ECG in 180 patients with STEMI. Interestingly,

ST-segment resolution was not associated with LV function, infarct size, transmurality indexes or microvascular injury in multivariable analysis [34] (Fig. 17.4a). A distortion of the terminal portion of the QRS complex was significantly associated with infarct size, impaired myocardial salvage and reperfusion injury in 572 patients with reperfused STEMI as assessed by cardiac magnetic resonance imaging (CMR). Moreover, this QRS modification was independently associated with MACE [35].

17.7.2 Echocardiography

Myocardial contrast echocardiography (MCE) is a bedside technique that can be used to assess microvascular perfusion (Fig. 17.4c). Echo contrast agents are microbubbles of inert gases of sizes and rheology similar to that of red blood cells and can be administered intravenously. Myocardial uptake of microbubbles is delayed in areas of "no-reflow" and MVO. MCE is able to detect only 1/3 of patients with a no-reflow phenomenon after ACS [36, 37]. However, widespread use of MCE has been hampered by a long learning curve for image acquisition and reporting,

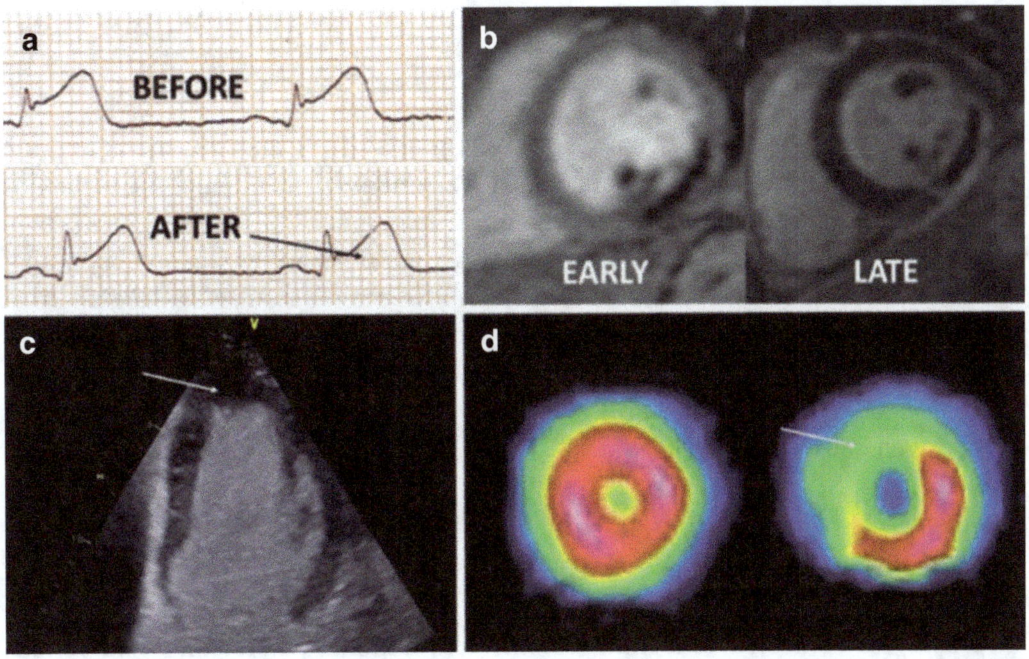

Fig. 17.4 Non-invasive tools to assess microvascular obstruction. (**a**) ST-segment resolution represents a useful tool of coronary microvascular obstruction after myocardial infarction. Black arrows showing absence of ST-segment resolution after artery recanalization. (**b**) Cardiac magnetic resonance. On late gadolinium enhancement, areas of microvascular obstruction are seen, hypoenhancement (so-called "dark zones") within an avidly enhancing site of myocardial infarction. (**c**) Myocardial contrast echocardiography showing lack of intra-myocardial contrast opacification (indicated by white arrow). (**d**) Single-photon emission computed tomography showing absent tracer uptake (white arrow, scintigraphic no-reflow phenomenon), as compared to normal uptake (left position). Adapted from Adjedj, J., et al. (2018). "Coronary microcirculation in acute myocardial ischaemia: From non-invasive to invasive absolute flow assessment." *Arch Cardiovasc Dis*

uncertain reproducibility, concerns over microbubble contrast safety. Moreover, MCE has some limitations such as operator skills, moderate spatial resolution, incomplete left ventricular coverage and semi-quantitative assessment of MVO.

17.7.3 Cardiac Magnetic Resonance

CMR is the non-invasive gold standard to assess MVO. It allows multislice imaging with high tissue contrast and high spatial resolution, enabling accurate quantification and localization of MVO and the infarct size relative to the entire left ventricle (Fig. 17.4b). CMR-defined MVO has been well correlated with MCE, angiographic and invasive indices used for the assessment of MVO [38]. Symons et al. demonstrated that early post-infarction CMR-based MVO was a strong independent predictor of MACE in reperfused STEMI patients at long-term follow-up. Remarkably, MVO extent ≥2.6% of LV was the strongest independent predictor of death and heart failure hospitalization, overriding the prognostic performance of traditional outcome predictors and leading to better long-term risk stratification [39].

17.7.4 Nuclear Imaging

Both single-photon emission computed tomography [40] and positron emission tomography (PET) [41] demonstrated the "no-reflow" phenomenon in humans could be detected by nuclear imaging. Nuclear imaging no-reflow phenomenon can occur in a subgroup of patients without angiographic no-reflow phenomenon, that the myocardial damage depends on the severity of microvascular damage and that prolonged ischemia time may increase the likelihood of "microvascular no-reflow phenomenon" (Fig. 17.4d) [42]. However, PET scanning is still underutilized in clinical practice, and its clinical use is limited to sites with PET scans and cyclotrons or generators.

Conclusion

Currently, there is still a lack of an optimal treatment for no-reflow phenomenon. Prevention is effective to reduce no-reflow occurrence with medical therapy and proper use of dedicated techniques such as rotational atherectomy and venous graft PCI. The diagnosis of no-reflow remains a challenge and, if not recognized, may be treated inadvertently by additional PCI which will only harm the situation. When no-reflow occurs, the main objective is to diagnose properly, stabilize the patient and treat this condition by sub selective administration of vasodilator drugs to "open" the microcirculation, avoiding a systemic effect on the blood pressure. No-reflow management aims to improve coronary blood flow at the level of microcirculation to reduce myocardial damage and improve clinical outcome.

References

1. Eeckhout E, Kern MJ. The coronary no-reflow phenomenon: a review of mechanisms and therapies. Eur Heart J. 2001;22:729–39.
2. Matsuo H, Watanabe S, Watanabe T, et al. Prevention of no-reflow/slow-flow phenomenon during rotational atherectomy—a prospective randomized study comparing intracoronary continuous infusion of verapamil and nicorandil. Am Heart J. 2007;154:994.e1–6.
3. Sharma SK, Dangas G, Mehran R, et al. Risk factors for the development of slow flow during rotational coronary atherectomy. Am J Cardiol. 1997;80:219–22.
4. Iwasaki K, Samukawa M, Furukawa H. Comparison of the effects of nicorandil versus verapamil on the incidence of slow flow/no reflow during rotational atherectomy. Am J Cardiol. 2006;98:1354–6.
5. Kaplan BM, Benzuly KH, Kinn JW, et al. Treatment of no-reflow in degenerated saphenous vein graft interventions: comparison of intracoronary verapamil and nitroglycerin. Catheter Cardiovasc Diagn. 1996;39:113–8.
6. Fischell TA, Carter AJ, Foster MT, et al. Reversal of "no reflow" during vein graft stenting using high velocity boluses of intracoronary adenosine. Catheter Cardiovasc Diagn. 1998;45:360–5.
7. Resnic FS, Wainstein M, Lee MK, et al. No-reflow is an independent predictor of death and myocardial infarction after percutaneous coronary intervention. Am Heart J. 2003;145:42–6.
8. Mehta RH, Harjai KJ, Boura J, et al. Prognostic significance of transient no-reflow during primary percutaneous coronary intervention for ST-elevation acute myocardial infarction. Am J Cardiol. 2003;92:1445–7.
9. Kunadian V, Harrigan C, Zorkun C, et al. Use of the TIMI frame count in the assessment of coronary artery blood flow and microvascular function over the past 15 years. J Thromb Thrombolysis. 2009;27:316–28.
10. Niccoli G, Cosentino N, Spaziani C, Fracassi F, Tarantini G, Crea F. No-reflow: incidence and detection in the cath-lab. Curr Pharm Des. 2013;19:4564–75.
11. Malmberg K, Ryden L, Efendic S, et al. Randomized trial of insulin-glucose infusion followed by subcutaneous insulin treatment in diabetic patients with acute myocardial infarction (DIGAMI study): effects on mortality at 1 year. J Am Coll Cardiol. 1995;26:57–65.
12. Iwakura K, Ito H, Ikushima M, et al. Association between hyperglycemia and the no-reflow phenomenon in patients with acute myocardial infarction. J Am Coll Cardiol. 2003;41:1–7.
13. Pantsios C, Kapelios C, Vakrou S, et al. Effect of elevated reperfusion pressure on "no reflow" area and infarct size in a porcine model of ischemia-reperfusion. J Cardiovasc Pharmacol Ther. 2016;21:405–11.
14. Li XD, Yang YJ, Hao YC, et al. Effect of pre-procedural statin therapy on myocardial no-reflow following percutaneous coronary intervention: a meta analysis. Chin Med J. 2013;126:1755–60.
15. Adgey AA. An overview of the results of clinical trials with glycoprotein IIb/IIIa inhibitors. Eur Heart J. 1998;19(Suppl D):D10–21.
16. Reisman M, Shuman BJ, Harms V. Analysis of heat generation during rotational atherectomy using different operational techniques. Cathet Cardiovasc Diagn. 1998;44:453–5.
17. Kini A, Reich D, Marmur JD, Mitre CA, Sharma SK. Reduction in periprocedural enzyme elevation by abciximab after rotational atherectomy of type B2 lesions: results of the Rota ReoPro randomized trial. Am Heart J. 2001;142:965–9.
18. Fischell TA, Maheshwari A. Current applications for nicardipine in invasive and interventional cardiology. J Invasive Cardiol. 2004;16:428–32.
19. Tomey MI, Kini AS, Sharma SK. Current status of rotational atherectomy. JACC Cardiovasc Interv. 2014;7:345–53.
20. Windecker S, Kolh P, Alfonso F, et al. 2014 ESC/EACTS Guidelines on myocardial revascularization: The Task Force on Myocardial Revascularization of the European Society of Cardiology (ESC) and the European Association for Cardio-Thoracic Surgery (EACTS) developed with the special contribution of the European Association of Percutaneous Cardiovascular Interventions (EAPCI). Eur Heart J. 2014;35:2541–619.

21. Mehta SK, Frutkin AD, Milford-Beland S, et al. Utilization of distal embolic protection in saphenous vein graft interventions (an analysis of 19,546 patients in the American College of Cardiology-National Cardiovascular Data Registry). Am J Cardiol. 2007;100:1114–8.
22. Kapoor N, Yalamanchili V, Siddiqui T, Raza S, Leesar MA. Cardioprotective effect of high-dose intragraft adenosine infusion on microvascular function and prevention of no-reflow during saphenous vein grafts intervention. Catheter Cardiovasc Interv. 2014;83:1045–54.
23. Ibanez B, James S, Agewall S, et al. 2017 ESC guidelines for the management of acute myocardial infarction in patients presenting with ST-segment elevation: the task force for the management of acute myocardial infarction in patients presenting with ST-segment elevation of the European Society of Cardiology (ESC). Eur Heart J. 2018;39(2):119–77.
24. Mahaffey KW, Puma JA, Barbagelata NA, et al. Adenosine as an adjunct to thrombolytic therapy for acute myocardial infarction: results of a multicenter, randomized, placebo-controlled trial: the acute myocardial infarction STudy of ADenosine (AMISTAD) trial. J Am Coll Cardiol. 1999;34:1711–20.
25. Ross AM, Gibbons RJ, Stone GW, Kloner RA, Alexander RW. A randomized, double-blinded, placebo-controlled multicenter trial of adenosine as an adjunct to reperfusion in the treatment of acute myocardial infarction (AMISTAD-II). J Am Coll Cardiol. 2005;45:1775–80.
26. Kloner RA, Forman MB, Gibbons RJ, Ross AM, Alexander RW, Stone GW. Impact of time to therapy and reperfusion modality on the efficacy of adenosine in acute myocardial infarction: the AMISTAD-2 trial. Eur Heart J. 2006;27:2400–5.
27. Niccoli G, Rigattieri S, De Vita MR, et al. Open-label, randomized, placebo-controlled evaluation of intracoronary adenosine or nitroprusside after thrombus aspiration during primary percutaneous coronary intervention for the prevention of microvascular obstruction in acute myocardial infarction: the REOPEN-AMI study (intracoronary nitroprusside versus adenosine in acute myocardial infarction). JACC Cardiovasc Interv. 2013;6:580–9.
28. Niccoli G, Spaziani C, Crea F. Left ventricular remodeling and 1-year clinical follow-up of the REOPEN-AMI trial. J Am Coll Cardiol. 2014;63:1454–5.
29. Kim JS, Kim J, Choi D, et al. Efficacy of high-dose atorvastatin loading before primary percutaneous coronary intervention in ST-segment elevation myocardial infarction: the STATIN STEMI trial. JACC Cardiovasc Interv. 2010;3:332–9.
30. Su Q, Li L, Liu Y. Short-term effect of verapamil on coronary no-reflow associated with percutaneous coronary intervention in patients with acute coronary syndrome: a systematic review and meta-analysis of randomized controlled trials. Clin Cardiol. 2013;36:E11–6.
31. Wang L, Cheng Z, Gu Y, Peng D. Short-term effects of verapamil and diltiazem in the treatment of no reflow phenomenon: a meta-analysis of randomized controlled trials. Biomed Res Int. 2015;2015:382086.
32. Su Q, Li L, Naing KA, Sun Y. Safety and effectiveness of nitroprusside in preventing no-reflow during percutaneous coronary intervention: a systematic review. Cell Biochem Biophys. 2014;68:201–6.
33. Zhao S, Qi G, Tian W, Chen L, Sun Y. Effect of intracoronary nitroprusside in preventing no reflow phenomenon during primary percutaneous coronary intervention: a meta-analysis. J Interv Cardiol. 2014;27:356–64.
34. Nijveldt R, van der Vleuten PA, Hirsch A, et al. Early electrocardiographic findings and MR imaging-verified microvascular injury and myocardial infarct size. JACC Cardiovasc Imaging. 2009;2:1187–94.
35. Rommel KP, Badarnih H, Desch S, et al. QRS complex distortion (grade 3 ischaemia) as a predictor of myocardial damage assessed by cardiac magnetic resonance imaging and clinical prognosis in patients with ST-elevation myocardial infarction. Eur Heart J Cardiovasc Imaging. 2016;17:194–202.
36. Dwivedi G, Janardhanan R, Hayat SA, Lim TK, Greaves K, Senior R. Relationship between myocardial perfusion with myocardial contrast echocardiography and function early after acute myocardial infarction for the prediction of late recovery of function. Int J Cardiol. 2010;140:169–74.

37. Galiuto L, Garramone B, Scara A, et al. The extent of microvascular damage during myocardial contrast echocardiography is superior to other known indexes of post-infarct reperfusion in predicting left ventricular remodeling: results of the multicenter AMICI study. J Am Coll Cardiol. 2008;51:552–9.
38. Nijveldt R, Beek AM, Hirsch A, et al. Functional recovery after acute myocardial infarction: comparison between angiography, electrocardiography, and cardiovascular magnetic resonance measures of microvascular injury. J Am Coll Cardiol. 2008;52:181–9.
39. Symons R, Pontone G, Schwitter J, et al. Long-term incremental prognostic value of cardiovascular magnetic resonance after ST-segment elevation myocardial infarction: a study of the collaborative registry on CMR in STEMI. JACC Cardiovasc Imaging. 2018;11(6):813–25. https://doi.org/10.1016/j.jcmg.2017.05.023.
40. Schofer J, Montz R, Mathey DG. Scintigraphic evidence of the "no reflow" phenomenon in human beings after coronary thrombolysis. J Am Coll Cardiol. 1985;5:593–8.
41. Jeremy RW, Links JM, Becker LC. Progressive failure of coronary flow during reperfusion of myocardial infarction: documentation of the no reflow phenomenon with positron emission tomography. J Am Coll Cardiol. 1990;16:695–704.
42. Kondo M, Nakano A, Saito D, Shimono Y. Assessment of "microvascular no-reflow phenomenon" using technetium-99m macroaggregated albumin scintigraphy in patients with acute myocardial infarction. J Am Coll Cardiol. 1998;32:898–903.

Medications in Cardiogenic Shock

18

Mei-Tzu Wang, Cheng Chung Hung, and Wei-Chun Huang

18.1 Introduction

Shock is circulatory failure with inadequate cellular oxygen utilization. Four potential pathophysiological mechanisms result in shock, including hypovolemic, cardiogenic, obstructive, and distributive factors. Cardiogenic shock (CS) decreases myocardial contractility and is the most common cause of death in patients with acute myocardial infarction (AMI). To differentiate the type and cause of shock, medical history, physical examination, and clinical investigations are important. Focused echocardiography offers advanced information for differentiation and should be performed as soon as possible in any shock patient.

AMI with subsequent ventricular dysfunction is the most frequent cause of CS accounting for about half of cases, and other causes of CS include end-stage cardiomyopathy, advanced valvular heart disease, myocarditis, and cardiac arrhythmias. Around 5–15% AMI patients complicated with CS. For AMI patient, early revascularization is the most important strategy [1]. In addition to percutaneous coronary intervention (PCI) or coronary artery bypass grafting (CABG), intra-aortic balloon pumping (IABP), active assist devices, inotropes, and vasopressors are widely used

M.-T. Wang · C. C. Hung
Department of Critical Care Medicine, Kaohsiung Veterans General Hospital, Kaohsiung, Taiwan

W.-C. Huang (✉)
Department of Critical Care Medicine, Kaohsiung Veterans General Hospital, Kaohsiung, Taiwan

School of Medicine, National Yang-Ming University, Taipei, Taiwan

Department of Physical Therapy, Fooyin University, Kaohsiung, Taiwan

Graduate Institute of Clinical Medicine, Kaohsiung Medical University, Kaohsiung, Taiwan

National Defense Medical Center, National Defense University, Taipei, Taiwan

T. J. Watson et al. (eds.), *Primary Angioplasty*,
https://doi.org/10.1007/978-981-13-1114-7_18

for CS management. Resuscitation should be started early and adequately to prevent organ dysfunction worsening. The basic resuscitation principles for patients with CS are based on the "VIP rule," including ventilate (oxygen administration), infuse (fluid resuscitation), and pump (vasoactive agents). The chapter focused on inotropic support in cardiogenic shock patient.

18.2 Definition and Initial Assessment

CS is a lethal disease and a state of reduced cardiac output and critical end organ hypoperfusion. It ranges from mild hypoperfusion to profound shock and multi-organ system dysfunction. Established criteria for the diagnosis of CS are (1) systolic blood pressure (SBP) <90 mmHg for >30 min, vasopressors required to achieve SBP ≥90 mmHg, or a reduction of cardiac index (<1.8 L/min/m^2 without support and less than 2.2 L/min/m^2 with support); (2) pulmonary congestion or elevated left ventricular filling pressures (pulmonary capillary wedge pressure > 18 mmHg); and (3) impaired organ perfusion. Inadequate organ perfusion contains at least one of the following criteria: (a) altered mental status; (b) cold, clammy skin; (c) oliguria; and (d) increased serum lactate. Clinical signs of tissue hypoperfusion are apparent through three "windows" of the body: (1) skin (cold and clammy skin, with vasoconstriction and cyanosis), (2) kidney (urine output of <0.5 mL per kilogram of body weight per hour), (3) and brain (altered mental state, which typically includes obtundation, disorientation, and confusion). Hyperlactatemia is typically present, indicating abnormal cellular oxygen metabolism. The normal blood lactate level is approximately 1 mmol per liter, but the level is increased (>1.5 mmol per liter) in acute circulatory failure. A full clinical assessment contains skin color and temperature, jugular venous distention, and peripheral edema. Point-of-care echocardiogram offers advanced information for diagnosis via the evaluations of pericardial effusion, left and right ventricular size and function, and respiratory variations in vena cava dimensions, the calculation of the aortic velocity–time integral, and a measure of stroke volume [1–3].

18.3 Initial Approach to the Patient in Cardiogenic Shock (VIP)

Irrespective of early revascularization by PCI or CABG, the basic principle of treatment for CS is "VIP rules" to maintain ventilation, obtain euvolemia with volume expansion, and administer vasopressors or inotropes for the prevention or treatment of multi-organ dysfunction.

18.3.1 Ventilation

Oxygen should be administered immediately to increase oxygen delivery. Pulse oximetry is not reliable due to peripheral vasoconstriction, and blood gas monitoring is required for precise determination of oxygen. For CS patients presenting with severe dyspnea, hypoxemia, persistent, or worsening acidemia (pH <7.30), symptoms could rapidly progress in respiratory failure and cardiac arrest, which prompted physicians to perform endotracheal intubation and invasive mechanical ventilation. Invasive mechanical ventilation also reduces the oxygen demand of respiratory muscles and decreases left ventricular afterload by increasing intrathoracic pressure. After the initiation of invasive mechanical ventilation, an abrupt decrease in arterial pressure implies hypovolemia, and sedative agents in minimum should be kept to avoid further decrease in arterial pressure and cardiac output.

18.3.2 Fluid Resuscitation and Objective Fluid Status Evaluation

The pragmatic endpoints for fluid resuscitation are to achieve the plateau portion of the Frank–Starling curve and become preload-independent status. In patients receiving mechanical ventilation, signs of fluid responsiveness could be identified directly from beat-by-beat stroke-volume measurements with the use of cardiac-output monitors or indirectly from observed variations in pulse pressure on the arterial-pressure tracing during the ventilator cycle. There are several limitations in such bedside inferences, including that patients must have no spontaneous breathing effort (usually requires the administration of sedatives or muscle relaxants), receive ventilation with relatively large tidal volumes, and be free of major arrhythmia and right ventricular dysfunction. A passive leg-raising test is an alternative method, but the effect is transient and requires a rapid response device.

Four elements are incorporated in fluid challenge, including (1) the type of fluid, (2) the rate of fluid administration, (3) the objective of fluid challenge, and (4) the safety limit. First, crystalloid solutions are the first choice, and the use of albumin to correct severe hypoalbuminemia may be reasonable in some patients. Second, fluids should be infused rapidly to achieve a quick response but not fast to develop an artificial stress response. (i.e., infuse 300–500 mL of fluid during a period of 20–30 min). Third, the objective of the fluid challenge contains an increase in SBP, a decrease in heart rate, or an increase in urine output. Finally, the safety limit is to avoid fluid infusion-associated pulmonary edema, and central venous pressure of a few millimeters of mercury above the baseline value is usually set to prevent fluid overload, although it is not a perfect guideline. Because hemodynamic management depends on optimal filling pressures, pulmonary artery catheters, Pulse Contour Cardiac Output (PiCCO), or other measure systems should be used in all complicated patients [4].

18.4 Vasoactive and Inotropic Agents

Catecholamines are used in near 90% CS patients, but there is limited evidence from randomized trials to compare different catecholamines. In SOAP II (Sepsis Occurrence in Acutely Ill Patients) trial, dopamine was shown to have higher rates of arrhythmias and mortality in CS subgroup [5]. Nevertheless, clinical and methodological concerns have raised questions about the external validity and applicability of the findings because SOAP II trial did not have an operationalized definition of CS. The predefined CS subgroup had lower mortality with norepinephrine [5]. Therefore, norepinephrine should be the first choice as vasopressor in patients with CS. European STEMI guidelines recommend dopamine (IIa/C recommendation) over norepinephrine (IIb/B recommendation), which are partly confusing and are in contrast to current evidence, but it is also stated that norepinephrine is preferred over dopamine when the blood pressure is low.

There are no clear SBP or mean arterial pressure (MAP) recommendations for CS patients. MAP targets are often extrapolated from non-CS populations and 65–70 mm Hg has been considered a reasonable target. However, higher blood pressure is not associated with beneficial outcome [6]. CS is a hemodynamically heterogeneous disorder; thus despite improvements in hemodynamic variables, microcirculatory dysfunction may persist. Inotropic and vasopressor agents have been recommended and used in the treatment of patients with shock. Despite the benefit of myocardial contractility, the pharmacodynamics of different inotropic agents and associated side effects (arrhythmias and increased myocardial oxygen consumption) may increase mortality [7]. The use of catecholamine and vasoconstrictors should be restricted to the shortest duration and the lowest possible dose. The ideal inotrope would increase cardiac output and reduce ventricular filling pressures and mortality without adverse effects. Several studies still continue to develop ideal inotrope for the treatment of CS [8]. Omecamtiv mecarbil is a promising new drug for stable heart failure that exerts inotropic effects by activating cardiac myosin [9]. Gene therapy is another area and further results of these new approaches are awaited [10]. Medications and their characteristics prescribed in CS patients are listed in Table 18.1 [11]. Initial vasoactive management strategies in different types of CS are presented in Table 18.2.

18.5 Vasoactive Agents

18.5.1 Norepinephrine

Norepinephrine is a naturally occurring catecholamine and acts mainly on α-adrenergic receptor but has small effect on beta receptor. Norepinephrine can increase blood pressure by constricting small vessels. The increasing blood pressure will stimulate the parasympathetic tone, with little change in heart rate or cardiac output. The well-known adverse effects are reduced renal and splanchnic blood flow, especially in patients needing volume expansion. Norepinephrine is associated with fewer arrhythmias and may be the vasopressor of choice in many patients with CS. However, in light of SOAP II trial limitations, the optimal first-line vasoactive medication in CS remains unclear, but norepinephrine should be considered as the vasopressor of first choice.

Table 18.1 Medications used in cardiogenic shock patients

Medication	Class	Mechanism of action	Receptor binding	Half-life	Usual infusion dose	Hemodynamic effect
Vasopressor/inotropes						
Dopamine (0.5–2 μg/kg/min)	Catecholamine	β- and α-adrenergic and dopaminergic agonist	α_1 (−) β_1 (+) β_2 (−) D (+++)	2 min	0.5–2 μg/kg/min	↑CO
Dopamine (5–10 μg/kg/min)	Catecholamine	β- and α-adrenergic and dopaminergic agonist	α_1 (+) β_1 (+++) β_2 (+) D (++)	2 min	5–10 μg/kg/min	↑↑CO, ↑SVR
Dopamine (10–20 μg/kg/min)	Catecholamine	β- and α-adrenergic and dopaminergic agonist	α_1 (+++) β_1 (++) β_2 (−) D (++)	2 min	10–20 μg/kg/min	↑↑SVR, ↑CO
Norepinephrine	Catecholamine	α-adrenergic agonist	α_1 (++++) β_1 (++) β_2 (+) D (−)	2–2.5 min	0.05–0.4 μg/kg/min	↑↑SVR, ↑CO
Epinephrine	Catecholamine	α- and β-adrenergic blockade	α_1 (++++) β_1 (++++) β_2 (+++) D (−)	2 min	0.01–0.5 μg/kg/min	↑↑CO, ↑↑SVR
Phenylephrine			α_1 (+++) β_1 (−) β_2 (−) D (−)	5 min	0.1–10 μg/kg/min	↑↑SVR

(continued)

Table 18.1 (continued)

Medication	Class	Mechanism of action	Receptor binding	Half-life	Usual infusion dose	Hemodynamic effect
Vasopressin	Vasopressor	Stimulate V_1 receptors in vascular smooth muscle	V_1 and V_2 vasopressin receptor agonist	10–20 min	0.02–0.04 U/min	↑↑SVR, ↔PVR
Inodilators						
Dobutamine	Catecholamine	β-adrenergic blockade	α_1 (+) β_1 (++++) β_2 (++) D (−)	2–3 min	2.5–20 μg/kg/min	↑↑CO, ↓SVR, ↓PVR
Isoproterenol			α_1 (−) β_1 (++++) β_2 (+++) D (−)	2.5–5 min	2.0–20 μg/min	↑↑CO, ↓SVR, ↓PVR
Milrinone	PDE inhibitor	Increases cAMP by inhibiting PDE3	PDE3	2 h	0.125–0.75 μg/kg/min	↑CO, ↓SVR, ↓PVR
Enoximone		PDE3 inhibitor	PDE3	3-6 h	2–10 μg/kg/min	↑CO, ↓SVR, ↓PVR
Levosimendan	Calcium sensitizer	Increases sensitivity of troponin C to intracellular Ca^{2+}	Myofilament Ca^{2+} sensitizer, PDE3 inhibitor	1 h (metabolites up to 80 h)	0.05–0.2 μg/kg/min	↑CO, ↓SVR, ↓PVR

cAMP cyclic adenosine monophosphate, *CO* cardiac output, *D* dopamine, *PDE* phosphodiesterase inhibitor, *PVR* pulmonary vascular resistance, *SVR* systemic vascular resistance

Table 18.2 Initial vasoactive management strategies in different types of cardiogenic shock

Cause or presentation	Vasoactive strategies	Hemodynamic rationale	Further management
Classic wet and cold (low CI and high SVR)	1. Norepinephrine or dopamine 2. Inotropic agent	1. Norepinephrine (↑HR or arrhythmias) 2. Dopamine (↓HR preferred but associated with higher risk of arrhythmias)	Inotropic agent when stabilized and after revascularization (MI only)
Euvolemic cold and dry (LVEDP may be low, and patients may tolerate fluid boluses)	1. Norepinephrine or dopamine 2. Inotropic agent 3. Small fluid boluses	1. Norepinephrine (preferred in ↑HR or arrhythmias) 2. Dopamine (↓HR preferred but associated with higher risk of arrhythmias)	Inotropic agent when stabilized and after revascularization (MI only)
Vasodilatory warm and wet or mixed cardiogenic and vasodilatory (low SVR)	Norepinephrine		Hemodynamics-guided therapy
RV shock	1. Fluid boluses 2. Norepinephrine, dopamine, or vasopressin 3. Inotropic agents 4. Inhaled pulmonary vasodilators	1. Maintaining preload 2. Lowering RV afterload 3. Treat absolute or relative bradycardias 4. Maintain atrioventricular synchrony	Inotropic agent after initial hemodynamic stabilization and revascularization
Normotensive shock (SBP >90 mm Hg and relatively high SVR)	Inotropic agent or vasopressor		
Aortic stenosis	1. Phenylephrine or vasopressin 2. In patients with reduced LVEF, echocardiography or PAC-guided dobutamine titration	1. An afterload-dependent state 2. Inotropy may not improve hemodynamics if LVEF is preserved	Surgical aortic valve replacement or balloon valvuloplasty and/or transcatheter aortic valve replacement
Aortic regurgitation	1. Dopamine 2. Temporary pacing	Maintaining an elevated HR may shorten diastolic filling time and reduce LVEDP	Surgical aortic valve replacement

(continued)

Table 18.2 (continued)

Cause or presentation	Vasoactive strategies	Hemodynamic rationale	Further management
Mitral stenosis	1. Phenylephrine or vasopressin 2. Esmolol or amiodarone	1. A preload-dependent state 2. Slowing the HR to increase diastolic filling time 3. Maintain atrioventricular synchrony to improve preload	Surgical mitral valve replacement or balloon valvuloplasty
Mitral regurgitation	1. Norepinephrine or dopamine 2. Inotropic agents 3. Temporary MCS, including IABP	1. Afterload reduction may help reduce LVEDP 2. IABP may reduce regurgitation fraction by reducing afterload and increasing CI	Surgical mitral Valve replacement/repair and percutaneous edge-to-edge repair
Post-infarction ventricular septal defect	1. Classic wet and cold considerations 2. Temporary MCS, including IABP	IABP reduces shunt fraction by reducing afterload and increasing CI	Cardiac surgical referral for repair or percutaneous interventional umbrella closure
Dynamic LVOT Obstruction	1. Fluid boluses 2. Phenylephrine or vasopressin 3. Avoid inotropic agents 4. Avoid vasodilating agents 5. Esmolol or amiodarone 6. RV pacing	1. Increasing preload and afterload reduces dynamic gradients 2. Reduce inotropy and ectopy 3. Maintain atrioventricular synchrony 4. Induce ventricular dyssynchrony	
Bradycardia	1. Chronotropic agents: atropine, isoproterenol, dopamine, dobutamine, and epinephrine 2. Temporary pacing	Identifying and treating underlying cause of bradycardia	
Pericardial tamponade	1. Fluid bolus 2. Norepinephrine		Pericardiocentesis or surgical pericardial window

CI cardiac index, *CS* cardiogenic shock, *HR* heart rate, *IABP* intra-aortic balloon pump, *LVEDP* left ventricular end-diastolic pressure, *LVEF* left ventricular ejection fraction, *LVOT* left ventricular outflow tract, *MCS* mechanical circulatory support, *MI* myocardial infarction, *PAC* pulmonary artery catheter, *PVR* pulmonary vascular resistance, *RV* right ventricular, *SBP* systolic blood pressure, *SVR* systemic vascular resistance

18.5.2 Epinephrine

Epinephrine is a naturally occurring catecholamine which acts on both α- and β-receptor. Epinephrine has predominantly β-adrenergic effects in lower dosage, which increases myocardial contraction and heart rate. In higher dosage, it acts on α-adrenergic receptor and constricts peripheral small vessels which can increase blood pressure. Epinephrine is associated with arrhythmia and decreases splanchnic blood flow. It also increases blood lactate levels, probably by increasing cellular metabolism. Prospective, randomized studies have not shown any beneficial effects of epinephrine over norepinephrine in septic shock. Therefore, epinephrine was considered as a second-line agent for severe cardiogenic shock.

18.5.3 Vasopressin

Vasopressin is a hormone that binds to its own receptors. Binding to V1 receptors leads to vasoconstriction due to contraction of the vascular smooth muscle, while V2 stimulation increases renal free water reabsorption. Norepinephrine is effective and safe for treating patients in septic shock and enables tapering down other vasopressors. Vasopressin deficiency can generate in those patients with severe distributive shock. Administration of low-dose vasopressin may result in substantial increases in arterial pressure. Addition of low-dose vasopressin to norepinephrine in the treatment of patients with septic shock was safe and may have been associated with a survival benefit for patients with forms of shock that were not severe and for those who also received glucocorticoids. Vasopressin should not be used at doses higher than 0.04 U per minute and should be administered only in patients with a high level of cardiac output [12, 13].

18.6 Inotropic Agents

18.6.1 Dopamine

Dopamine is a natural precursor of norepinephrine and epinephrine. Its effects are dose-dependent: at low doses (1–2 μg/kg/min), it binds to dopaminergic receptors and has a vasodilatory effect, while at higher doses (5–10 μg/kg/min), it acts as a β1 receptor agonist and thus has inotropic effects. At even higher levels (>10 μg/kg/min), dopamine stimulates α-adrenergic receptors, leading to vasoconstriction and an increase in BP. Previously, dopaminergic effects at very low doses (<3 μg/kg/min) may selectively dilate the hepatosplanchnic and renal circulations, of which the protective effect on renal function was not supported by controlled trials, and its routine use for this purpose is no longer recommended [14]. Dopaminergic stimulation may be associated with undesired endocrine effects on the hypothalamic–pituitary system and reduction of the release of prolactin, resulting in immunosuppression.

18.6.2 Dobutamine

Dobutamine acts on the myocardium by stimulating β1-adrenergic receptors to increase heart rate and enhance myocardial contractility, and it also acts on smooth muscle via β2 receptors to induce system vasodilation and lower blood pressure. As a result, dobutamine can increase cardiac output and reduce LV filling pressures. Dobutamine may be given simultaneously with norepinephrine to improve cardiac contractility. It may improve capillary perfusion in patients with septic shock, independent of its systemic effects. For CS patients, dobutamine is less likely to induce tachycardia than isoproterenol. Intravenous doses in excess of 20 μg/kg/min could not provide additional benefit. Dobutamine has limited effects on arterial pressure, although pressure may increase slightly in patients with myocardial dysfunction or decrease slightly in patients with underlying hypovolemia.

18.6.3 Levosimendan

Levosimendan increases the myocardium sensitivity of troponin C to intracellular calcium and thus has inotropic and lusitropic properties. It also acts on ATP-dependent potassium channels, making the relaxation of vascular smooth muscle associated with coronary and peripheral vasodilation. Levosimendan induces vasodilation and improves myocardial contractility without increasing oxygen requirements and affecting blood pressure or heart rate. Compared to enoximone, levosimendan showed a borderline survival benefit in AMI complicated by cardiogenic shock or low cardiac output syndrome (hazard ratio 0.33; 95% confidence interval 0.11–0.97) and had only small differences in hemodynamics and length of hospital stay [15]. This study also showed that there was no difference between levosimendan and dobutamine in cardiogenic shock. Furthermore, levosimendan has a half-life of several days, which limits the practicality of its use in acute shock states.

18.6.4 Phosphodiesterase Inhibitors (Milrinone and Enoximone)

By inhibiting PDE3, milrinone prevents degradation of cyclic adenosine monophosphate (cAMP) and increases cAMP levels, which promotes calcium uptake by cardiomyocytes and increases myocardial contractility without affecting heart rate. In vascular smooth muscle, it reduces the degradation of cAMP and accelerates the removal of intracellular calcium, leading to relaxation and vasodilation. These agents reinforce the effects of dobutamine by decreasing the metabolism of cyclic AMP. Milrinone may also be useful in patients recently treated with beta-blockers or when β-adrenergic receptors are downregulated. However, phosphodiesterase type III (PDE III) inhibitors have long half-lives (4–6 h) and may complicate with unacceptable adverse effects in patients with hypotension. Thus, intermittent and short-term infusions of small doses of PDE III inhibitors may be preferable to a continuous infusion in shock states.

18.7 Outcome

CS remains the leading cause of in-hospital mortality in the setting of an acute MI. Most longitudinal studies and registries have reported a decline in MI-associated CS mortality. The prevalence of CS from 6 to 10% in the overall population and from 7 to 12% among patients >75 years of age presenting with STEMI was reported in an analysis of the Nationwide Inpatient Sample Database between 2003 and 2010 [16]. In-hospital mortality decreased from 45 to 34% over the same time frame, although mortality rates remained high (55%) in patients >75 years of age. In the IABP-SHOCK II trial, despite inotropic and vasopressor therapy, in addition to the benefit of intra-aortic balloon counterpulsation, mortality in patients with CS complicating AMI was still around 40%. Mortality in CS patients occurs mainly in the first 3 days. Thus, besides medical therapy, mechanical circulatory support devices should be considered as soon as possible in CS patients [2].

18.8 Conclusion

CS decreases myocardial contractility and represents the majority causes of death in patients with AMI. It can result in both acute and subacute derangements to the entire circulatory system, including the peripheral vasculature. A full clinical assessment and point-of-care echocardiogram offer more information for differentiation of different mechanisms of shock. The initial approach and basic principle of treatment for CS are "VIP rules" to maintain ventilation, obtain euvolemia with volume expansion, and administer vasopressors or inotropes for the prevention or treatment of multi-organ dysfunction. Stimulation of each type of adrenergic receptor has potentially beneficial and harmful effects. For example, β-adrenergic stimulation increases blood flow but also increases heart rate and elevates the risk of myocardial ischemia; hence, the use of pure β-adrenergic agent (i.e., isoproterenol) is limited for patients with severe bradycardia. At the other extreme, α-adrenergic stimulation increases vascular tone but decreases cardiac output and impairs tissue blood flow, especially in the hepatosplanchnic region. For this reason, phenylephrine is rarely indicated. Adrenergic agonists characterize rapid onset of action, high potency, and short half-life and thus are the first-line vasopressors. In order to prevent tissue hypoperfusion and organ dysfunction, inotropes and vasopressors are essential in the management of patients in CS to maintain a mean arterial pressure of 65–70 mmHg. Physicians should keep in mind to administer vasopressor temporarily while fluid resuscitation is ongoing and discontinue it as soon as possible after hypovolemia has been corrected.

18.9 Case Example: Successful Medical Management of Cardiogenic Shock

Cheng Chung Hung and Wei-Chun Huang

18.9.1 Case Example

A 58-year-old male suffered from inferior wall STEMI. His blood pressure was low before primary PCI, which was shown as 90/60 mmHg. Fluid challenge was provided. During primary PCI, his blood pressure dropped to 80/50 mmHg with junctional rhythm, while blood clot was aspirated (Figs. 18.1 and 18.2). Therefore, atropine 1 mg was injected immediately, but in vain. Norepinephrine 100 mcg were injected directly via the coronary artery (Fig. 18.3). After 10 s, sinus tachycardia regained, and his blood pressure increased to 120/80 mmHg. Norepinephrine 10 mcg/kg/min was used to infuse continuously via the peripheral vein, and his vital sign remained stable with inotropic agents support (Figs. 18.4 and 18.5).

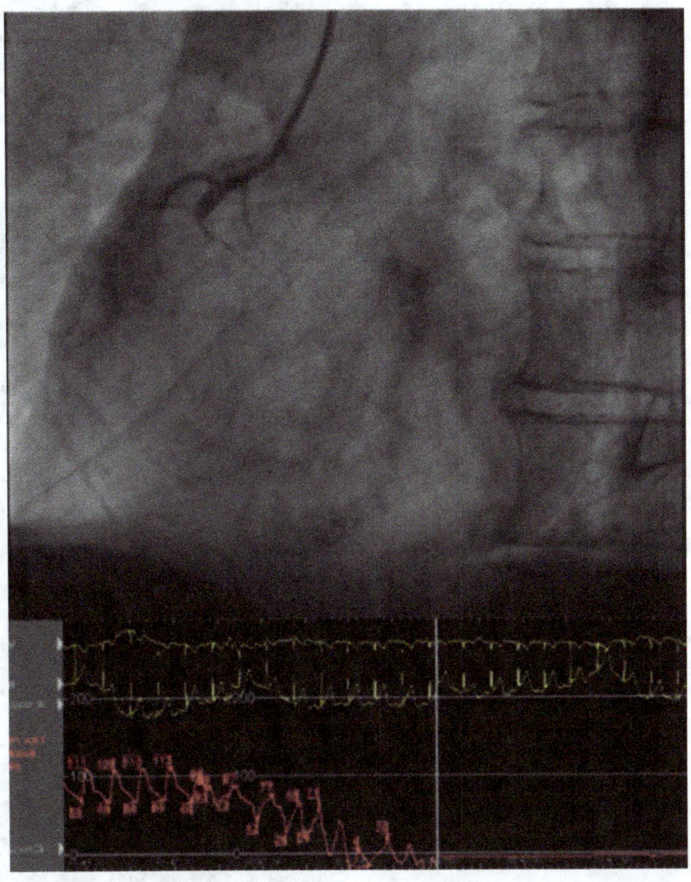

Fig. 18.1 Coronary image before percutaneous coronary intervention

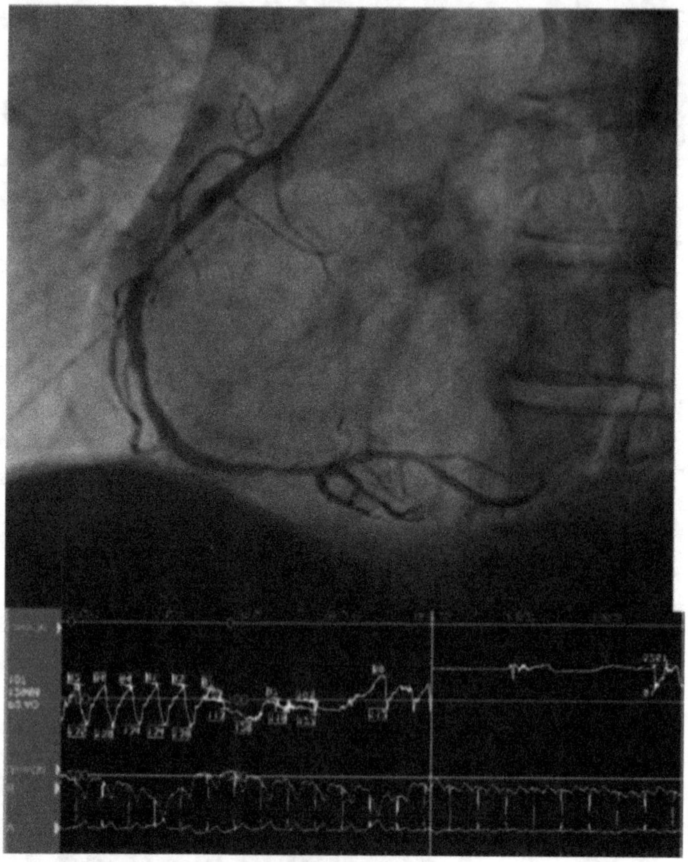

Fig. 18.2 Coronary image after thrombus aspiration

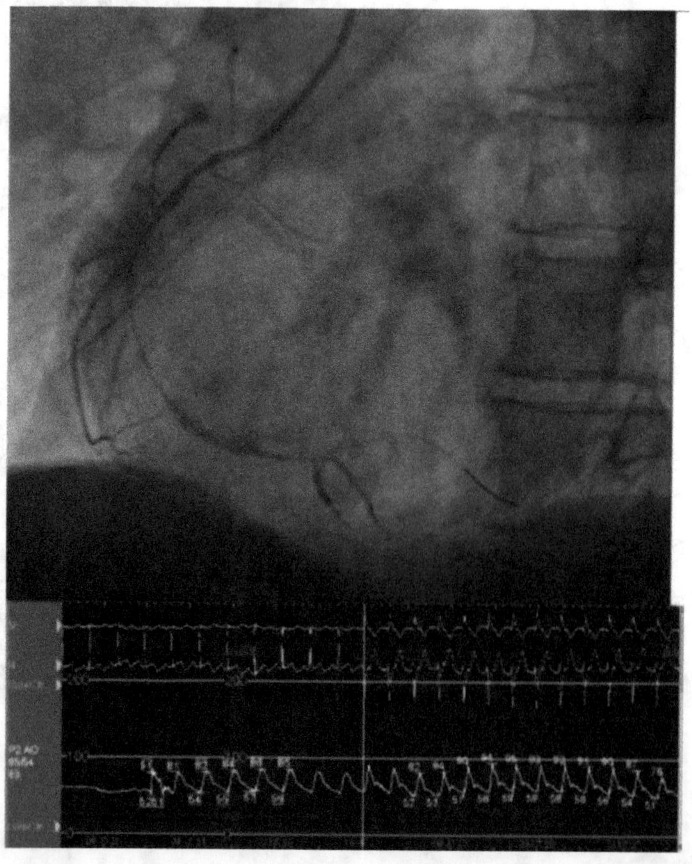

Fig. 18.3 Norepinephrine was used due to low blood pressure

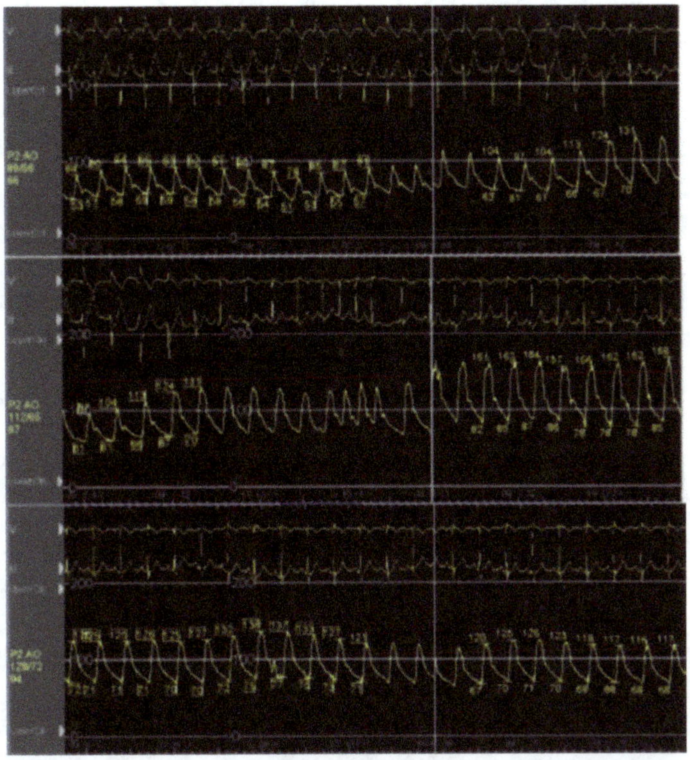

Fig. 18.4 After norepinephrine infusion, blood pressure increases rapidly

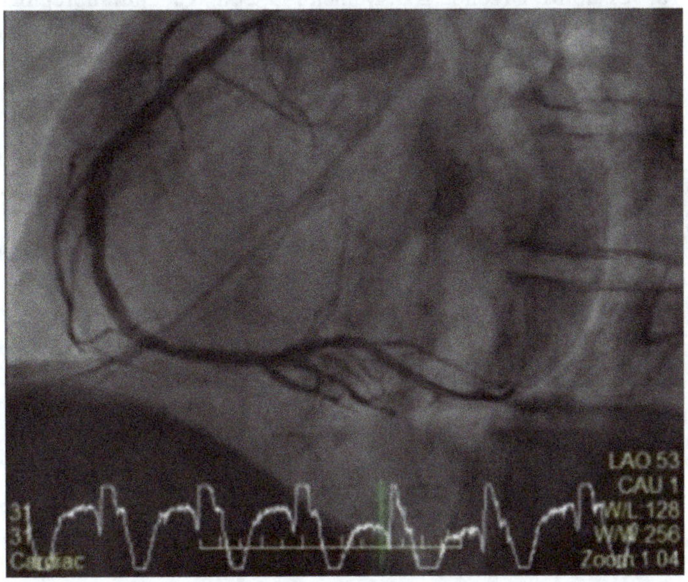

Fig. 18.5 Final images

References

1. Hochman JS, Sleeper LA, Webb JG, et al. Early revascularization in acute myocardial infarction complicated by cardiogenic SHOCK. SHOCK investigators. Should we emergently revascularize occluded coronaries for cardiogenic shock. N Engl J Med. 1999;341:625–34.
2. Thiele H, Zeymer U, Neumann FJ, Ferenc M, Olbrich HG, Hausleiter J, Richardt G, Hennersdorf M, Empen K, Fuernau G, Desch S, Eitel I, Hambrecht R, Fuhrmann J, BoÅNhm M, Ebelt H, Schneider S, Schuler G, Werdan K, IABPSHOCK II Trial Investigators. Intraaortic balloon support for myocardial infarction with cardiogenic shock. N Engl J Med. 2012;367:1287–96. https://doi.org/10.1056/NEJMoa1208410.

3. Ponikowski P, Voors AA, Anker SD, Bueno H, Cleland JG, Coats AJ, Falk V, GonzaÅLlez-Juanatey JR, Harjola VP, Jankowska EA, Jessup M, Linde C, Nihoyannopoulos P, Parissis JT, Pieske B, Riley JP, Rosano GM, Ruilope LM, Ruschitzka F, Rutten FH, van der Meer P. 2016 ESC guidelines for the diagnosis and treatment of acute and chronic heart failure: the Task Force for the Diagnosis and Treatment of Acute and Chronic Heart Failure of the European Society of Cardiology (ESC) [published correction appears in *Eur Heart J*. 2016;38:ehw383]. Eur Heart J. 2016;37:2129–200. https://doi.org/10.1093/eurheartj/ehw128.
4. Vincent JL, De Backer D. Circulatory shock. N Engl J Med. 2013;369(18):1726–34.
5. De Backer D, Biston P, Devriendt J, Madl C, Chochrad D, Aldecoa C, Brasseur A, Defrance P, Gottignies P, Vincent JL, SOAP II Investigators. Comparison of dopamine and norepinephrine in the treatment of shock. N Engl J Med. 2010;362:779–89. https://doi.org/10.1056/NEJMoa0907118.
6. Werdan K, Russ M, Buerke M, Delle-Karth G, Geppert A, SchoÅNndube FA, German Cardiac Society, German Society of Intensive Care and Emergency Medicine, German Society for Thoracic and Cardiovascular Surgery, Austrian Society of Internal and General Intensive Care Medicine; German Interdisciplinary Association of Intensive Care and Emergency Medicine, Austrian Society of Cardiology, German Society of Anaesthesiology and Intensive Care Medicine, German Society of Preventive Medicine and Rehabilitation. Cardiogenic shock due to myocardial infarction: diagnosis, monitoring and treatment: a German- Austrian S3 Guideline. Dtsch Arztebl Int. 2012;109:343–51. https://doi.org/10.3238/arztebl.2012.0343.
7. Amado J, Gago P, Santos W, Mimoso J, de Jesus I. Cardiogenic shock: inotropes and vasopressors. Rev Port Cardiol. 2016;35(12):681–95.
8. Arrigo M, Mebazaa A. Understanding the differences among inotropes. Intensive Care Med. 2015;41(5):912.
9. Francis GS, Bartos JA, Adatya S. Inotropes. J Am Coll Cardiol. 2014;63:2069–78.
10. Jessup M, Greenberg B, Mancini D, et al. Calcium upregulation by percutaneous administration of gene therapy in cardiac disease (CUPID): a phase 2 trial of intracoronary gene therapy of sarcoplasmic reticulum Ca2+-ATPase in patients with advanced heart failure. Circulation. 2011;124:304–13.
11. van Diepen S, Katz JN, Albert NM, Henry TD, Jacobs AK, Kapur NK, Kilic A, Menon V, Ohman EM, Sweitzer NK, Thiele H, Washam JB, Cohen MG. Contemporary management of cardiogenic shock: a scientific statement from the American Heart Association. Circulation. 2017;136(16):e232–68.
12. Russell JA, Walley KR, Singer J, et al. Vasopressin versus norepinephrine infusion in patients with septic shock. N Engl J Med. 2008;358:877–87.
13. Russell JA, Walley KR, Gordon AC, et al. Interaction of vasopressin infusion, corticosteroid treatment, and mortality of septic shock. Crit Care Med. 2009;37:811–8.
14. Bellomo R, Chapman M, Finfer S, Hickling K, Myburgh J. Low-dose dopamine in patients with early renal dysfunction: a placebo-controlled randomised trial. Lancet. 2000;356:2139–43.
15. Unverzagt S, Wachsmuth L, Hirsch K, Thiele H, Buerke M, Haerting J, Werdan K, Prondzinsky R. Inotropic agents and vasodilator strategies for acute myocardial infarction complicated by cardiogenic shock or low cardiac output syndrome. Cochrane Database Syst Rev. 2014;1:CD009669.
16. Kolte D, Khera S, Aronow WS, Mujib M, Palaniswamy C, Sule S, Jain D, Gotsis W, Ahmed A, Frishman WH, Fonarow GC. Trends in incidence, management, and outcomes of cardiogenic shock complicating ST-elevation myocardial infarction in the United States. J Am Heart Assoc. 2014;3:e000590. https://doi.org/10.1161/JAHA.113.000590.

Further Readings

Amado J, Gago P, Santos W, Mimoso J, de Jesus I. Cardiogenic shock: inotropes and vasopressors. Rev Port Cardiol. 2016;35(12):681–95.

van Diepen S, Katz JN, Albert NM, Henry TD, Jacobs AK, Kapur NK, Kilic A, Menon V, Ohman EM, Sweitzer NK, Thiele H, Washam JB, Cohen MG. Contemporary Management of

Cardiogenic Shock: a scientific statement from the American Heart Association. Circulation. 2017;136(16):e232-e268.

Ponikowski P, Voors AA, Anker SD, Bueno H, Cleland JG, Coats AJ, Falk V, GonzaÅLlez-Juanatey JR, Harjola VP, Jankowska EA, Jessup M, Linde C, Nihoyannopoulos P, Parissis JT, Pieske B, Riley JP, Rosano GM, Ruilope LM, Ruschitzka F, Rutten FH, van der Meer P. 2016 ESC guidelines for the diagnosis and treatment of acute and chronic heart failure: the Task Force for the Diagnosis and Treatment of Acute and Chronic Heart Failure of the European Society of Cardiology (ESC) [published correction appears in Eur Heart J. 2016;38:ehw383]. Eur Heart J. 2016;37:2129–200. https://doi.org/10.1093/eurheartj/ehw128.

Thiele H, Ohman EM, Desch S, Eitel I, de Waha S. Management of cardiogenic shock. Eur Heart J. 2015;36(20):1223–30.

Vincent JL, De Backer D. Circulatory shock. N Engl J Med. 2013;369(18):1726–34.

19 Mechanical Circulatory Support in ST-Elevation Myocardial Infarction

Nathan Lo and E. Magnus Ohman

19.1 Introduction

Cardiogenic shock (CS) occurs in approximately 8–10% of patients with ST-elevation myocardial infarction (STEMI). While immediate percutaneous coronary intervention (PCI) continues to be the mainline treatment strategy, mortality remains as high as 40% before hospital discharge. Even after hospital discharge, survivors of cardiogenic shock complicating myocardial infarction (CSMI) often suffer from severe heart failure and its consequences, including repeated hospitalization and high mortality. Mechanical circulatory support (MCS) devices during CSMI PCI can be lifesaving by supporting poor ventricular function while decreasing myocardial wall stress and relieving ischemia. In this chapter, we review the definition and pathophysiology of CSMI, the major ventricular support devices, an algorithm for MCS use in STEMI, relevant data, and a prototypic case that illustrates CSMI management augmented by MCS.

19.2 Definition and Identification of Cardiogenic Shock

Cardiogenic shock is typically defined as a cardiac index <2.2 L/min/m^2 and systolic blood pressure <90 mmHg with signs of impaired organ perfusion such as decreased urine output, altered mental status, or cool extremities. Initial evaluation of a patient with STEMI suspected to be in CS should rely on clinical bedside evaluation (Table 19.1). Generally, the focused evaluation should determine clinical stability and whether the patient exhibits signs of low cardiac

N. Lo · E. Magnus Ohman (✉)
Duke University Medical Center, Duke Clinical Research Institute, Durham, NC, USA
e-mail: erik.ohman@duke.edu

T. J. Watson et al. (eds.), *Primary Angioplasty*,
https://doi.org/10.1007/978-981-13-1114-7_19

Table 19.1 Important physical examination findings in patients with ST-elevation myocardial infarction suspected to be in cardiogenic shock

Intravascular volume status—“wet”	Cardiac output—“cold”
↑ Jugular venous pressure	Cool extremities
Rales	Hypotension
S_3 gallop	Narrow pulse pressure
Orthopnea	Altered mental status

output and high intravascular volume. The Killip classification score combines assessment of cardiac output and intravascular volume and can be helpful to quickly assess patients suffering from heart failure after myocardial infarction. Killip Class I patients show no signs of heart failure; Class II patients have rales, S_3 gallop, and venous hypertension; Class III patients have severe heart failure with pulmonary edema; and Class IV patients are in cardiogenic shock with hypotension and evidence of poor perfusion. Higher Killip score has been shown to be an independent predictor of mortality in STEMI patients and may be useful for quick risk stratification in the emergency department in patients presenting with acute coronary syndrome. This initial evaluation is vital as it guides further therapy and whether vasopressors, inotropes, or MCS need to be started concurrent with or even prior to PCI.

19.3 Pathophysiology of Cardiogenic Shock Complicating Myocardial Infarction

CS begins with pump failure but soon becomes systemic, multiorgan failure. Pump failure begins a “downward spiral” which—if unchecked—potentiates itself as worsened ischemia, causing progressive myocardial dysfunction and eventually death (Fig. 19.1). Pump failure leads to decreased cardiac output, reduced systemic perfusion, fluid retention, elevated cardiac filling pressures, decreased coronary perfusion, worsened ischemia, multiorgan failure, worsened myocardial dysfunction, and death. Pressure-volume loops provide a useful construct in visualizing the pathophysiology of CS (Fig. 19.2), as well as the effects of MCS in CS (Fig. 19.3). The rationale for mechanical support in CSMI is to (1) support pump failure and provide increased cardiac output and systemic perfusion, (2) alleviate myocardial ischemia and limit infarct size (after STEMI, a large region of myocardium is often stunned, which may regain function after revascularization with PCI, and MCS can serve to decrease myocardial wall stress and demand while bridging the time for the myocardium to recover function), and (3) delay or halt the “downward spiral.”

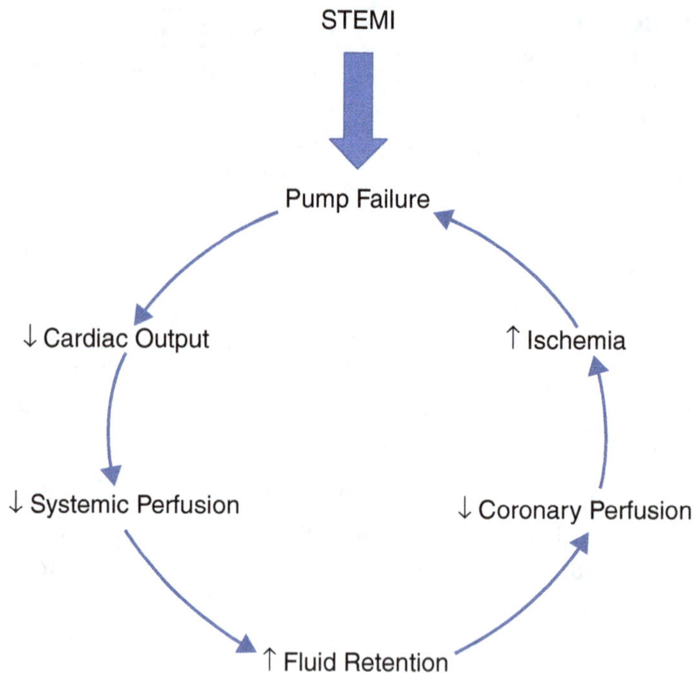

Fig. 19.1 "Downward spiral" in cardiogenic shock complicating myocardial infarction. STEMI causes left ventricular dysfunction that begets a "downward spiral" that potentiates itself. Pump failure leads to decreased cardiac output and systemic perfusion, causing increased fluid retention and elevated cardiac filling pressures, decreasing coronary perfusion, and worsening existing myocardial ischemia, which in turn worsens pump function. *STEMI* ST-elevation myocardial infarction

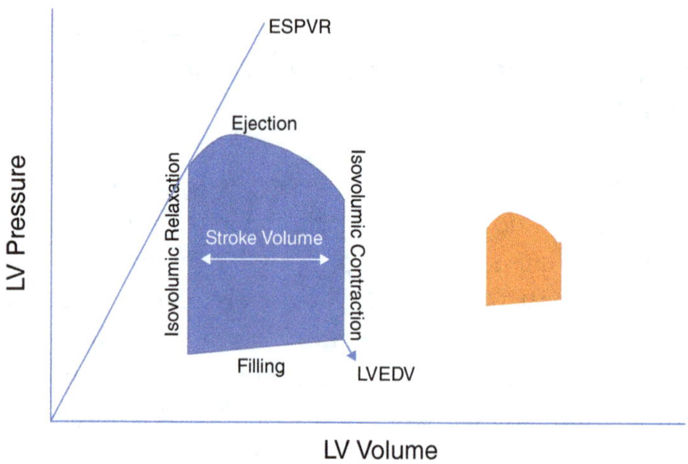

Fig. 19.2 Pressure-volume loops in normal conditions and in cardiogenic shock complicating myocardial infarction. The blue loop represents a pressure-volume loop in normal conditions, and the orange loop represents a pressure-volume loop in CSMI. Stroke volume is represented by the width of the loop, preload is represented by LVEDV, and myocardial contractility is represented by the slope of ESPVR. Compared to normal conditions, CSMI patients have lower stroke volume (decreased width of the loop), higher LVEDV, and reduced contractility (decreased ESPVR slope). *LV* left ventricle, *LVEDV* left ventricular end-diastolic volume, *ESPVR* end-systolic pressure-volume relationship

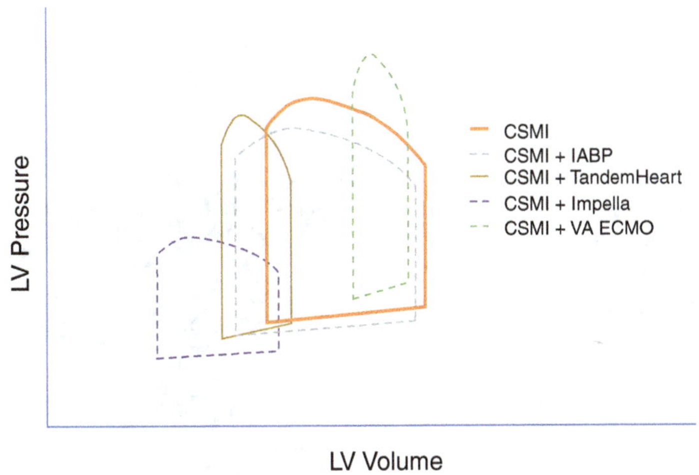

Fig. 19.3 Pressure-volume loops in cardiogenic shock and various mechanical ventricular support devices. The orange loop represents a pressure-volume loop in a patient with CSMI, while the other loops represent pressure-volume loops in patients with CSMI supported by various MCS. IABP reduces LVEDP and increases stroke volume. Both Impella and TandemHeart reduce LVEDP. Notably, VA ECMO increases LVEDP, which increases wall stress and myocardial oxygen demand. *LV* left ventricle, *CSMI* cardiogenic shock complicating myocardial infarction, *MCS* mechanical circulatory support, *IABP* intra-aortic balloon pump, *LVEDP* left ventricular end-diastolic pressure, *VA ECMO* venoarterial extracorporeal membrane oxygenation

19.4 Intra-aortic Balloon Pump

19.4.1 Introduction

The intra-aortic balloon pump (IABP) is the most widely used mechanical support device (Fig 19.4). The IABP is usually inserted via the femoral artery through a 7.5–8.0 French (Fr) sheath (Table 19.2). It is a polyethylene balloon mounted on a catheter that is inserted into the descending aorta, with the tip ideally positioned ~1–2 cm distal to the origin of the left subclavian artery. The catheter itself is connected to a console that controls timed inflation of the balloon during the cardiac cycle. Different sizes of the IABP balloon exist and should usually be chosen based on patient height:

- 4′10″–5′4″ height should receive 30 mL IABP balloon.
- 5′4″–6′0″ height should receive 40 mL IABP balloon.
- >6′0″ height should receive 50 mL IABP balloon.

19.4.2 Hemodynamic Effect

IABP works by counterpulsation in which the balloon is inflated by helium during diastole and deflated during systole. In diastole, inflation of the balloon increases aortic diastolic pressure, which enhances coronary and systemic blood flow. In

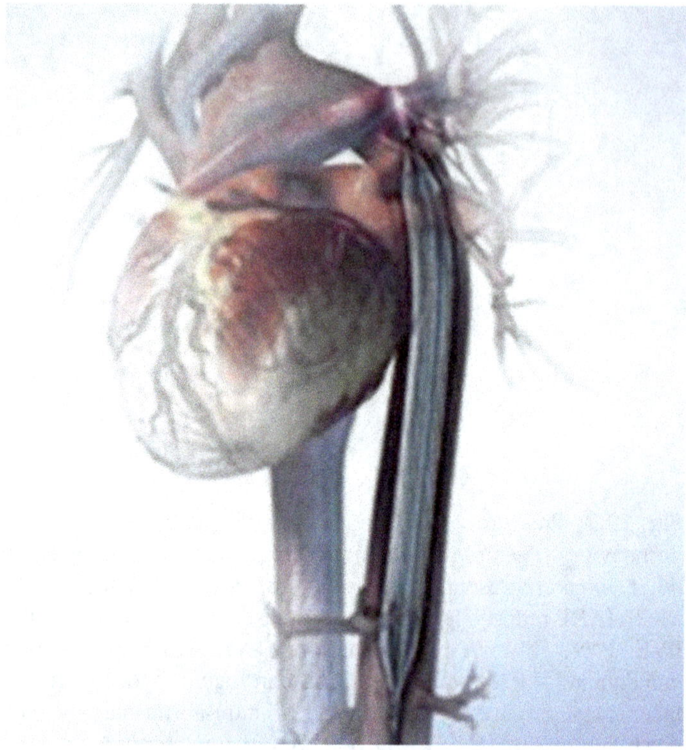

Fig. 19.4 Intra-aortic balloon pump. The intra-aortic balloon pump consists of a polyethylene balloon mounted on a catheter that is inserted into the descending aorta with the tip ~1–2 cm distal to the origin of the left subclavian artery (Image used with permission from Getinge)

Table 19.2 Comparison of mechanical circulatory support devices

	IABP	Impella 2.5, CP, 5.0	TandemHeart	VA ECMO
Pump mechanism	Pneumatic	Axial	Centrifugal	Centrifugal
Sheath size	7.5–8.0 Fr	13 Fr (2.5); 14 Fr (CP); 21 Fr (5.0)	15–19 Fr arterial; 21 Fr venous	15–17 Fr arterial; 18–21 Fr venous
Hemodynamic support	0.5 L/min	2.5 L/min (2.5); 4.0 L/min (4.0); 5.0 L/min (5.0)	3.5–5.0 L/min	4.0–6.0 L/min
Afterload	↓	↓	↑	↑↑↑
Risk of limb ischemia and bleeding	↑	↑↑	↑↑↑	↑↑↑
Complexity of insertion	↑	↑↑	↑↑↑↑	↑↑↑

IABP intra-aortic balloon pump, *VA ECMO* venoarterial extracorporeal membrane oxygenation, *Fr* French

systole, deflation of the balloon reduces left ventricle (LV) afterload and increases cardiac output (Fig. 19.5). The net effect is an increase in mean arterial pressure (MAP), reduction of LV end-diastolic volume and LV end-diastolic pressure, and decreased myocardial oxygen demand (Fig. 19.3). The hemodynamic support provided is ~0.5 L/min (Table 19.2).

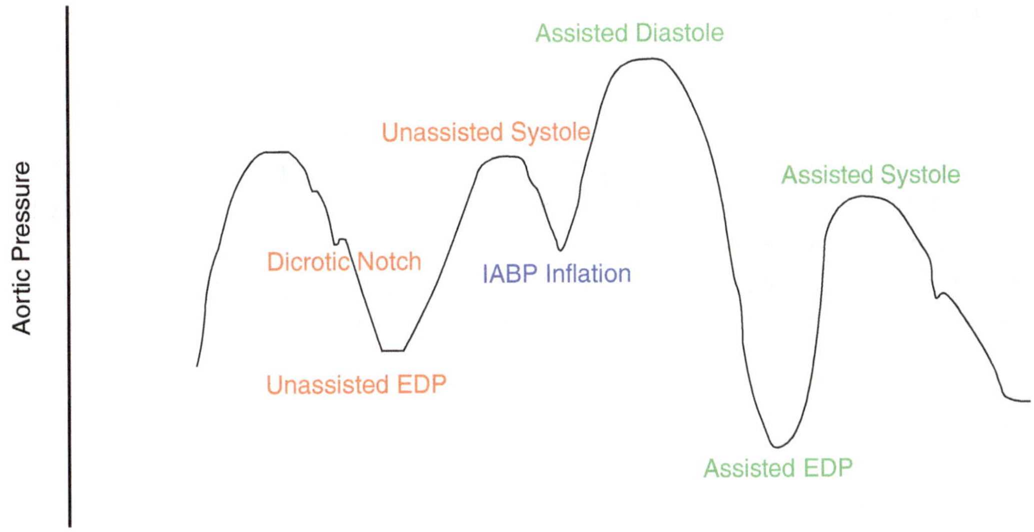

Fig. 19.5 Intra-aortic balloon pump aortic waveform. The IABP inflates at the timing of aortic valve closure or the dicrotic notch on the aortic pressure waveform. Inflation results in diastolic augmentation that is higher pressure than unassisted systole, which results in increased coronary blood flow and MAP. IABP deflates just prior to systole, resulting in a lower assisted aortic EDP and lower assisted systolic pressure. This decrease in afterload decreases myocardial demand and workload. *IABP* intra-aortic balloon pump, *MAP* mean arterial pressure, *EDP* end-diastolic pressure

19.4.3 Data

Clinical studies have failed to consistently show benefit of IABP in CSMI. While some retrospective studies and meta-analyses have shown mortality benefit with IABP in CSMI, these studies were often confounded by higher rates of revascularization in patients who received IABP. The most important study of IABP in CSMI was the IABP SHOCK II study published in 2012. This was a multicenter, open-label trial of 600 patients with CSMI receiving early revascularization who were randomized 1:1 to use of IABP or no IABP. There was no difference in the primary endpoint of 30-day all-cause mortality (39.7% in IABP group vs. 41.3% in control group; $p = 0.69$), and subsequent studies of the cohort failed to show differences in 6- and 12-month mortality. Furthermore, no difference was seen in subgroup analysis or secondary safety endpoints such as bleeding, peripheral complications, sepsis, and stroke. Critics of the study note that 10% of patients from the control group crossed over to the IABP group, some of the control group patients received left ventricular assist devices, and the vast majority of the patients received the IABP after PCI. Proponents of IABP in CSMI claim that IABP placement may be most beneficial prior to PCI to halt the progression of the "downward spiral" and to reduce infarct size. However, the CRISP AMI (Counterpulsation to Reduce Infarct Size Pre-PCI Acute Myocardial Infarction) multicenter, randomized trial failed to show that the use of IABP prior to PCI reduced infarct size measured by MRI in patients presenting with anterior STEMI without CS. The secondary endpoint of all-cause mortality at 6 months was also not statistically different between groups.

19.4.4 Guidelines

The ACC/AHA guidelines give a Class IIa (level of evidence [LOE] B) recommendation for the use of IABP in CSMI who do not stabilize with pharmacologic therapy. ESC guidelines are more stringent in their recommendation for the use of IABP in STEMI, giving a Class IIa (LOE C) recommendation only in CSMI patients who have a mechanical complication, such as papillary muscle rupture with severe mitral regurgitation or ventricular septal defect. Otherwise, ESC guidelines give IABP a Class III recommendation (LOE B) for routine use in STEMI patients (Table 19.3).

19.4.5 Contraindications

- Severe aortic regurgitation
- Aortic dissection
- Severe aortic-iliac-femoral vascular disease
- Severe thrombocytopenia
- Abdominal aortic aneurysm
- Sepsis

19.4.6 Complications

The incidence of complications is ~7% based on outcomes data from the Benchmark Counterpulsation Outcomes Registry of 16,909 patients undergoing IABP therapy between 1996 and 2000. Independent risk factors for major complications of IABP

Table 19.3 ACC/AHA and ESC guidelines for use of mechanical support in ST-elevation myocardial infarction

Mechanical assist device	ACC/AHA guidelines		ESC guidelines	
IABP	Class IIa (LOE B)	CSMI that does not stabilize quickly with pharmacological therapy	Class IIa (LOE C)	CSMI due to mechanical complications
			Class III (LOE B)	Routine use in STEMI
Impella/TandemHeart/ECMO	Class IIb (LOE C)	May be considered in refractory CSMI	Class IIb (LOE C)	Short-term use may be considered in refractory CSMI

ACC/AHA American College of Cardiology/American Heart Association, *ESC* European Society of Cardiology, *IABP* intra-aortic balloon pump, *LOE* level of evidence, *CSMI* cardiogenic shock complicating myocardial infarction, *STEMI* ST-elevation myocardial infarction, *ECMO* extracorporeal membrane oxygenation were peripheral vascular disease, female sex, body surface area < 1.65 m^2, and age ≥ 75 years. Complications of IABP include:

- Severe bleeding
- Limb ischemia
- Stroke
- Balloon leak or rupture
- Thrombocytopenia
- Hemolysis
- Aortic dissection
- Renal artery, mesenteric artery, or left subclavian artery obstruction
- Infection/sepsis

19.5 Axial-Flow Pump (Impella)

19.5.1 Introduction

The Impella consists of a miniature axial-flow pump system that continuously pulls blood from the LV into the ascending aorta, thus augmenting cardiac output (Fig. 19.6). The pump is mounted on a catheter that is inserted retrograde across

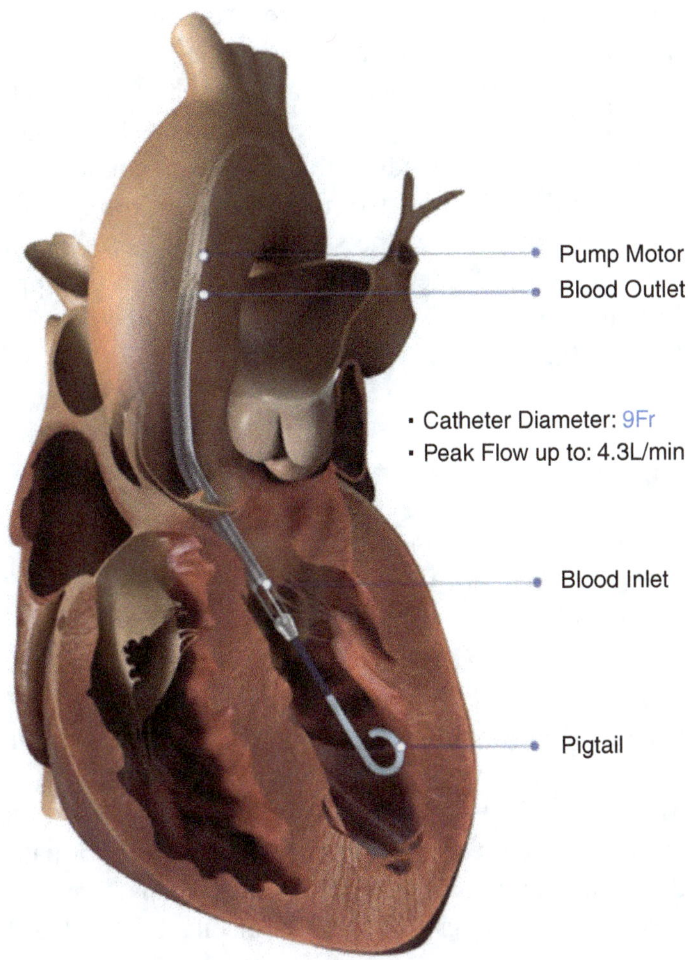

Fig. 19.6 Impella CP. The Impella is placed retrograde across the aortic valve, with the pigtail and inlet area in the left ventricle and the outlet area in the ascending aorta. Blood is continuously pulled from the left ventricle into the ascending aorta. *CP* cardiac power (© 2018 Abiomed, Inc, image used with permission)

the aortic valve, usually via the femoral artery. The tip of the catheter is in the shape of a pigtail for stabilization and safety of the device in the LV. Near the tip of the catheter is an inlet area, from which blood is pulled to be expelled through the outlet area into the aorta. While three versions of the device are available, Impella 2.5 and the Impella cardiac power (CP) are most commonly used in STEMI since they can both be inserted percutaneously. The third version, Impella 5.0, requires surgical cutdown. Although all three devices have a 9 Fr catheter, the size of the femoral artery sheath varies due to different sizes of the pump motor (Table 19.2):

- Impella 2.5: 12 Fr pump motor requiring a 13 Fr femoral arterial sheath
- Impella CP: 14 Fr pump motor requiring a 14 Fr femoral arterial sheath
- Impella 5.0: 21 Fr pump motor requiring a 22 Fr femoral arterial sheath

Similar to the IABP, the Impella is connected to a console outside of the body that powers and regulates its function.

19.5.2 Hemodynamic Effect

By directly removing blood from the LV, the Impella reduces LV end-diastolic volume and end-diastolic pressure. The blood is expelled into the ascending aorta, which increases aortic root pressure and increases coronary perfusion during diastole. The net effect is an increase in cardiac output, MAP, and coronary perfusion, with a decrease in wall stress. The Impella more markedly reduces LV volumes and preload compared with an IABP, thus reducing myocardial oxygen demands of the LV which can be visualized as the area inside the loop (Fig. 19.3). It is also important to note that the width of the pressure-volume loop only shows the stroke volume produced by the heart and not by the contributions of the Impella. Hemodynamic support is ~2.5 L/min for the Impella 2.5, ~4.0 L/min for the Impella CP, and ~5.0 L/min for the Impella 5.0 (Table 19.2).

19.5.3 Data

The most important study evaluating the use of Impella in CSMI is the ISAR-SHOCK (Efficacy Study of LV Assist Device to Treat Patients with Cardiogenic Shock) trial, which tested whether Impella 2.5 provided superior hemodynamic support in CSMI compared with IABP. This prospective trial randomized 26 patients presenting with CSMI to either IABP or Impella 2.5 implantation after PCI. The primary endpoint of hemodynamic improvement after 30 minutes of device implantation was significantly better in patients receiving the Impella 2.5 versus IABP (Δcardiac index = 0.49 ± 0.46 L/min/m^2 vs. 0.11 ± 0.31 L/min/m^2; $p = 0.02$). Overall 30-day mortality was 46% in both groups. However, the study had a small number of patients and was not powered to detect mortality differences between groups. Similar to criticisms of the IABP SHOCK II trial, proponents of Impella 2.5 in CSMI note that the patients in

ISAR-SHOCK received the mechanical devices only after revascularization, when the expected benefit may not be as large. Indeed, an observational study evaluating 154 consecutive unselected patients from the USpella Registry who received Impella 2.5 in CSMI found that the patients who received Impella 2.5 prior to PCI had significantly better survival to hospital discharge compared with patients who received Impella 2.5 after PCI (65.1 vs. 40.7%; $p = 0.003$). In the interval following the publication of the ISAR-SHOCK results, the Impella CP became available, which can also be placed percutaneously and should provide greater hemodynamic support in CSMI. However, no randomized trials have evaluated the Impella CP or 5.0 in CSMI.

19.5.4 Guidelines

Both ACC/AHA and ESC guidelines give Impella a Class IIb (LOE C) indication for use in refractory CSMI (Table 19.3).

19.5.5 Contraindications

- Mechanical aortic valve
- Critical severe aortic stenosis
- Moderate to severe aortic regurgitation
- LV thrombus
- Ventricular septal defect
- Severe peripheral arterial disease
- Severe sepsis

19.5.6 Complications

The most common complication of Impella is bleeding, given the need for anticoagulation and the 13–22 Fr size catheters needed for arterial access. In the Impella-EUROSHOCK-registry that retrospectively evaluated 120 patients receiving Impella 2.5 for CSMI, bleeding requiring transfusion occurred in 24.2% of patients, and bleeding requiring surgery occurred in 4.2% of patients. Other complications of Impella include:

- Limb ischemia
- Stroke
- LV injury or perforation
- Cardiac tamponade
- Hemolysis
- Arrhythmias
- Acquired von Willebrand syndrome
- Mitral regurgitation secondary to chordal rupture
- Functional mitral stenosis

19.6 Extracorporeal Left Heart Bypass (TandemHeart)

19.6.1 Introduction

The TandemHeart is an extracorporeal left atrial to arterial assist device (Fig. 19.7). Unlike the IABP and Impella that require only arterial access, the TandemHeart requires both venous and arterial access. It is inserted by first creating a transseptal puncture from the right atrium into the left atrium. After a guidewire is passed into the left atrium and the transseptal opening is sufficiently dilated, a 21 Fr cannula is inserted via the femoral vein, up the inferior vena cava, through the right atrium, and into the left atrium. The cannula has a large end-hole and multiple side holes that

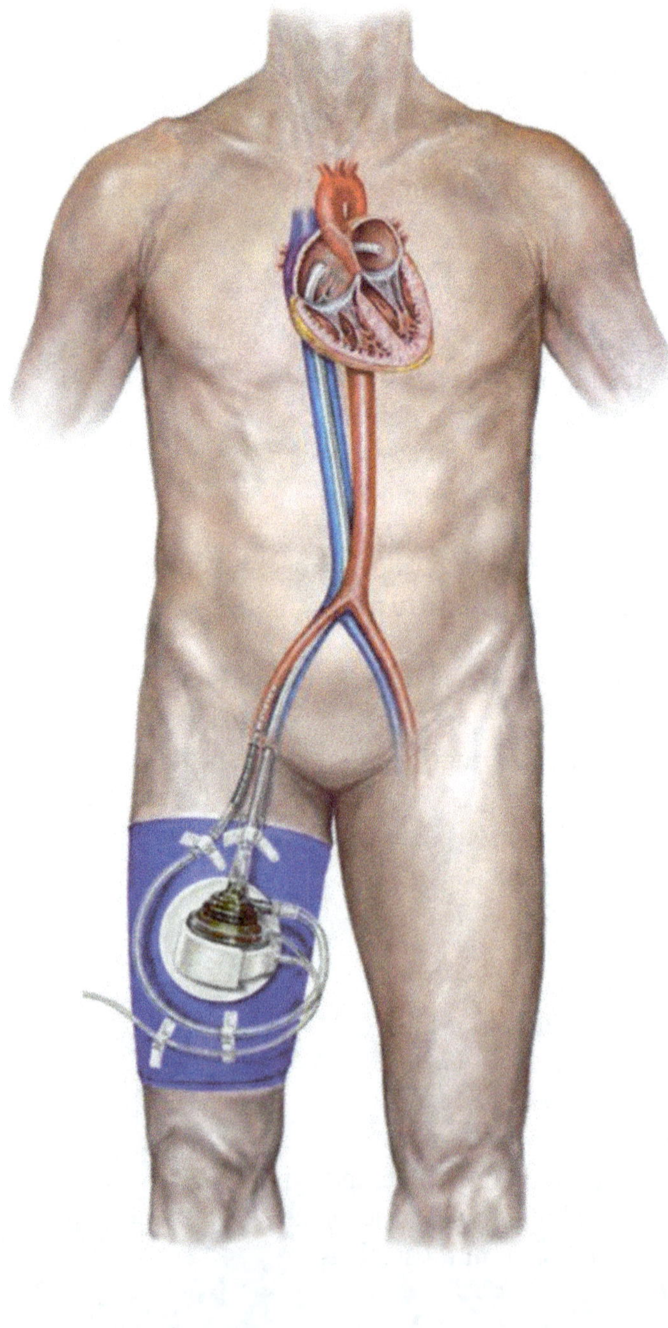

Fig. 19.7 TandemHeart. The TandemHeart is a left atrial to arterial extracorporeal device that requires atrial transseptal puncture. A cannula is situated into the left atrium and aspirates oxygenated blood, which is delivered to the body by a femoral artery outflow cannula (Image used with permission from CardiacAssist)

allow for aspiration of oxygenated left atrial blood. The aspirated blood is pulled into an extracorporeal centrifugal pump that pumps the blood into a 15 Fr–19 Fr arterial outflow cannula in the femoral artery. An external console controls the pump.

19.6.2 Hemodynamic Effect

By taking blood from the left atrium, the TandemHeart directly reduces left atrial pressure, which reduces LV end-diastolic volume and LV end-diastolic pressure (Fig. 19.3). Afterload is mildly increased due to the blood flow into the large outflow cannula in the femoral artery. The net effect is an increase in cardiac output, MAP, and coronary perfusion, with a decrease in wall stress. The TandemHeart works in "tandem" with the native heart; therefore, the aorta is still perfused via the native LV pump as well as the TandemHeart pump. However, due to the decrease in preload and increase in afterload associated with the TandemHeart, the contribution to cardiac output from the native heart usually falls. It is not uncommon to have a flat, non-pulsatile arterial waveform on the display console showing little contribution of pulsatile blood flow from heart. Hemodynamic support is ~3.5–5.0 L/min, mostly depending on the size of the femoral artery outflow cannula (Table 19.2).

19.6.3 Data

The most important study evaluating TandemHeart in CSMI was a prospective, single-center, randomized trial published in 2005 comparing IABP to TandemHeart in the setting of intended PCI of the infarct artery in 41 patients. The primary outcome of improvement in cardiac power index was much greater for the TandemHeart group compared with the IABP group (0.22–0.37 W/m^2 vs. 0.22–0.28 W/m^2; $p = 0.004$). Pulmonary capillary wedge pressure and serum creatinine levels also decreased. However, 30-day mortality was similar between the two groups (IABP 45% vs. TandemHeart 43%; $p = 0.86$). Complications such as severe bleeding and limb ischemia were seen much more frequently in the TandemHeart patients. Limitations of the study included its lack of power to detect mortality differences as well as the lack of generalizability since >50% of study patients were excluded from the study.

19.6.4 Guidelines

Both ACC/AHA and ESC guidelines give TandemHeart a Class IIb (LOE C) indication for use in refractory CSMI (Table 19.3).

19.6.5 Contraindications

- Bleeding diathesis
- Severe peripheral vascular disease

- Severe right ventricular dysfunction
- Severe aortic regurgitation
- Ventricular septal defect

19.6.6 Complications

The major complications of the TandemHeart are severe bleeding and limb ischemia. In the randomized trial in 2005 noted above, 19 of the 21 patients randomized to TandemHeart required blood transfusions. Most of the patients had bleeding at the arterial access site. Seven of the 21 patients developed limb ischemia that either required surgical or percutaneous revascularization. Other complications of TandemHeart include:

- Atrial perforation
- Cardiac tamponade
- Thromboembolism
- Infection/sepsis/systemic inflammatory response syndrome
- Stroke

19.7 Extracorporeal Membrane Oxygenation

19.7.1 Introduction

Venoarterial extracorporeal membrane oxygenation (VA ECMO) can be percutaneously placed at the bedside or catheterization laboratory table, providing not only circulatory support but also gas exchange (Fig. 19.8). An 18–21 Fr inflow cannula is placed via the femoral vein into the right atrium. A 15–17 Fr outflow cannula is placed via the femoral artery into the aorta (Table 19.2). Deoxygenated blood is removed from the right atrium by an extracorporeal centrifugal pump into a membrane oxygenator for gas exchange, and the oxygenated blood is then pumped back into the patient via the femoral artery cannula. A perfusionist is needed to assemble and manage the circuit.

19.7.2 Hemodynamic Effect

Although VA ECMO directly removes blood from the right atrium, it does not decrease LV preload. This is due to pulmonary and bronchial venous return to the LV. VA ECMO also increases afterload due to the retrograde flow via the femoral artery cannula into the aorta. The combined effect of both increased preload and afterload of the LV results in an overloaded LV with elevated LV end-diastolic volume and LV end-diastolic pressure (Fig. 19.3), causing increased wall stress and myocardial oxygen consumption. In CSMI, this increase in wall stress can worsen ischemia and LV function, as well as decrease the likelihood of stunned

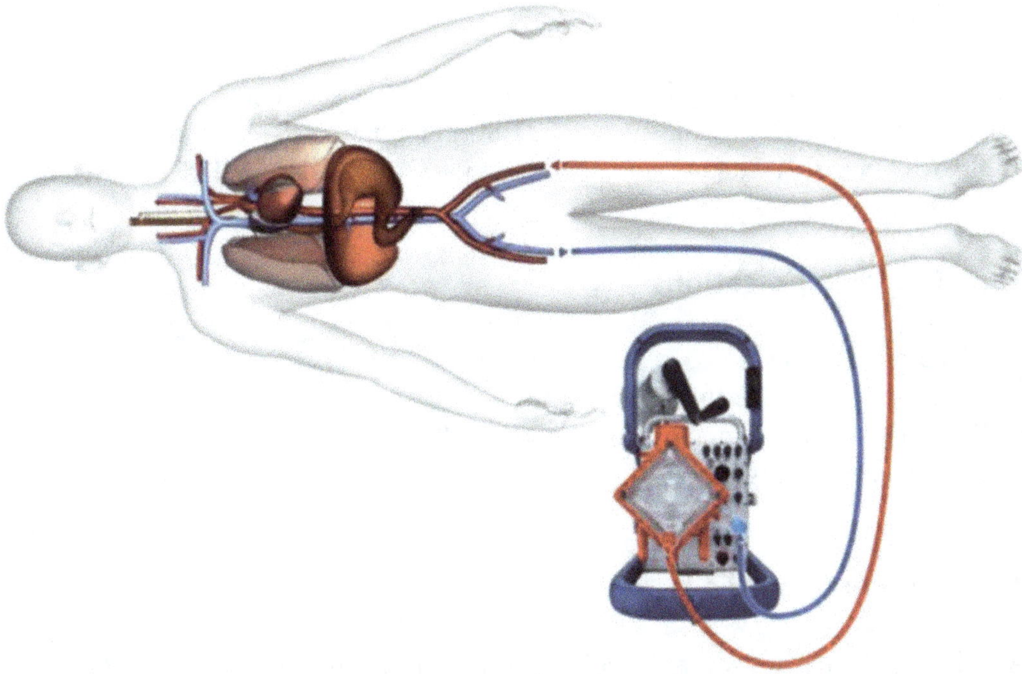

Fig. 19.8 Venoarterial extracorporeal membrane oxygenation. Venoarterial extracorporeal membrane oxygenation is a unique MCS device that provides both circulatory support and gas exchange. Deoxygenated blood is removed from the right atrium by a large venous cannula and pumped through a membrane oxygenator for gas exchange, and the oxygenated blood is delivered to the body through a large outflow femoral artery cannula. *MCS* mechanical circulatory support (Image used with permission from Getinge)

myocardium to recover. Hemodynamic support is ~4.0–6.0 L/min, with significant increases in MAP and total cardiac output (Table 19.2).

19.7.3 Data

The data for ECMO in CSMI are from retrospective, small studies. One single-center study evaluated 30-day outcomes in patients with STEMI complicated by profound CS, defined as systolic blood pressure $\leq$ 75 mmHg after IABP and inotrope agents. This study compared 46 patients with profound CSMI treated with primary PCI and ECMO between 2002 and 2009 with a historical control group of 25 patients with profound CSMI treated with primary PCI without ECMO between 1993 and 2002. Thirty-day mortality in the group treated with ECMO and PCI was significantly lower than the historical group (72 vs. 32%, RRR 46%; $p = 0.003$). However, results may be confounded due to the large temporal differences between the groups, as some of the improvement in mortality may be due to improved adjunctive pharmacotherapy, equipment, and technique. Other retrospective studies have suggested that VA ECMO may be particularly beneficial in CSMI patients with cardiac arrest, with improvements in short- and mid-term survival. No randomized controlled trials exist for ECMO in CSMI.

19.7.4 Guidelines

Both ACC/AHA and ESC guidelines give ECMO a Class IIb (LOE C) indication for use in refractory CSMI (Table 19.3). The ESC guidelines also recommend considering ECMO in CSMI patients who continue to deteriorate despite IABP.

19.7.5 Contraindications

- Bleeding diathesis
- Severe peripheral vascular disease
- Prolonged cardiopulmonary resuscitation (CPR)
- Severe aortic regurgitation

19.7.6 Complications

As with TandemHeart, severe bleeding and limb ischemia are major complications of ECMO. Unique to ECMO among the mechanical support devices, however, are the complications resulting from LV overload. Over time, LV dilatation, LV thrombus, pulmonary edema, and pulmonary venous hypertension may occur. Strategies to "vent" the LV such as IABP, Impella, atrial septostomy, or direct LV decompression may decrease complications from LV overload. Other complications of ECMO include:

- Acquired von Willebrand deficiency
- Hemolysis
- Thrombocytopenia
- Infection/sepsis/systemic inflammatory response syndrome
- Coronary and cerebral hypoxia
- Renal insufficiency
- Stroke

19.8 Practical Approach to the Use of Mechanical Support Devices in STEMI

The main decision points for use of mechanical support in STEMI are (1) when to initiate MCS and (2) which device to use. MCS needs to be carefully selected in STEMI patients. First, an evaluation based on vital signs, physical examination, and available data needs to be conducted. If the patient exhibits no evidence of cardiogenic shock, then prompt revascularization without planned MCS should be the initial strategy. An algorithm for MCS in STEMI is shown in Fig. 19.9.

For patients who initially present in shock, either immediate revascularization or early use of MCS with prompt revascularization is the preferred strategy. As

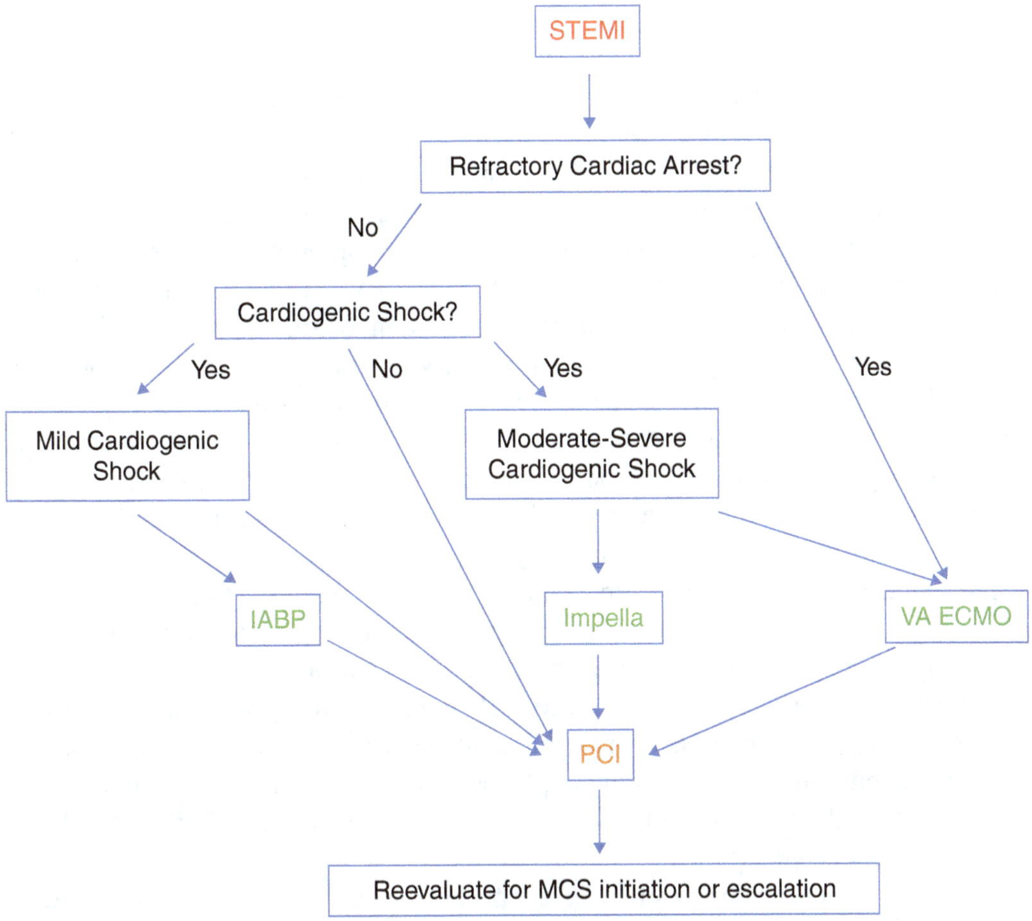

Fig. 19.9 Algorithm for mechanical circulatory support in STEMI. *STEMI* ST-elevation myocardial infarction, *IABP* intra-aortic balloon pump, *VA ECMO* venoarterial extracorporeal membrane oxygenation, *PCI* percutaneous coronary intervention

discussed earlier in this chapter, there is no clear evidence that MCS should be routinely used in CSMI. Despite the benefits of MCS, the use of support devices exposes the patient to more complications—especially bleeding—and may also delay door-to-device time. Prompt revascularization in CSMI continues to be the ultimate goal, with Class I indications from both AHA and ESC. The randomized SHOCK trial in 1999 showed that patients presenting with CSMI had statistically significant improved survival at 6 months with emergency revascularization compared with initial medical stabilization, despite a high use of IABP in both groups. Regardless of the initial strategy chosen, once stabilized in the emergency department, patients with CSMI should be immediately rushed to the cardiac catheterization laboratory, at which point the operator can proceed with either primary PCI or MCS with subsequent PCI. If the patient cannot be stabilized in the emergency department and has refractory cardiac arrest despite high-quality advanced cardiovascular life support, then consideration should be given for ECMO.

If the patient with CSMI requires no inotropic or vasopressor therapy, or only low-dose therapy, and signs of only mild CS (wedge <20, normal mental status), then we generally proceed with immediate PCI. However, if the patient is requiring either increasing doses of adjunctive pharmacologic therapy or is already on multiple inotropes or vasopressors and has signs of moderate to severe CS (wedge >20, altered mental status, cool extremities, elevated serum lactate), then MCS should first be initiated prior to PCI in the cardiac catheterization laboratory. Pharmacological therapy such as inotropes and vasopressors may be used to stabilize the patient, but these agents may actually be harmful over time. Vasopressors increase MAP and improve hypotension but at the cost of increased LV afterload, which increases myocardial work and demand, leading to worsened myocardial ischemia. Similarly, inotropes improve pump function but directly increase myocardial work and demand, again leading to worsened myocardial ischemia. Furthermore, these drugs are often proarrhythmic and inadequately support a failing heart pump. Thus, while a patient may initially be "stable" on vasopressor and inotrope therapy, the increased myocardial workload and ischemia with these agents may hasten the "downward spiral" of cardiogenic shock. Conversely, mechanical ventricular support devices can provide greater circulatory support, reduce filling pressures, reduce myocardial wall stress and demand, increase coronary perfusion, and even limit infarct size. Therefore, for patients in moderate to severe CS with moderate or high doses of inotropes or vasopressors, MCS prior to PCI should be strongly considered to support the patient and to relieve myocardial demand and ischemia. Similarly, if a STEMI patient who initially received planned PCI without MCS deteriorates and develops CS, then strong consideration should be given for immediate MCS implantation.

Consideration of which mechanical support device to be used is mostly based on the amount of hemodynamic support needed, risk of bleeding, ease and rapidity of placement, and contraindications (Table 19.2). Immediate measurement of LV end-diastolic pressure and the performance of a left ventriculogram should be done to help assess the severity of CS, dysfunction of the LV, and any possible mechanical complications. Additionally, if concern for peripheral arterial disease exists, ilio-femoral angiography should be quickly done via a femoral artery sheath to help determine whether the femoral artery is suitable for an MCS device. In general, the favored MCS devices should be the IABP and Impella CP. While the IABP is relatively inexpensive, generally safe, and straightforward to implant, the tradeoff is that it provides only modest hemodynamic support. Impella CP provides much greater hemodynamic support and is a better choice for patients in severe CS. It can still be inserted percutaneously, and provides greater hemodynamic support than the Impella 2.5, with a femoral artery sheath only 1 Fr size larger. It can provide nearly the same forward cardiac output as the TandemHeart without the technical challenges associated with the latter device (the larger femoral artery sheath and the need for a transseptal puncture). Finally, while VA ECMO can effectively provide complete cardiopulmonary support, it also increases afterload and can worsen myocardial ischemia. Thus, generally patients in mild CS should receive IABP with frequent reevaluation for device escalation (replacement with Impella or VA ECMO), and those with moderate to severe CS should receive Impella CP. VA ECMO should be reserved for those patients in cardiac arrest.

19.9 Summary

MCS in STEMI can be useful in carefully selected patients with cardiogenic shock. Early identification of CS is paramount, and early initiation of MCS can help support a failing LV, reduce filling pressures, improve coronary perfusion, relieve myocardial ischemia, and ultimately prevent the "downward spiral" of CS that leads to multiorgan failure and death. An algorithm for use of MCS in STEMI patients helps select which patients may benefit from MCS and which ventricular support device may be optimal. Ultimately, a multidisciplinary team approach to patients with CSMI is vital, as quick action and communication from EMS, emergency medicine physicians, interventional cardiologists, cardiac surgeons, nurses, and technicians can stabilize and identify the patients who are best candidates for mechanical ventricular support devices.

19.10 Case Report: Severe Cardiogenic Shock in Context of Cardiac Arrest

Nathan Lo and E. Magnus Ohman

19.10.1 Case Report

A 66-year-old female with history of hypertension, hyperlipidemia, and smoking abuse presented with chest pain at home prompting a call to emergency medical services (EMS). Upon EMS arrival, she was hypotensive with electrocardiogram (ECG) showing sinus bradycardia and ST-elevations in leads II, III, and AVF. On arrival to the emergency department, she sustained a pulseless electrical activity (PEA) arrest requiring CPR, epinephrine administration, and intubation. She regained return of spontaneous circulation (ROSC) after several minutes, but she remained hypotensive requiring norepinephrine drip at a low dose. Physical examination was notable for elevated JVP of ~16 mmHg, S3 gallop, and no rales. She was given IV heparin and PO aspirin via an orogastric tube. She was quickly taken to the cardiac catheterization laboratory.

On the catheterization laboratory table, she had a bradycardic cardiac arrest requiring CPR, atropine, and epinephrine. She regained ROSC after several minutes. We obtained access in the right femoral artery with a 6 Fr sheath and performed diagnostic angiograms of the left and right coronary arteries. This revealed three-vessel disease with a culprit proximal 95% dominant RCA thrombotic occlusion, 80% mid-LAD lesion, and 90% large ramus lesion (Fig. 19.10). A pigtail catheter was used to cross the aortic valve revealing LVEDP of 19 mmHg and akinetic inferior and apical walls with LV ejection fraction ~40% on left ventriculogram. Arterial blood gas showed a pH of 7.07, PCO_2 of 63, and PO_2 of 154, and the tidal volume and respiratory rate were increased on the ventilator.

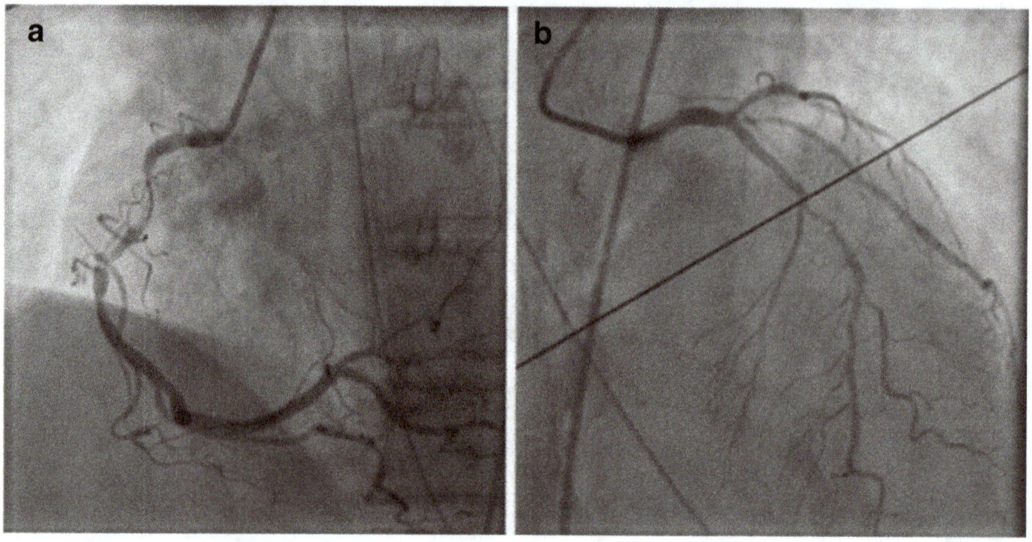

Fig. 19.10 Severe three-vessel disease in a patient with cardiogenic shock complicating STEMI. Angiography reveals a dominant RCA with culprit 95% lesion (**a**), 80% mid-LAD lesion, and 90% ostial ramus lesion (**b**). *STEMI* ST-elevation myocardial infarction, *RCA* right coronary artery, *LAD* left anterior descending artery

We decided to proceed directly with PCI of her culprit RCA lesion without upfront MCS due to her mild cardiogenic shock and low vasopressor requirements, although upfront IABP placement could arguably have been better. Eptifibatide bolus and drip was started. On balloon inflation of her RCA occlusion, the patient became bradycardic and hypotensive, requiring further brief CPR, atropine, and epinephrine administration. Angiography of her RCA showed slow flow. We immediately proceeded to IABP placement via the left femoral artery. She had excellent diastolic augmentation with MAP in the 90s. Flow in her RCA improved, and we proceeded to stent her RCA with a 3.0 × 38 mm drug-eluting stent, with distal embolization to a posterolateral branch (Fig. 19.11). Her MAP decreased to 70s despite the IABP and vasopressor support. A Swan-Ganz catheter was placed via her right femoral vein which showed mean RA pressure of 16 mmHg, RV pressure of 33/15 mmHg, PA pressure of 33/21 mmHg with mean of 26 mmHg, and wedge of 19 mmHg. PA saturations were 52 and 54% in duplicate, and Fick CO was 2.2 L/min with index of 1.4 L/min-m^2. We considered MCS device escalation to Impella and further revascularization of her other coronary disease, but given her relative stability, we decided to transfer her to the CCU and closely watch her over the next several hours. Her right femoral artery sheath was left in place in case ECMO was required. Transthoracic echocardiogram showed LVEF of 35% with akinetic inferior and posterior walls and hypokinetic anterior, lateral, and apical walls. RV was mildly enlarged with moderate global dysfunction. Over the next 36 h, her vasopressors were weaned off, she was extubated, and the IABP removed. Her Fick CO improved to 4.2 L/min with index of 2.6 L/min-m^2. She was discharged home in stable condition with plan for elective revascularization of her LAD and ramus. This case illustrates several important points: (1) MCS can be very effective in conjunction with PCI in the treatment of CSMI; (2) even in cases where MCS is not placed

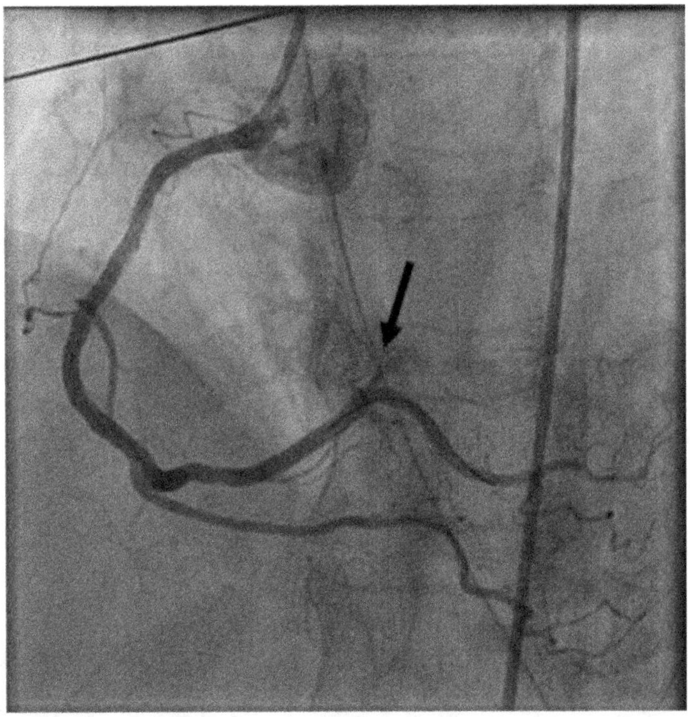

Fig. 19.11 RCA after stent placement. A long 3.0 × 38 mm drug-eluting stent was placed with excellent angiographic result in the proximal to middle RCA. Due to distal embolization, there was initially loss of flow to a posterolateral branch (arrow). *RCA* right coronary artery

upfront prior to PCI, it is important to always reevaluate whether MCS should be initiated or whether device escalation is necessary; and (3) a clear algorithm can help guide device initiation and selection in CSMI.

Further Readings

Atkinson TM, Ohman ME, O'Neill WW, et al. A practical approach to mechanical circulatory support in patients undergoing percutaneous coronary intervention. J Am Coll Cardiol Intv. 2016;9:871–83.

Burkhoff D, Sayer G, Doshi D, et al. Hemodynamics of mechanical circulatory support. J Am Coll Cardiol. 2015;66:2663–74.

Doll JA, Ohman EM, Patel MR, et al. A team-based approach to patients in cardiogenic shock. Catheter Cardiovasc Interv. 2016;88(3):424–33.

Ferguson JJ, Cohen M, Freedman RJ, et al. The current practice of intra-aortic balloon counterpulsation: results from the benchmark registry. J Am Coll Cardiol. 2001;38:1456–62.

Ibanez B, James S, Agewall S, et al. 2017 ESC Guidelines for the management of acute myocardial infarction in patients presenting with ST-segment elevation: the task force for the management of acute myocardial infarction in patients presenting with ST-segment elevation of the European Society of Cardiology (ESC). Eur Heart J. 2018;39(2):119–77.

Lauten A, Engstrom AE, Jung C, et al. Percutaneous left-ventricular support with the Impella-2.5-assist device in acute cardiogenic shock: results of the Impella-EUROSHOCK-registry. Circ Heart Fail. 2013;6:23–30.

O'Gara PT, Kushner FG, Ascheim DD, et al. 2013 ACCF/AHA Guideline for the management of ST-elevation myocardial infarction. Circulation. 2013;127:e362–425.

Patel M, Smalling R, Thiele H, et al. Intra-aortic balloon counterpulsation and infarct size in patients with acute anterior myocardial infarction without shock: the CRISP AMI randomized trial. JAMA. 2011;306(12):1329–37.

Rihal CS, Naidu SS, Givertz MM, et al. 2015 SCAI/ACC/HFSA/STS clinical expert consensus statement on the use of percutaneous mechanical circulatory support devices in cardiovascular care. J Am Coll Cardiol. 2015;65:e7–26.

Sayfarth M, Sibbing D, Bauer I, et al. A randomized clinical trial to evaluate the safety and efficacy of a percutaneous left ventricular assist device versus intra-aortic balloon pumping for treatment of cardiogenic shock caused by myocardial infarction. J Am Coll Cardiol. 2008;52:1584–8.

Shah P, Cowger JA. Cardiogenic shock. Crit Care Clin. 2014;30:391–412.

Sheu J, Tsai T, Lee F, et al. Early extracorporeal membrane oxygenator-assisted primary percutaneous coronary intervention improved 30-day clinical outcomes in patients with ST-segment elevation myocardial infarction complicated with profound cardiogenic shock. Crit Care Med. 2010;38:810–1817.

Thiele H, Sick P, Boudiot E, et al. Randomized comparison of intra-aortic balloon support with a percutaneous left ventricular assist device in patients with revascularized acute myocardial infarction complicated by cardiogenic shock. Eur Heart J. 2005;26:1276–83.

Thiele H, Zeymer U, Neumann F, et al. Intra-aortic balloon counterpulsation in acute myocardial infarction complicated by cardiogenic shock (IABP-SHOCK II): final 12 month results of a randomised, open-label trial. Lancet. 2013;382(9905):1638–45.

Thiele H, Zeymer U, Neumann F, et al. Intraaortic balloon support for myocardial infarction with cardiogenic shock. N Engl J Med. 2012;367:1287–96.

20 Mechanical Complications of Acute Myocardial Infraction

Wei Wang and Anson Cheung

20.1 Introduction

With timely reperfusion, myocardial loss following myocardial infarction (MI) can be significantly reduced and may limit the incidence of mechanical complications. However, with improving treatment of those with larger or delayed presentation MI, appropriate management of mechanical complications remains a key consideration for those working in heart attack centers.

20.2 Ischemic Ventricular Septal Defect

20.2.1 Incidence and Pathophysiology

The incidence of post-infarction ventricular septal defect (VSD) is reported as 1–2% after acute myocardial infarction (MI). However, the true incidence may be decreasing in modern era with the advancement of early interventions after acute myocardial infarction including thrombolytic treatment, early revascularization with percutaneous coronary angioplasty, or stenting and coronary bypass grafting. Nonetheless, timely and appropriate management of this important complication of MI can be lifesaving.

The timing to develop post-infarction VSD is variable, in a few hours and up to 2 weeks with an average time of 2–4 days after acute MI. It is usually associated with complete occlusion of a single coronary artery with poor collateral vessels. About 2/3 of post-infarction VSDs are located in the anteroapical septum, while the

W. Wang · A. Cheung (✉)
University of British Columbia, Vancouver, BC, Canada
e-mail: wwang7@providencehealth.bc.ca; acheung@providencehealth.bc.ca

T. J. Watson et al. (eds.), *Primary Angioplasty*,
https://doi.org/10.1007/978-981-13-1114-7_20

remaining in the posterior septum, from acute left anterior artery (LAD) and dominant right coronary artery (RCA) or circumflex artery (LCx) occlusions, respectively.

The natural history of untreated VSD is extremely poor, carrying a mortality rate of 25% within 24 h and 80% within 4 weeks. The early development of congestive heart failure (CHF) leading to cardiogenic shock is the primary cause of death. Ventricular dysfunction can be primarily left or right, depending on the territory infracted and the location of the septal rupture. Especially in posterior infarct, significant mitral valve regurgitation (MR) can play an important role in the development of heart failure, resulting in elevated left ventricular end-diastolic pressure (LVEDP) and pulmonary edema. The degree of left-to-right shunt depends on the size of the VSD and pressure gradient across the septum. If the shunt is large, the normally compliant right ventricle (RV) will not tolerate the sudden increase in load, and the development of significant RV failure pursues. As a result, severe biventricular failure is not uncommon in patients with post-infarction VSD.

20.2.2 Presentation and Diagnosis

Typical presentation of post-infarction VSD includes the presence of a new holosystolic murmur radiating to the axilla a few days post MI. It is often accompanied by an abrupt hemodynamic deterioration, i.e., signs of CHF and cardiogenic shock.

Electrocardiography (ECG) may show ST elevation and/or Q wave in accordance with location of transmural MI. Chest radiography (CXR) often shows acute pulmonary edema. Currently, transthoracic echocardiography (TTE) with color Doppler is the quickest and most definitively diagnostic method for post-infarction VSD. It can delineate the size, location, presence, and degree of shunt. In addition, TTE can identify and quantify the degree of MR and rule out other causes of MR, such as secondary to papillary muscle rupture and primary MR. Other valuable information include the presence of other valvular pathology, the degree of ventricular dysfunctions, free wall rupture, cardiac infront of tamponade, pulmonary embolism, and aortic dissection/rupture. As many patients now undergo rapid left heart catheterization to permit primary percutaneous coronary intervention (PCI)—even increasingly among late presenters—the finding of a compatible murmur during clinical evaluation may prompt left ventriculography which may prove diagnostic for VSD. The role of primary PCI or concomitant coronary artery bypass grafting in the setting of VSD is debatable as myocardial damage is already transmural and residual viability therefore questionable.

Right heart catheterization is usually not required, but a step-up in the oxygen saturation between the right atrium (RA) and pulmonary artery (PA) indicates left-to-right shunt. The right heart catheterization can also calculate the pulmonary to systemic flow ratio (Qp/Qs).

20.2.3 Timing of Surgery

The natural history of untreated post-infarction VSD is very poor with a 25% mortality within 24 h, 50% mortality within 1 week, 80% within 1 month, and 97% at 1 year [1]. The presence of post-infarction VSD is therefore an indication for urgent interventions. Intervention includes definitive surgical correction, mechanical circulatory support (MCS), and device closure of VSD. Cardiogenic shock in the setting of post-infarction VSD is a surgical emergency. In patients with cardiogenic shock, early MCS using extracorporeal membrane oxygenation (ECMO) or other short-term devices should be initiated to stabilize hemodymics and correct metabolic derangements. Furthermore, it can bridge the patient to decision regarding the best therapeutic option. Percutaneous device closure rarely works in the acute setting as the VSD is frequently serpentines, the infarcted and peri-infarct myocardium is necrotic and fragile. Given friable myocardium at the rim of the VSD, the use of percutaneous closure device can result in significant residual shunt and device embolization.

20.2.4 Preoperative Care

Medical management is aimed to improve cardiac output and reduce the left-to-right shunt by reducing systemic vascular resistance and LV pressure. Inotropes and diuretics are often used. Placement of an intra-aortic balloon pump (IABP) and other short-term MCS device can be helpful.

20.2.5 Surgical Techniques

Surgical principles include elimination of left-to-right shunt, preservation of LV function, and revascularization when possible. Small anterior and apical defects can be closed by suturing the free wall of the RV and LV, sandwiching the septum. For larger defects, generally the two commonly employed surgical techniques are infarctectomy and infarct exclusion. Infarctectomy technique involves removal of left ventricular infarction area and closure of VSD without tension. Infarct exclusion technique, on the other hand, does not remove any infarct tissue. Principles of both techniques include good myocardial protection during the operation, suture placement through non-infarcted tissue to maximize suture line integrity, and minimizing tension with the use of large prosthetic patches. Infarct exclusion techniques are more popular and thought to have the advantages of preserving left ventricular geometry and function. Meticulous medical management intraoperatively is critical, and intraoperative transesophageal echo (TEE) is mandatory. After the establishment of cardio-pulmonary bypass (CPB) and arresting the heart, the heart is inspected and the infarcted area exposed. In primary infarctectomy repair, the infarcted wall is incised (Fig. 20.1). After the resection of necrotic septal myocardium, pledgeted interrupted horizontal mattress sutures are placed around the defect. Subsequently, sutures are then passed through the septum from right to left through a felt strip. Closure of the ventriculotomy is reinforced with felt strips. Infarctectomy may also be performed with bovine pericardial patch repair (Fig. 20.2). As previously described, after the resection of infarcted tissue, pledgeted interrupted horizontal mattress sutures are placed around the defect. Sutures are then passed through a large bovine pericardial patch. All sutures are pledgeted once again and then tied down. The edges of the ventriculotomy are reapproximated with a double-layer buttressed closure with Teflon felt. Biological glue is often used to ensure complete hemostasis.

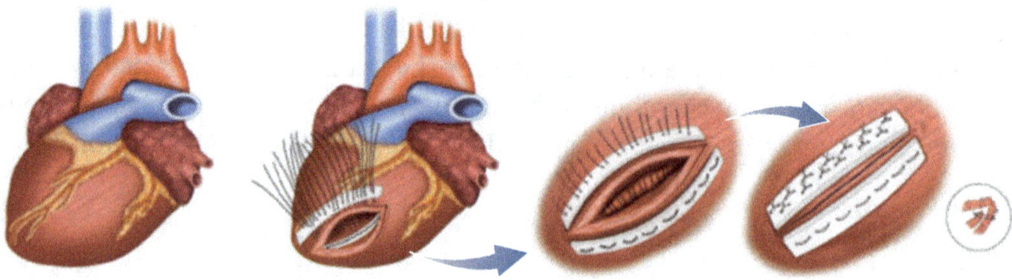

Fig. 20.1 Infarctectomy technique for anterior VSD repair with primary closure. [Courtesy of Miss Christina YS Wong]

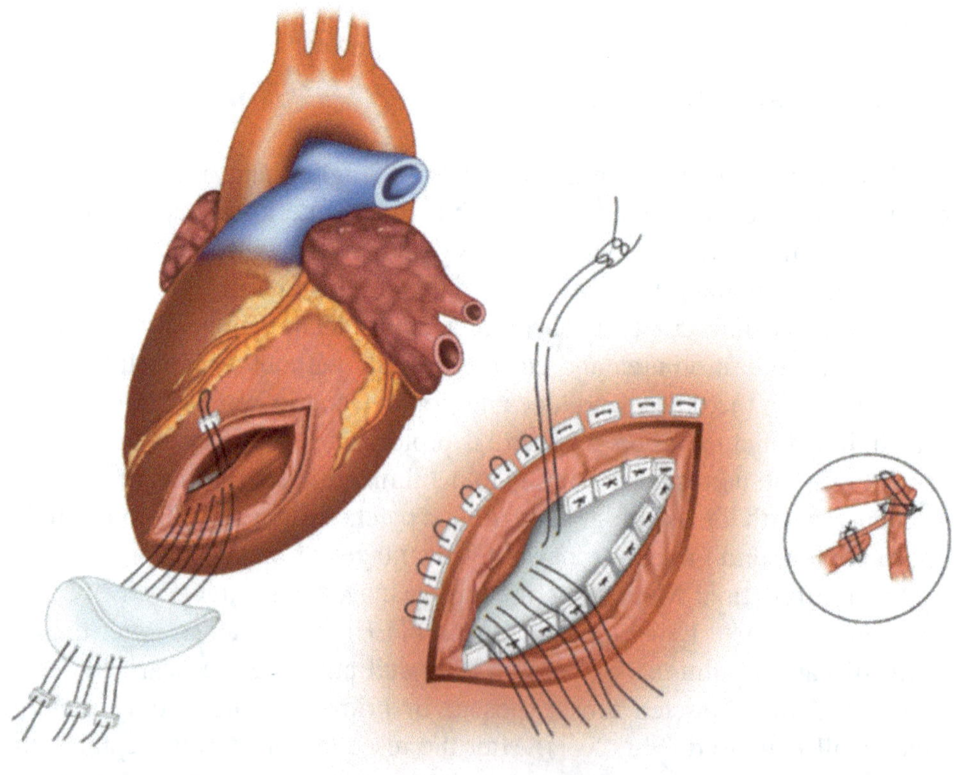

Fig. 20.2 Infarctectomy with bovine pericardial patch. [Courtesy of Miss Christina YS Wong]

Infarct exclusion techniques differ from infarctectomy where no infarcted tissue is being removed (Fig. 20.3). A trans-infarct incision is made and the extent of the infarct inspected. A large bovine pericardial patch covering is used to exclude defect from LV cavity; placements of suture onto healthy septal tissue are crucial in the integrity of the repair. Closure of the ventriculotomy is then closed as previously described. Repair of posterior ischemic VSD can sometimes be technically more challenging than anterior as exposure is less ideal. The infarct exclusion technique can provide a more tension-free repair and is believed to be better in preserving LV and RV geometry and function.

A third surgical technique, the right atrium approach, has been described for the post-infarction VSD (Fig. 20.4). It is used more commonly in posterior VSD repair. It has the benefit of not performing a left ventriculotomy. Repair is done through the tricuspid valve as performed in congenital ventricular septal defect patients [2]. However, this technique has not gained popularity for a number of reasons. Firstly,

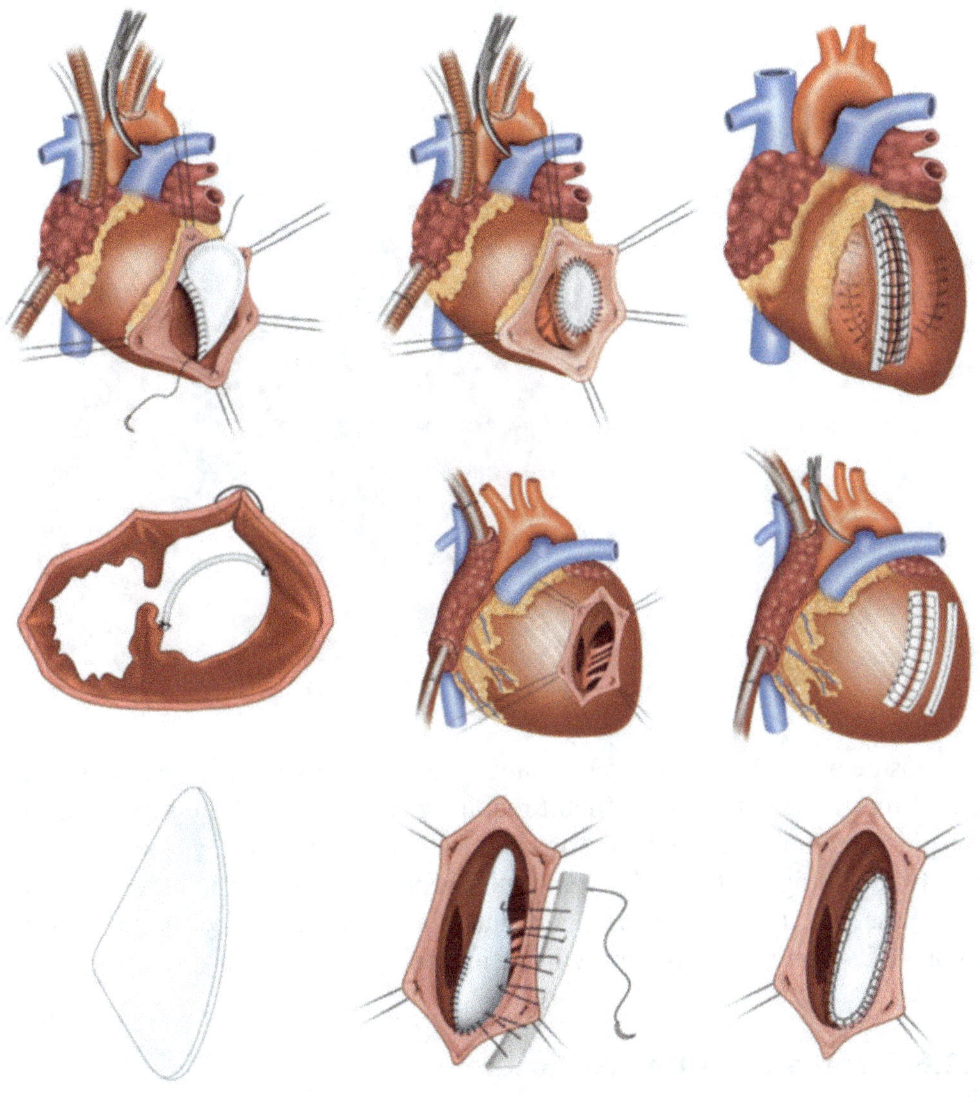

Fig. 20.3 Infarct exclusion for anterior (left) and posterior (right) post-infarction VSD. [Courtesy of Miss Christina YS Wong]

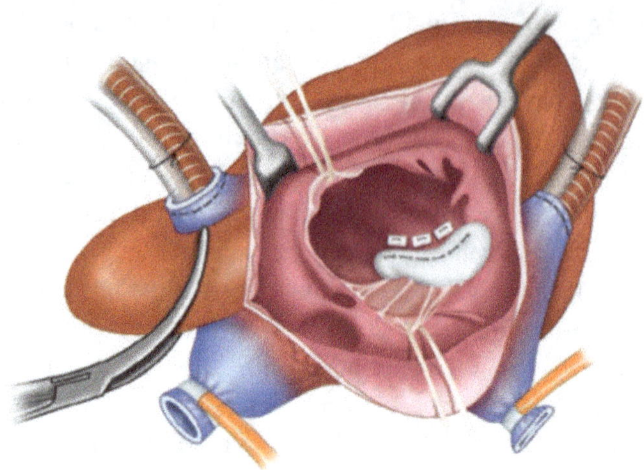

Fig. 20.4 Right atrium approach for posterior VSD repair. [Courtesy of Miss Christina YS Wong]

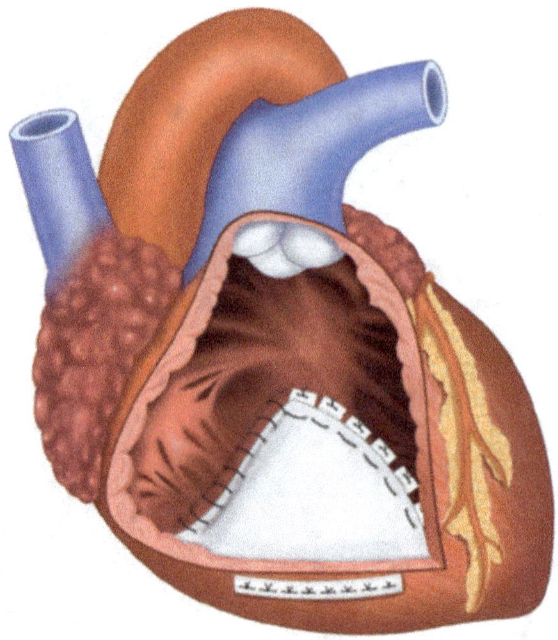

the exposure of VSD through the right atrium is often suboptimal. Secondly, placement of repair sutures can be difficult requiring detachment of the septal leaflet of tricuspid valve and the need for tricuspid valvuloplasty. Thirdly, putting a large patch from the right side of the ventricular septum can be difficult, especially in acute phase. This technique is best performed in patients 2–4 weeks after presentation of VSD, where a fibrotic rim will often develop.

20.2.6 Transcatheter Device Closure

Transcatheter device is widely used in patients with congenital VSD. However, the role of transcatheter device in post-infarction VSD is unclear. Limited data is available and most of the case studies had small number of patients. When device closure is

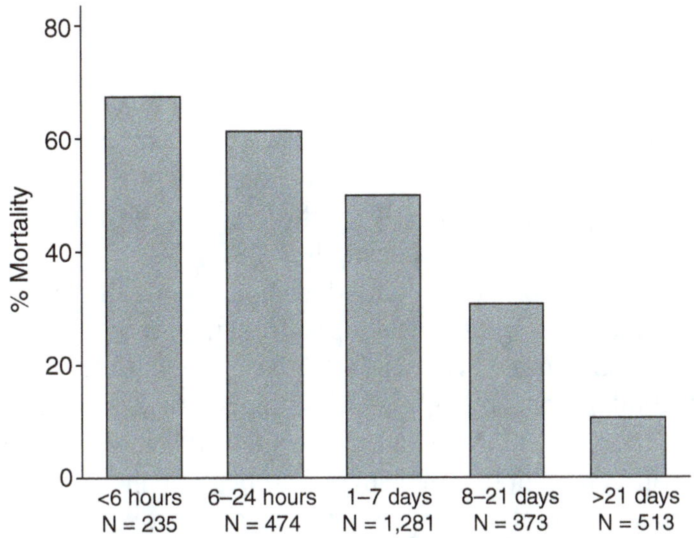

Fig. 20.5 Operative mortality rate stratified by timing of VSD repair [5]

performed in acute phase of post-infarction VSD, the 30-day mortality can be as high as 65% [3]. A study from Mayo Clinic also showed the predictors of adverse events from transcatheter device closure of post-infarction VSD included cardiogenic shock and acute phase post MI. At present, device closure is limited in selected patients 4–6 weeks after post-infarction VSD, with the fibrotic rim is well developed.

20.2.7 Mechanical Circulatory Support Involvement (ECMO, LVAD)

With the advancement of mechanical circulatory support, patients with severe end-organ damage deemed too sick to undergo operative repair may be candidates for a delayed repair. Interval treatment which may involve placement of short-term MCS devices will help improve end-organ dysfunction and allow for maturation of the infarcted tissue. Durable MCS devices can be used, however, not encouraged, due to complexity of the implant procedure, the high mortality associated with postinfarct VSD, and the cost of the device (Fig. 20.5).

20.2.8 Postoperative Management and Surgical Results

Postoperative care centers on ensuring adequate cardiac output for end-organ perfusion and correcting metabolic derangements. Pharmacologic agents such as epinephrine and milrinone may help to augment contractility. After separating from CPB, right-sided heart failure is common; inhaled nitric oxide, prostaglandin, and milrinone can be helpful in this setting. Some patients may require temporary right ventricular assist device postoperatively. The utility and effectiveness of IABP in this setting are not well established, and its use in cardiogenic shock is not recommended [4].

20.2.9 Outcome

Operative mortality is relatively high which ranges from 30 to 50%. Risk factors for early mortality after surgical intervention include persistent low cardiac output state and recurrent or residual VSD. While a residual defect with a significant shunt in an unstable patient should be imminently addressed, delayed repair is favored in a hemodynamically stable patient with a residual VSD.

Arnaoutakis et al. analyzed and reported the outcome of 2876 patients with post-infarction VSD who underwent surgical repair from the Society of Thoracic Surgery database. The operative mortality was 54.1% when repair occurred within 7 days from myocardial infarction, and only 18.4% when repair was performed more than 7 days from infarction [5]. These results may suggest mechanical circulatory support could play an important role in delaying surgical repair to achieve much better outcome in hemodynamically unstable patients. Alternatively, this finding can be explained by selection bias.

20.3 Acute Mitral Valve Regurgitation Secondary to Papillary Muscle Rupture

20.3.1 Pathophysiology

Acute mitral valve regurgitation secondary to papillary muscle rupture is a catastrophic complication after acute MI. Approximately 1–5% of death after acute MI is due to acute mitral valve regurgitation as a result of papillary muscle rupture. As in post-infarction VSD, the incidence of acute papillary muscle rupture is decreasing with early reperfusion interventions. Typically, the anterolateral papillary muscle has dual blood supply by the LAD and LCx, whereas the posteromedial papillary muscle has single blood supply by either the dominant RCA or the circumflex artery in a left dominant circulation. Hence the posteromedial papillary muscle is more susceptible to ischemia and consequent rupture accounting for 2/3 of all cases and are more commonly associated with an acute inferior STEMI.

20.3.2 Presentation and Diagnosis

Post-infarction acute MR usually occurs 2–7 days after MI. It carries a very high mortality of 50–75% without surgical intervention and 20–25% with surgical intervention. A new holosystolic murmur in conjunction with cardiovascular collapse several days after MI should raise the suspicion of papillary muscle rupture. The major differential is post-infarction VSD. Unlike an acute VSD, MR is best heard at the apex rather than the left sternal border and does not have an associated thrill. Papillary muscle rupture results in mitral valve flail leaflet and severe mitral valve regurgitation. In a normal left atrium (LA) with a relatively low compliance, acute mitral regurgitation results in sudden elevation of LA pressure leading to rapid development of pulmonary edema and cardiogenic shock.

EKG may show signs of an inferior MI, and chest radiography may demonstrate severe pulmonary edema. TTE with color Doppler is the golden standard for diagnosis. It can confirm mitral valve prolapse with flailing chordae or papillary muscle, quantify the degree of MR and ventricular function, and rule out post-infarction VSD. Development of multi-organ failure is common in patients with acute MR.

20.3.3 Preoperative Considerations

Acute MR often results in rapid hemodynamic collapse. Intubation and mechanical ventilation may be required for respiratory failure. Inotropes and diuretics can stabilize some patients; however, in unstable patients with evidence of cardiogenic shock or severe end-organ failure, early MCS with short-term devices can be lifesaving.

20.3.4 Operative Techniques

Emergent mitral valve replacement (MVR) is most commonly undertaken with concomitant coronary revascularization. Even in patients who received satisfactory percutaneous coronary interventions, isolated MVR should be performed emergently in papillary muscle rupture cases. Successful MV repair cases have been reported with reimplantation of papillary muscle, chordal transfer, and artificial chord implantation; however, repair is not recommended as the early failure rate is very high in the acute setting.

Surgical technique emphasizes on a swift operation with good myocardial protection, and MVR is generally performed via a median sternotomy. Arterial and vein graft conduits are harvested if concomitant CABG is needed. Routine cardiopulmonary bypass cannulation and antegrade and retrograde cardioplegia are routinely used. For patients with concomitant CABG, distal coronary anastomoses are performed first. Mitral valve exposure can be difficult in acute setting as the LA is often small and not dilated. Both mechanical and tissue valve may be used. It is important to preserve the chordae and leaflets (especially posterior leaflet) as much as possible to better preserve the left ventricular geometry.

20.3.5 Results

The surgical mortality of MVR in patients with acute MR secondary to papillary muscle rupture can be as high as 30%. Literature-supported concomitant CABG with MVR has an improved long-term survival compared to MVR alone [6].

20.4 Left Ventricular Free Wall Rupture

20.4.1 Pathophysiology

Free wall ventricular rupture occurs in 2–4% of patients presenting with an acute MI. Autopsy data showed the incidence could be as high as 11% [1]. Like ventricular septal defect, patients with LV free wall rupture commonly have transmural ST elevation MI. Rupture tends to occur at the junction of viable and necrotic myocardium when the infarction expands. Early thrombolytic therapy is associated with decreased incidence of free wall rupture after acute MI.

LV free wall rupture can be classified as acute, subacute, and chronic. Acute LV free wall rupture may cause severe hemodynamic compromise secondary to cardiac tamponade, often leading to sudden death. Subacute rupture indicates a small tear on LV free wall that may be temporarily clotted, contained, and not leading to immediate death. Chronic LV free wall ruptures commonly occur in the posterior wall. It is associated with very small leakage of blood that is walled-off by pericardium and the subsequent formation of a false aneurysm. Surgical interventions are indicated in subacute and chronic LV free wall ruptures.

20.4.2 Presentation and Diagnosis

Cardiac tamponade and cardiogenic shock are the most common presentations in patients with LV free wall rupture. Patients can have signs of tamponade including increased in jugular venous pressure and pulsus paradoxus. An urgent echocardiography is the choice for diagnosis in unstable patient. In stable and chronic patients, cardiac CT with contrast can provide better anatomical information and may aid surgical planning.

20.4.3 Surgical Techniques for Repair

Subacute LV free wall rupture requires emergency surgical repair. Pericardiocentesis might be helpful to stabilize patient's hemodynamic status while preparing an operating room. An IABP or other short-term MCS device is commonly necessary for preoperative stabilization. A variety of repair techniques have been described. Rupture closure with horizontal mattress sutures buttressed with Teflon felts is widely used. An additional bovine pericardial, Dacron, or PTFE patch can also be used to reinforce the suture line. Simple placement of a large pericardial patch on the ruptured surface with Bio-glue can be an option in cases where the myocardial tissue is too fragile to be repaired safely.

Chronic LV free wall rupture with false aneurysm does not require emergency surgery. Cardiac CT and MRI can better delineate the anatomical defect. The aneurysm neck can be identified readily and contains fibrotic scar tissue; primary closure can be performed on an elective basis. Reconstruction with Dacron or bovine pericardial patch can also be used.

20.4.4 Results

LV free wall rupture is usually lethal, and many diagnoses are only established by postmortem. Thus only small series studies have been reported in patients with LV free wall rupture who were able to undergo surgery. Operative mortality can be as high as 30% in patients with contained rupture. Haddadin et al. showed the simple glued patch covering technique is superior than direct suture closure technique (hospital mortality 12% vs. 36%) [7].

20.5 Case Reports: Mechanical Complications of Acute Myocardial Infraction

Wei Wang and Anson Cheung

20.5.1 Clinical Case 1

A 55-year-old male with no previous cardiac history presented late with an inferior STEMI. The patient developed acute heart failure and cardiogenic shock requiring intubation in emergency department. TTE showed a large posterior VSD involving the base of mitral valve and extending downward toward the apex. The patient had moderate to severe left ventricular dysfunction with an ejection fraction of 35%.

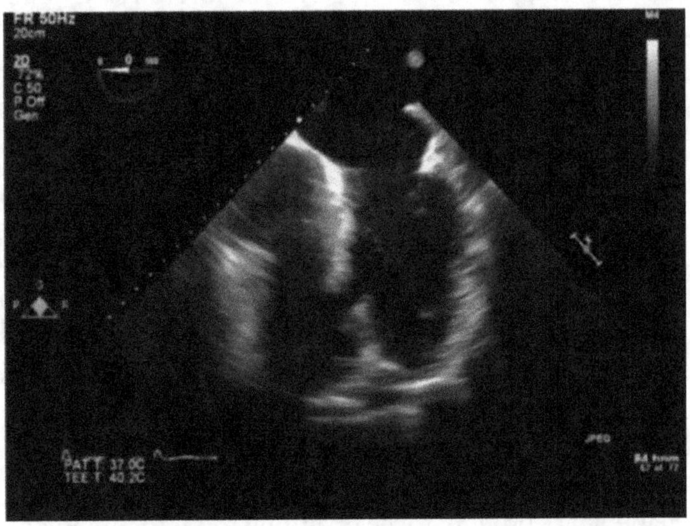

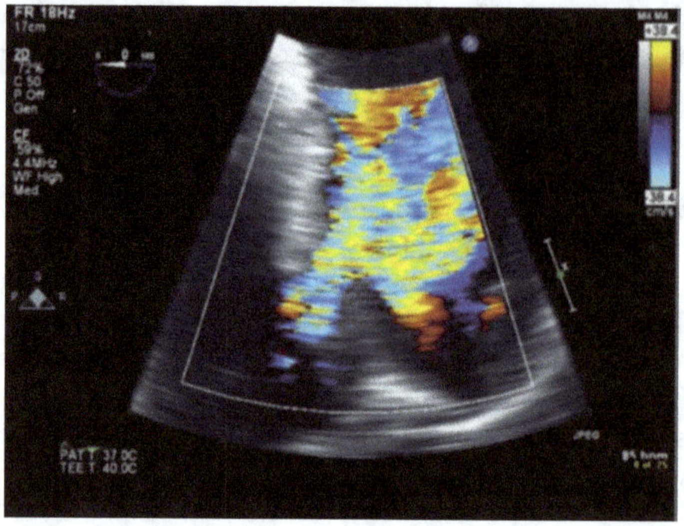

Coronary angiography showed an occluded RCA with no visible vessels distally, a small and diffusely diseased LAD, and LCx without any critical lesions. IABP was inserted in coronary suite. Despite escalating dosage of vasopressor and inotropes, the patient developed persistent cardiogenic shock with severe metabolic acidosis with a pH of 6.85. Short-term MCS was initiated percutaneously in the form of VA ECMO via femoral vessels.

Metabolic derangement and hemodynamic was corrected with ECMO support in the next 3 days. Subsequently, the patient was taken to the operating theatre for VSD repair. Intraoperative findings include infarction of the entire inferior wall with involvement of the RV and an extensive VSD extending from the base of mitral annulus to the apex. A successful VSD repair using infarct exclusion technique with large bovine pericardial patches was carried out. There was no residual shunt detected post repair, and only mild MR was seen by transesophageal echocardiogram (TEE) postoperatively. Unfortunately, the patient was unable to be weaned from cardiopulmonary bypass due to moderate to severe RV dysfunction and pulmonary dysfunction. VA ECMO was reinitiated, and further support was required for another 8 days with eventual successful wean from ECMO.

20.5.2 Clinic Case 2

A 62-year-old female, who had missed acute STEMI 5 days previously, presented with cardiogenic shock and was brought to catheter laboratory. The coronary angiogram showed occluded LAD and left circumflex with LVEF 15%. Balloon angioplasty was performed, but it was unable to restore LAD flow. The patient was hemodynamically unstable despite intubation, IABP, and high dose of norepinephrine and dobutamine. Echocardiogram showed severe MR and signs of tamponade secondary to large amount of pericardial fluid. Cardiac surgery was emergently consulted, and the patient was brought to the operating room for emergency ECMO. The patient had a cardiac arrest before cutting the skin. Stat cardiopulmonary bypass was established via median sternotomy. There was a lot of blood found in the pericardial cavity and LV free wall rupture was identified. The LV tissue around rupture area was necrotic, which made it impossible to sew on the fragile tissue. A large bovine pericardium patch was glued on the LV free wall. The patient was then placed on central ECMO and chest left open and was listed for high status heart transplant candidate. Fortunately, 3 days later a donor heart became available, and the patient received orthotopic heart transplant successfully. Posttransplant course was uneventful and she was discharged from hospital 3 weeks later.

References

1. Lawrence HC. Cardiac surgery in the adult. NY: McGraw-Hill Education; 2011.
2. Massetti M, et al. Postinfarction ventricular septal rupture: early repair through the right atrial approach. J Thorac Cardiovasc Surg. 2000;119(4 Pt 1):784–9.
3. Thiele H, et al. Immediate primary transcatheter closure of postinfarction ventricular septal defects. Eur Heart J. 2009;30(1):81–8.
4. Thiele H, et al. Intraaortic balloon support for myocardial infarction with cardiogenic shock. N Engl J Med. 2012;367(14):1287–96.
5. Arnaoutakis GJ, et al. Surgical repair of ventricular septal defect after myocardial infarction: outcomes from the Society of Thoracic Surgeons National Database. Ann Thorac Surg. 2012;94(2):436–43.
6. Lorusso R, Gelsomino S, De Cicco G, et al. Mitral valve surgery in emergency for severe acute regurgitation: analysis of postoperative results from a multicentre study. Eur J Cardiothorac Surg. 2008;33(4):573–82.
7. Haddadin S, et al. Surgical treatment of postinfarction left ventricular free wall rupture. J Card Surg. 2009;24(6):624–31.

Time to Reperfusion, Door-to-Balloon Times, and How to Reduce Them

21

Margot M. Sherman Jollis and James G. Jollis

21.1 Introduction

Time to reperfusion and first-medical-contact-to-balloon times are key parameters in assessing efficiency of the primary PCI pathway while also being powerful predictors of outcome. This chapter discusses the role of these measures and how improvements may impact clinical outcomes.

21.2 Does Time Matter?

The time-dependent nature of myocardial injury following coronary artery occlusion has been consistently documented in the literature and runs congruent with clinical experience. Reimer and Jennings first documented an "ischemic wavefront" after transient ligation of the circumflex coronary artery in open-chested dogs, followed by reperfusion for 2–4 days (Fig. 21.1) [1]. Examining transmural slices of the posterior papillary muscle, they identified a subepicardial zone of ischemic but viable myocardium which is available for salvage for at least 3 and perhaps 6 h following circumflex occlusion in the dog. Thus, the time-critical nature of coronary artery reperfusion was established.

Numerous observational studies have concurred with this relationship. Combining data from 22 fibrinolysis trials involving 50,246 patients, Boersma and colleagues found the number of lives saved per 1000 patients treated to be

M. M. Sherman Jollis
Department of Biology, Denison University, Granville, OH, USA

J. G. Jollis (✉)
Department of Medicine, Duke University, Durham, NC, USA
e-mail: james.jollis@duke.edu

T. J. Watson et al. (eds.), *Primary Angioplasty*,
https://doi.org/10.1007/978-981-13-1114-7_21

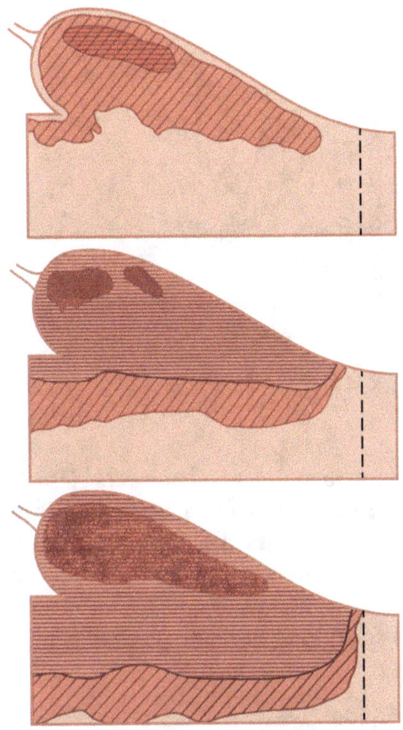

Fig. 21.1 Progression of the wavefront of ischemic cell death [1]. All shaded areas, necrosis; dotted areas, necrotic muscle; horizontal cross hatching, microvascular injury; dashed line, anatomic border between ischemic circumflex coronary and nonischemic left anterior descending coronary arteries

greatest for patients presenting within the first hour, with an inflection point for less benefit for patients presenting beyond 2 h (Fig. 21.2) [2]. This relationship between time and treatment has been documented in additional studies, with the greatest time benefit seen among patients with the highest-risk clinical presentations such as cardiogenic shock [3–5]. One notable exception to this relationship involved a manuscript by Menses et al. that showed no change in 30-day mortality for Medicare (over age 65) patients recorded in the CathPCI Registry, despite a fall in door-to-balloon (D2B) time from 83 to 67 min [6]. However, the finding was refuted in a subsequent publication that used the same data and shared two co-authors, showing that shorter patient-specific D2B times were consistently associated with lower mortality over time [7].

Most recently, data involving the coordination of ST-elevation myocardial infarction (STEMI) care in 12 regions across the United States in the Accelerator-2 project resulted in modest improvement in treatment times for patients transported by ambulance, with an increase from 67 to 74% of patients meeting the goal of first medical contact (FMC) to device within 90 min. This improvement in treatment time was associated with a relatively large and statistically significant decline in mortality compared to patients treated at the same time without such coordination [8] (Fig. 21.3). This finding suggests that time serves as a process measure that reflects coordination of care. Likely activities involved in such coordination lead to improved mortality beyond that is expected by time metrics alone such as better paramedic training and enhanced ability of emergency physicians to move the sickest patients to coronary intervention quickly (Fig. 21.3).

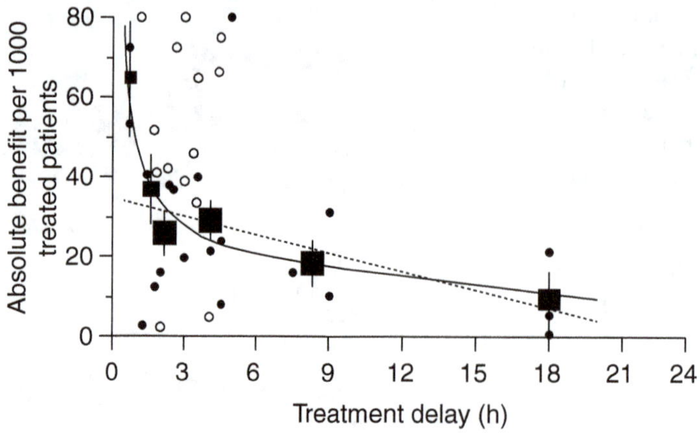

Fig. 21.2 A 35-day mortality reduction versus treatment delay [2]. Small closed dots, information from trials included in FTT analysis; open dots, information from additional trials; small squares, data beyond scale of *x*/*y* cross. The linear (34·7–1·6*x*) and nonlinear (19·4–0·6*x* + 29·3*x*1) regression lines are fitted within these data, weighted by inverse of the variance of the absolute benefit in each datapoint. Black squares, average effects in six time-to-treatment groups (areas of squares inversely proportional to variance of absolute benefit described)

Fig. 21.3 In-hospital mortality according to hospital participation in Accelerator-2 with overall improvements in timely treatment versus hospitals not involved in the project without significant improvement in treatment times [8]

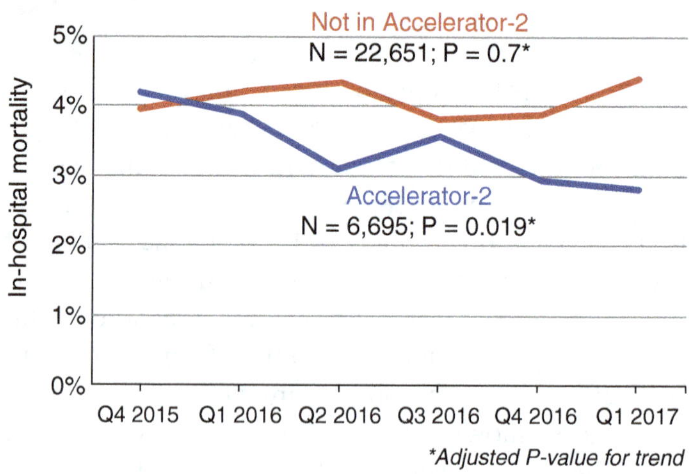

21.3 How to Reduce Time

The overall goal of efforts to expedite coronary reperfusion is to shorten the time from artery occlusion to resumption of normal flow. Initial efforts in the United States concentrated on a "door-to-needle" time of less than 30 min for patients treated with fibrinolysis and a "door-to-balloon" time of less than 90 min. Recognizing that treatment times could be accelerated with involvement of emergency medical services (EMS) and transferring hospitals, the standard was moved to an earlier starting point, "first medical contact," maintaining the same overall goal of 90 min. In the case of EMS-transported patients, FMC represents the time paramedics are "eyeball to eyeball" with the patient, and in the case of inter-hospital transfer, FMC is the time the patient arrives at the first hospital. To further encompass emergency response and treat patients sooner, the Los Angeles STEMI system starts the reperfusion clock at EMS dispatch time, and Dallas starts with symptom onset to arterial reperfusion (SOAR) time. The earlier processes are included in systematic measurements, the greater opportunity for process improvement.

In order to expedite coronary reperfusion, one needs to take a systemic survey of existing patterns of care, ideally considered separately according to the point of entry of the patient. Generally, patients present by one of four scenarios: walking into an emergency department, arriving by ambulance, transferring from another hospital emergency department, or experiencing a STEMI while hospitalized for some other condition. The latter group represents one of the most challenging with the highest mortality. Below, we will discuss approaches to accelerating coronary reperfusion according to each of these four presentation scenarios. Other tenets to improving care include data collection and feedback on a prompt and ongoing basis; establishing treatment plans agreed upon by all participating providers; establishing and maintaining treatment systems with the aid of dedicated coordinators; working across all disciplines involved in the diagnosis and treatment of acute myocardial infarction; developing as broad of a network as possible with the inclusion of competing hospitals, physician groups, and EMS agencies within a region; and recognizing that most opportunities, barriers, and solutions vary by region and can be overcome with local expertise and solutions. Our approach to organizing and transforming myocardial infarction care is summarized in Fig. 21.4. We first develop leadership, establish funding, and implement a data system. Leadership is best composed of passionate healthcare providers that span multiple disciplines and institutions. Funding is reserved to support regional coordinators, data analyses and feedback, and local and regional meetings. Once

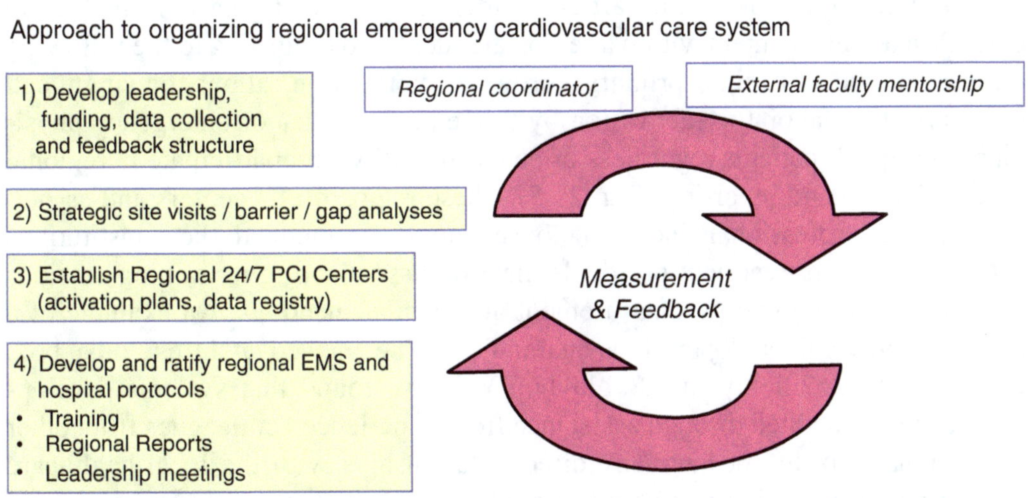

Fig. 21.4 Approach to organizing regional emergency cardiovascular care system [8]

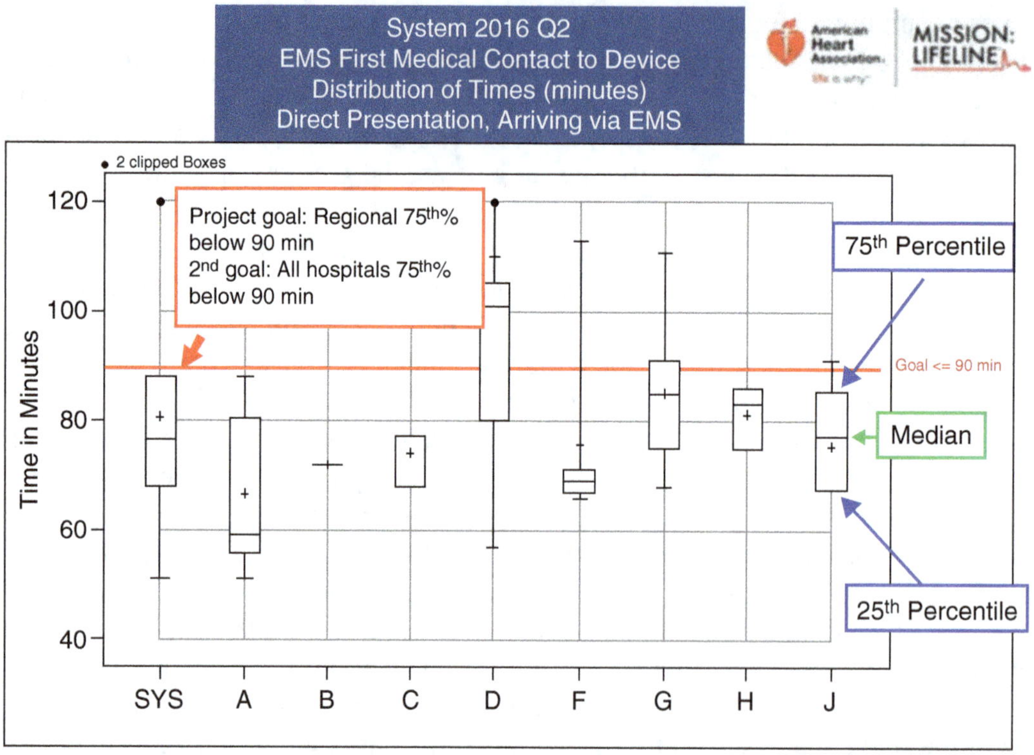

*Transferred from outside facility = No; Means transport to first facility = Ambulance; First EKG obtained = Pre-hospital or after arrival*32*

Fig. 21.5 Mission: lifeline regional report example. De-identified example of quarterly mission: Lifeline regional report used in system measurement and feedback to hospitals and emergency medical services. Bar and whisker plots. Whiskers represent ranges; bars represent interquartile range. Left hand bar is summary for region. Bars to right represent individual letter-coded hospitals. Goal of system is for each hospital to have 75% of EMS-transported patient treated within 90 min, depicted by the top of the bar graph lying at or below the 90 min red line goal [8]

these are established, our leadership team assesses the current system for diagnosing and treating STEMI with particular attention to existing barriers that delay care. Primary PCI centers within a region are identified according to the following criteria: provide full-time primary coronary intervention, allow for single-call catheterization laboratory activation by trained paramedics or emergency physicians, accept all patients regardless of bed availability, and participate in regional data collection and reporting (Fig. 21.5). These regional PCI centers and associated medical professionals including those who refer patients to these institutions establish regional treatment protocols that are disseminating in training sessions and supported by ongoing measurement and regular meetings. An example of a common protocol or "operations manual" can be viewed at https://duke.box.com/s/ks6ipcc262illo8jyethbst8bblqybcj. We have found that systems development can be expedited through assistance from experienced colleagues from other institutions who do not have any direct relationships with the local healthcare system and can be viewed as neutral advisors, termed "external faculty" in our organizational framework.

21.4 Expediting Care According to Point of Entry

Each of the four entry scenarios described above requires solutions specific to each setting. While each system and setting has unique challenges and opportunities, there are a number of common approaches that have been identified and are listed below, organized by point of entry (Table 21.1). Many of these approaches have been demonstrated to expedite treatment. For example, Fordyce showed significantly faster treatment times for hospitals that adopted paramedic catheterization lab pre-activation, single-call hospital transfer protocols, and emergency department bypass when the lab was prepared to accept an anticipated patient on hospital arrival [9]. In related work, Glickman demonstrated sequentially faster "door-in, door-out" times according to the number of eight recommended processes implemented by transferring hospitals [10]. Our work has associated paramedic prehospital activation with both faster treatment times and substantially lower mortality [10] (Fig. 21.6).

Table 21.1 Processes and protocols to expedite coronary artery reperfusion according to point of patient entry [8, 10]

Walk-in	
Key process measures: *Door to ECG time* *ECG to cath lab activation time*	Measures efficiency of identifying patients with STEMI and initiating reperfusion
Door-to-ECG target of 10 min	
"Nurse first"	Asking patients about possible cardiac symptoms prior to registration
Dedicated area for ECG	
Standard rules for ECG performance	ECG for all patients over age 30 with typical cardiac symptoms and for patients over age 50 with atypical cardiac symptoms such as shortness of breath or nausea
Hand ECG to emergency physician	
Standard plan for ST-elevation myocardial infarction reperfusion	
Emergency physician activates reperfusion plan	
Reperfusion inclusion and contraindication checklist	
If part of treatment plan, fibrinolytic medication stored in emergency department	
Imaging the infarct-suspected infarct-related artery first using a guide catheter and opening the vessel if appropriate prior to imaging the other coronary arteries or performing ventriculography	
Arrival by ambulance	
Key process measure: *Emergency department dwell time*	Systems with shorter times (less than 20 min) have successful pre-activation protocols

Table 21.1 (continued)

Medical leadership	
Standard plan for ST-elevation myocardial infarction reperfusion	This plan should include symptom, ECG, and exclusion criteria for catheterization lab activation by paramedics. Activation should have a regionally recognized designated term such as "code STEMI" or "level 1 heart alert"
Dispatch of 12-lead ECG and personnel trained to diagnose STEMI to patients with cardiac symptoms	
Standard rules for ECG performance	
EMS personnel perform and read ECG	
Single-call catheterization lab activation	
15 min scene time	
Diversion of STEMI patients directly to full-time PCI hospitals if additional transport time less than 30–45 min.	
Emergency department bypass when possible	Proceed directly to the catheterization laboratory if staffed and ready
Training of paramedics on diagnosis and treatment of STEMI	
Feedback within 24 h to all involved personnel including treatment times, catheterization findings, and patient outcomes	Health information privacy rules in the United States allow for exchange of patient-identified data between entities caring for the same patients and accrediting organizations requiring such communication
Regular interdisciplinary meetings to review STEMI cases	
Inter-hospital transfer	
Key process measure: *Door-in door-out time from first hospital*	Systems with shorter times (less than 40 min) have successful protocols for diagnosis and transfer of patients
Similar emergency department processes to those described for "walk-in" patients above	Nurse first, ECG area, ECG rules, immediate availability of technician, handing tracing to emergency physician, emergency physician activating reperfusion system
Standard plan for ST-elevation myocardial infarction reperfusion	120 min from first hospital door threshold PCI reliably available within 120 min, transfer to PCI hospital PCI not reliably available within 120 min fibrinolysis preferred
Nursing-led reperfusion protocols	
Use local ambulance for transfer when available	
Identify a primary and backup method of transfer	
Leave the patient on the stretcher	Patients with likely STEMI should be evaluated on the stretcher and rapidly moved back to the ambulance for transfer when appropriate

(continued)

Table 21.1 (continued)

Avoid intravenous drips	Aspirin, heparin bolus, and topical nitrates should be sufficient. Platelet inhibitors such as ticagrelor or cangrelor can be added according to local and regional preferences
Do not delay transfer for copying of medical records	Records can be transmitted by facsimile to the receiving hospital after patient departure
Single-call catheterization lab activation	
Feedback within 24 h to all involved personnel including treatment times, catheterization findings, and patient outcomes	
Regular interdisciplinary meetings to review STEMI cases	
STEMI in patient already hospitalized for another condition	
Key process measure: *Rapid response team can diagnose STEMI and activate reperfusion protocol*	
Standard plan for ST-elevation myocardial infarction reperfusion	
Rapid-response team responds to patients with acute cardiac symptoms and trained to recognize and diagnose	
Nurse leader or hospitalist authorized to activate reperfusion plan	
In hospitals without full-time PCI facilities, transfer to PCI hospital for patients with contraindications to fibrinolysis such as recent surgery, gastrointestinal bleeding, or recent non-compressible arterial access site	
Feedback within 24 h to all involved personnel including treatment times, catheterization findings, and patient outcomes	
Regular interdisciplinary meetings to review STEMI cases	

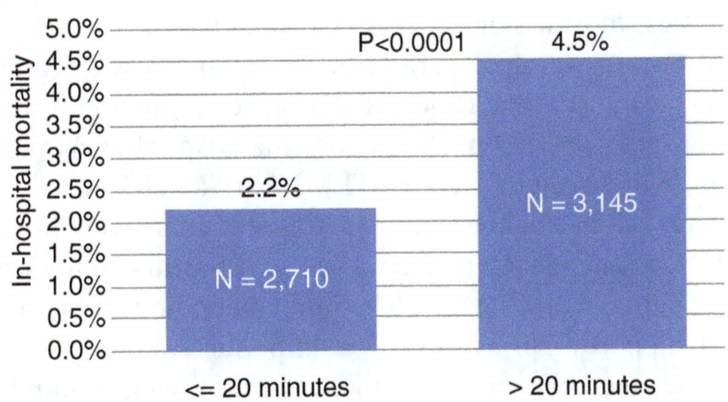

Fig. 21.6 First-medical-contact time to catheterization-activation time and in-hospital mortality [8]

21.5 Walk-In

Identifying and treating STEMI patients in the emergency department has been the focus of coordinated care efforts for decades, starting with the "door-to-needle" focus of the National Registry of Myocardial Infarction and culminating in the "door-to-balloon" projects of the last decade [11]. Approximately 2 in 100 patients presenting to an emergency department with chest pain are having an acute myocardial infarction, and the process mirrors that of "finding a needle in a haystack" in often crowded emergency departments. Successful approaches have included a target door-to-electrocardiogram (ECG) time of 10 min, asking patients about possible cardiac symptoms prior to registration, maintaining a dedicated area for rapid ECG performance, having standard rules for when to obtain an ECG, handing the ECG to the emergency physician, maintaining a standard approach to urgent coronary reperfusion most suitable to local resources and expertise, and allowing emergency physicians to activate the reperfusion plan, sometimes described as pressing the "easy button." In the catheterization laboratory, reperfusion can be accelerated by imaging the infarct-suspected infarct-related artery first using a guide catheter and opening the vessel if appropriate prior to imaging the other coronary arteries or performing ventriculography. The trade-off of treating the infarct artery first is that important lesions in other vessels may not be taken into account prior to intervention, and the rare patient with a mechanical complication such as ventricular septal rupture may undergo coronary intervention prior to urgent surgery. Using these approaches, most patients can be treated within 30 min of hospital arrival with fibrinolysis and within 60 min with primary angioplasty.

21.6 Arrival by Ambulance

Likely the ideal and most expedient process for rapid diagnosis and treatment of STEMI involves patient transport by ambulance. This process includes EMS dispatch, diagnosis at the patient location by symptoms and ECG, and pre-activation of the cardiac catheterization laboratory prior to hospital arrival. In the United States, most major systems dispatch emergency technicians with advanced levels of training termed "paramedics" to patients with cardiac symptoms. These paramedics perform a 12-lead ECG on scene, interpret the tracings, and activate cardiac catheterization labs prior to the hospital using prespecified terminology such as "STEMI alert," "code STEMI," or "level 1 heart alert." The process expedites care, and in ideal instances, infarct-related arteries are opened within 1 h of activating the emergency medical system, "aborting" a myocardial infarction before significant damage ensues. The implementation of pre-activation involves a number of supporting processes. Most importantly, strong medical leadership from emergency medicine or interventional cardiology is required to support paramedics and maintain a system of accurate diagnoses. Prior to initiation of prehospital activation, cardiologists and emergency medical leadership should agree to a common threshold of symptoms, ECG findings, and exclusions to activate. A reasonable approach differentiates a "definite" from a "possible" STEMI, reserving the former for activation and the latter for additional consultation with emergency medicine and cardiology, ideally supported with ECG transmission. Systems vary in ECG criteria for activation, from 1 mm of ST elevation in two contiguous leads to requiring 2 mm of ST elevation in precordial leads. Some systems include additional support from machine interpretation, with vendor-specific statements like "meets STEMI criteria" or "acute MI suspected" resulting in lab activation. In well-performing systems, cancellation rates of 20% are reasonable and can be lowered to 10–15% with focused paramedic training and ongoing feedback. Additional processes include standard rules for ECG performance similar to the emergency department, limiting "ambulance scene time" to 15 min with a "load and go" focus, the ability of medics to direct patients to hospitals that perform percutaneous coronary intervention (PCI) on a 24-h basis, an expectation that catheterization laboratories will be ready to begin procedures within 30 min or less of activation, and feedback to all involved personnel within 24 h and at regular multidisciplinary meetings to review cases. In the best situation, when a catheterization laboratory is fully staffed and ready to accept patients on hospital arrival, the emergency department is bypassed rather than required to partake in patient registration as they pass quickly through the area. Similar to patients with major trauma going directly to an awaiting operating room or women in childbirth proceeding directly to labor and delivery, there is no mandate for STEMI patients to be evaluated in the emergency department if they can be treated immediately in the catheterization lab. The emergency department remains an important component of rapid reperfusion systems, holding patients who arrive before the lab is ready and assisting in triage of questionable cases. Bagai found that emergency department bypass significantly lowered FMC-to-device times by 20 min [12].

21.7 Inter-Hospital Transfer

Timely treatment of patients requiring inter-hospital transfer remains one of the most challenging scenarios, with almost half of patients treated beyond 2 h of first hospital arrival. The delays are attributable to geographic challenges and the difficulty of coordinating patient care in referring hospitals that are often small, rural, and challenged with busy emergency departments. The same tenets that assist the treatment of patients who walk into PCI hospitals apply to emergency departments that must transfer patients for treatment including a "nurse first" query of symptoms before registration and a dedicated ECG area and personnel who are immediately available to obtain ECGs, handing the tracing to the emergency physician and relying on the emergency physician to activate the coronary reperfusion plan without cardiology consultation for obvious cases. As smaller hospitals may staff their emergency departments with itinerant emergency physicians, the system and plan for treatment should heavily rely on nursing leadership and guidance. Prespecified reperfusion plans should be developed with the input of local experts and be guided by available resources and geography. For locations where patients can be reliably transferred for PCI within 120 min to the hospital, transferring all patients for PCI is a reasonable approach. In our experience in published data, on average, ground transport by local ambulance is as fast as helicopter transport at any distance, and ground transport is not subject to weather restrictions often faced in air travel. Effective ground transport requires the willingness of local emergency medical or critical-care transport services to convey patients to PCI hospitals, a system for rapid dispatch of transport such as the use of terms "code STEMI patient" to prioritize ambulance resources, avoiding intravenous drips with a reliance on aspirin, heparin bolus, and topical nitrates during transfer, obtaining "mutual aid" from neighboring EMS when patient transport will leave large geographies without emergency responders, and transferring patients before records and Emergency Medical Treatment and Active Labor Act (EMTALA) forms are copied with routine facsimile of records to the receiving cath lab after the patient leaves the first hospital. Having two transport alternatives for transfer patients avoids unanticipated delays. For patients arriving at the first hospital by ambulance who appear likely to have a STEMI, leaving the patient on the stretcher for ED evaluation will preclude potentially long delays in procuring a second ambulance. Transfer systems are aided by EMS that will transport STEMI patients directly to PCI hospitals from the field when geographically feasible, avoiding the delays of inter-hospital transfer.

For emergency departments that cannot reliably transfer patients to PCI hospitals for device activation within 120 min of first hospital arrival, fibrinolysis remains an important and timely intervention. Again, protocols should be designed to provide lytics within 30 min of arrival to include standard criteria for STEMI diagnosis, systematic exclusion of contraindications, and the availability for fibrinolytic drugs in the emergency department. For the 20% of patients who are ineligible for fibrinolysis, and the 25% of patients who do not show signs of clinical reperfusion according to symptom relief and ST-segment elevation resolution, protocols for rapid transfer to PCI hospitals still need to be established.

21.8 STEMI in Patients Already Hospitalized for Another Condition

The highest-risk STEMI involves those that occur in patients who are already hospitalized for another condition. In California discharge data, Kaul and colleagues identified a threefold higher mortality for patients with inpatient-onset STEMI [13]. While some of the higher mortality may be attributed to age and comorbid illness, significant delays in the identification and treatment of these patients likely lead to worse outcomes. Recent efforts have focused on the systematic identification and treatment of these patients. Similar to other settings, a prespecified, in-hospital STEMI plan can increase treatment rates and reduce delays. In the hospital setting, "rapid-response teams" should be dispatched to patients who are possibly experiencing an acute coronary syndrome, and these teams should be trained in the recognition and diagnosis of STEMI. Nursing leadership or hospitalists who routinely respond to these patients should be authorized to activate the cardiac catheterization laboratory according to standard criteria and protocols. For hospitals lacking full-time PCI facilities, a plan should be in place for rapid transfer to a PCI hospital. Hospitalized patients with recent surgery, gastrointestinal bleeding, or non-compressible arterial access sites are not eligible for fibrinolysis and merit rapid transfer. In-hospital STEMI patients should be included in reporting and quality review efforts involving other STEMI settings.

21.9 Case Reports: Time to Reperfusion, Door-to-Balloon Times, and How to Reduce Them

Margot M. Sherman Jollis and James G. Jollis

21.9.1 Case Study

A 66-year-old man with the onset of chest pain while walking his dog in the evening. He called 911, paramedics were dispatched, and an anterior ST-elevation myocardial infarction was diagnosed at his house. The catheterization laboratory was activated while he was being transported to the hospital.

21.9.2 EMS Narrative

"A 66-year-old male lying on his couch. The patient stated he was out walking with his family dog and started to feel pressure across his chest. The patient was pale in color but not diaphoretic. He had already taken 325 mg of aspirin prior to EMS arrival. A 12-lead ECG showed anterior-septal STEMI. The patient was given 0.4 mg of nitroglycerine sublingually and moved to a stretcher and secured for transport to local ED per patient's choice. IV access was established, and the patient was placed on 3L O_2 due to room air saturation of 94%. STEMI alert to local ED and 12-lead ECG was transmitted. Upon arrival at ED, the patient had two 5–8 s runs of V-Tach that were self-corrective. Patient care was transferred to ED nursing staff and physician by verbal report, and EMS went with patient to cath lab. 100% LAD blockage noted in cath. END OF REPORT"

21.9.3 Cardiac Catheterization Report and Images

Once radial access was obtained with a Glidesheath Slender 6f radial introducer sheath, heparin 70 units per kilogram was administered. Verapamil 3 mg intra-arterial was infused through the sheath. A VL 3.5 guide catheter was advanced to the left main and a guiding angiogram was performed. Ticagrelor 180 mg was administered. A 0.014, 180-cm Extra Floppy Runthrough guidewire was advanced across the left anterior descending occlusion, and TIMI 1 flow was restored. The stenosis was pre-dilated with a 2.5 × 15-mm monorail balloon. The lesion was at the bifurcation of the first diagonal. A Forte Xsupport, 185-cm wire was placed into the diagonal to protect the side branch. A Synergy, 3.5 × 16-mm coronary stent was advance across the lesion. Angiography confirmed adequate coverage of the stenosis. The stent was deployed at 16 ATM and post-dilated with the same balloon to 17 ATM. An angiogram showed the proximal portion stent was slightly undersized. The stent was post-dilated with a Quantum 3.75-mm balloon to 16 ATM. A final angiogram showed no residual stenosis and TIMI 3 flow into the distal vessel. Ventriculography performed after coronary angiography showed anterior and apical hypokinesis and ejection fraction of 45% (Figs. 21.7, 21.8, 21.9, 21.10, 21.11, 21.12, 21.13, and 21.14).

Date of Service: 12/27/1 22:09
Time Code STEMI Activated: 22:01
EMS Team: W H ,KS
ED Physician: A
ED Nurse: R
Cardiologist: S
Cath Lab Team: Jennifer R, Amanda H, Seth S, Michelle B
Lesion: LAD
Comments:

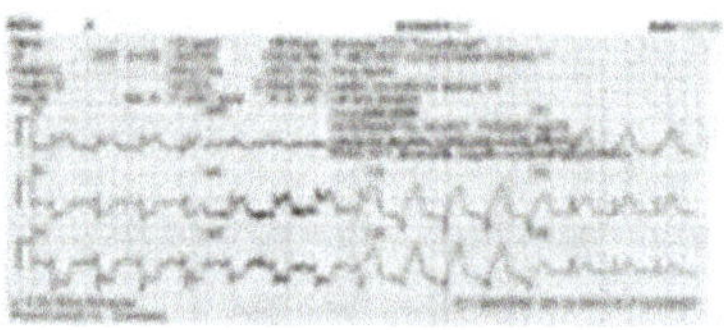

Incident #	Recommended Targets (mins)	Actual Date
EMS ECG Time	10	21:49
EMS ECG Received to Activation		2
EMS on Scene time	15	8
ED Door to ECG	10	NA
ECG to Activation	5	PTA
Total Time in ED	30	27
Activation to Cath Team Ready	30	25
Activation to MD Arrive in Cath Lab	30	30
Door to Device	60	40
FMC to Device	90	63

Fig. 21.7 STEMI Feedback Report. Returned to all involved providers including EMS, emergency department, catheterization laboratory, critical care transport, and STEMI team 1 day after catheterization. Case is also reviewed in biweekly multidisciplinary team review

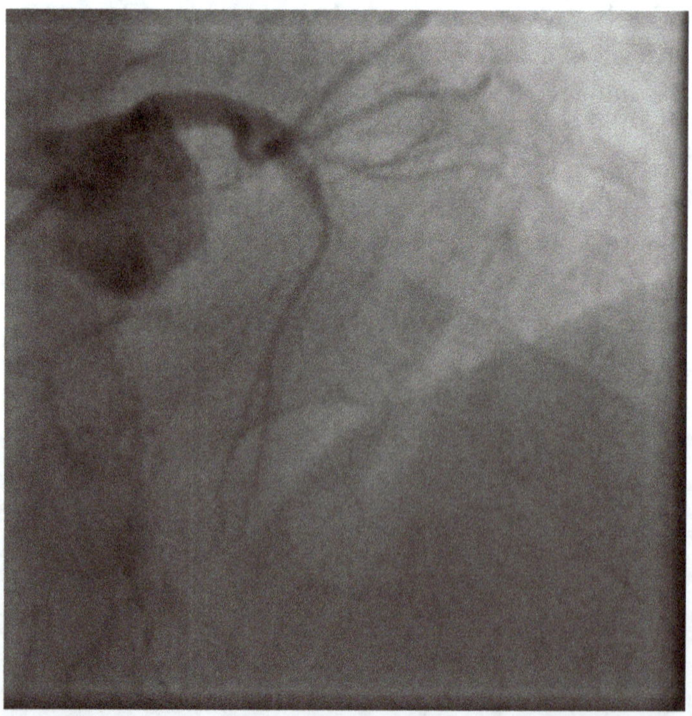

Fig. 21.8 Initial image, AP cranial view, radial access, guide catheter VL 3.5, 100% proximal LAD, TIMI 0 flow

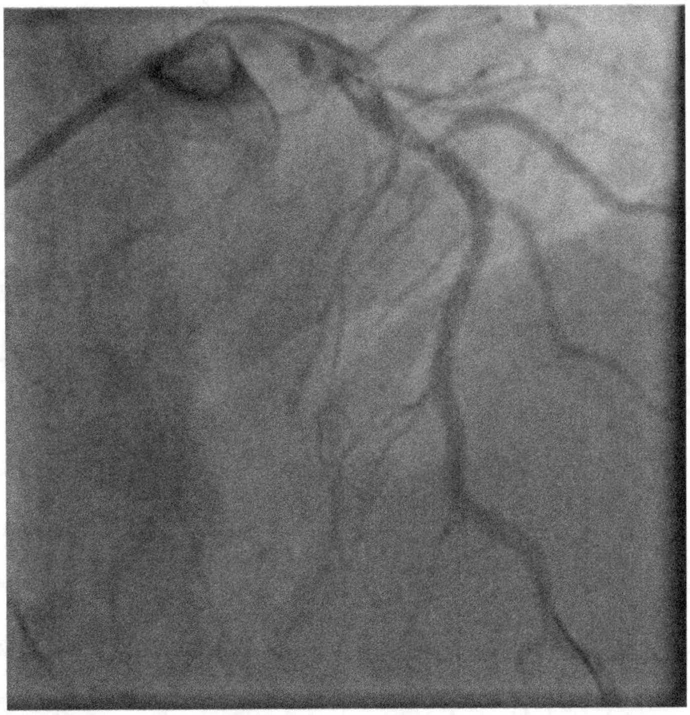

Fig. 21.9 Crossed with 0.014 guidewire and pre-dilated with a 2.5-mm balloon

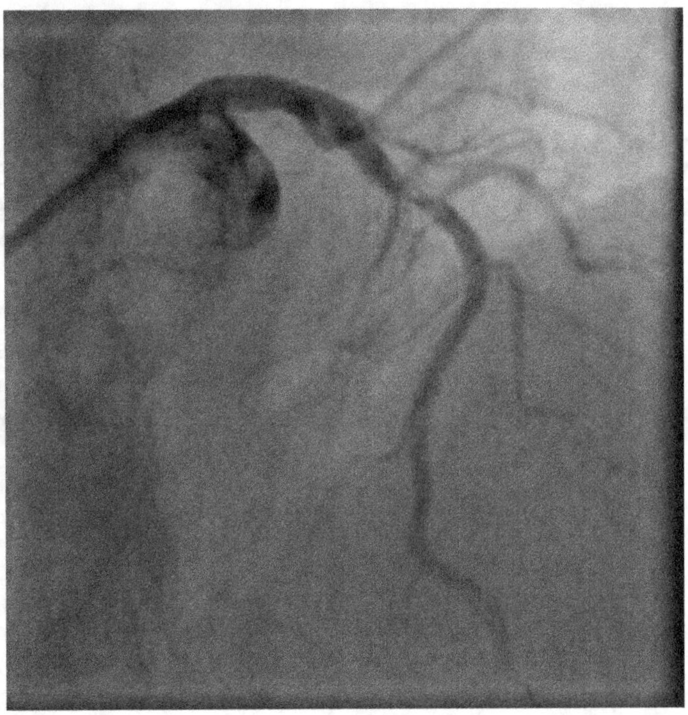

Fig. 21.10 Post initial dilation, residual filling defects, TIMI 3 flow

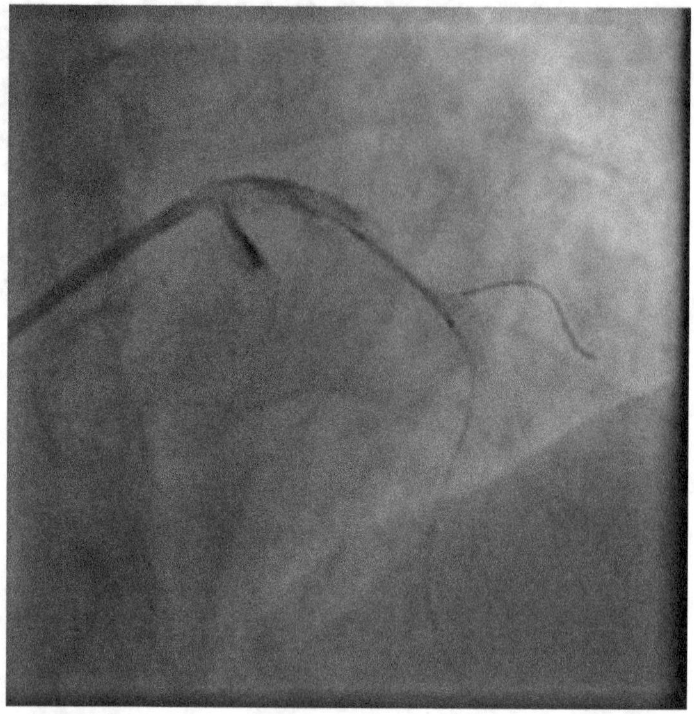

Fig. 21.11 Forte wire placed in diagonal branch for protection. 3.5 × 16-mm Synergy drug-eluting stent advanced across lesion

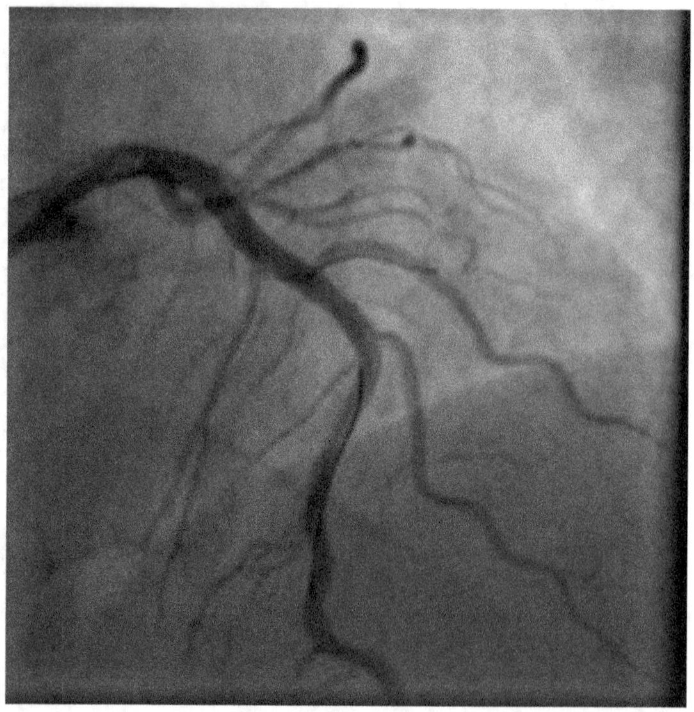

Fig. 21.12 Final images before wire pull. Stent deployed 16 ATM, post-dilated 17 ATM. Proximal portion post-dilated with Quantum 3.75-mm balloon to 16 ATM

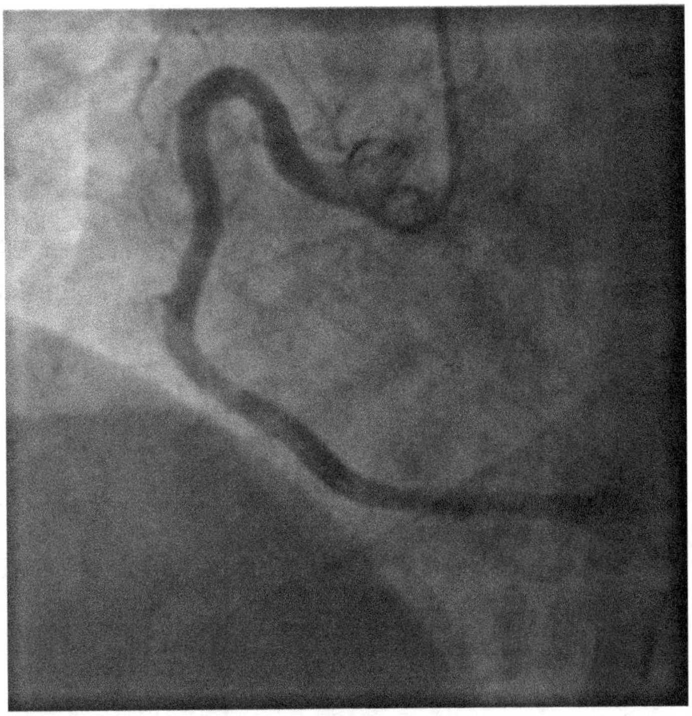

Fig. 21.13 RCA imaged after LAD opened. No stenosis

Report status:	Complete
Cumulative fluoroscopy time:	7.7 min
Cumulative DAP (fluoroscopy):	17473 mGycm²
Cumulative DAP (exposure):	24788 mGycm²
Total DAP:	42262 mGycm²
Cumulative Air Kerma:	1,113.87 mGy
Total number of acquired runs:	16
Total number of acquired images:	694
Total number of acquired exposure images:	694

Run no.	No. of images	Procedure	Speed fr/sec	kV	mA mAs	ms	DAP [mGycm²]	AK [mGy]	Rotation	Angulation	SID [cm]
1	40	Left Coronary 15 fps	15	82	869	7	1190	34.07	LAO4	CRAN36	119
2	31	Left Coronary 15 fps	15	92	775	8	1064	31.24	LAO3	CRAN37	120
3	38	Left Coronary 15 fps	15	92	781	8	1241	36.13	LAO3	CRAN37	120
4	34	Left Coronary 15 fps	15	87	825	8	1041	30.80	LAO3	CRAN37	120
5	8	Left Coronary 15 fps	15	87	823	8	252	7.80	LAO3	CRAN37	120
6	43	Left Coronary 15 fps	15	99	720	8	1519	45.34	LAO3	CRAN37	120
7	49	Left Coronary 15 fps	15	102	698	9	1796	53.20	LAO3	CRAN37	120
8	55	Left Coronary 15 fps	15	111	645	9	1879	67.28	LAO30	CRAN30	113
9	41	Left Coronary 15 fps	15	125	572	10	2437	67.91	LAO37	CAUD24	116
10	50	Left Coronary 15 fps	15	89	802	8	1792	49.24	RAO24	CAUD29	118
11	9	Left Coronary 15 fps	15	80	896	7	290	7.46	RAO24	CAUD10	111
12	6	Left Coronary 15 fps	15	79	900	7	191	4.98	RAO24	CAUD10	111
13	46	Left Coronary 15 fps	15	96	741	8	1410	41.79	0	CRAN36	119
14	69	Left Coronary 15 fps	15	94	758	8	2277	69.47	LAO35	CAUD5	107
15	83	Left Coronary 15 fps	15	78	916	7	2618	63.59	RAO21	CRAN3	110
16	92	Left Ventricle 15 fps	15	72	675	6	2487	33.78	RAO21	CRAN3	107

Fig. 21.14 Fluoroscopy report and camera angles

21.9.4 Summary

This patient was found to have total occlusion of the left anterior descending artery with TIMI 0 flow. This was opened with a 3.5-mm stent, and the first balloon inflation happened 63 min after the paramedics were "on scene" or arrived to the location of the patient. This case demonstrates how an ideal system for prehospital diagnosis and coordination between emergency medical services and hospitals serves to rapidly treat patients and thus how this translates into optimal outcomes.

References

1. Reimer KA, Lowe JE, Rasmussen MM, Jennings RB. The wavefront phenomenon of ischemic cell death. 1. Myocardial infarct size vs duration of coronary occlusion in dogs. Circulation. 1977;56:786–94.
2. Boersma E, Maas AC, Deckers JW, Simoons ML. Early thrombolytic treatment in acute myocardial infarction: reappraisal of the golden hour. Lancet. 1996;348:771–5.
3. Weaver WD. Time to thrombolytic treatment: factors affecting delay and their influence on outcome. J Am Coll Cardiol. 1995;25(Suppl 7):3S–9S.
4. Brodie BR, Stuckey TD, Muncy DB, Hansen CJ, Wall TC, Pulsipher M, Gupta N. Importance of time-to-reperfusion in patients with acute myocardial infarction with and without cardiogenic shock treated with primary percutaneous coronary intervention. Am Heart J. 2003;145:708–15.
5. Cannon CP, Gibson CM, Lambrew CT, Shoultz DA, Levy D, French WJ, Gore JM, Weaver WD, Rogers WJ, Tiefenbrunn AJ. Relationship of symptom-onset-to-balloon time and door-to-balloon time with mortality in patients undergoing angioplasty for acute myocardial infarction. JAMA. 2000;283:2941–7.
6. Menees DS, Peterson ED, Wang Y, Curtis JP, Messenger JC, Rumsfeld JS, Gurm HS. Door-to-balloon time and mortality among patients undergoing primary PCI. N Engl J Med. 2013;369:901–9.
7. Nallamothu BK, Normand S-LT, Wang Y, Hofer TP, Brush JE, Messenger JC, Bradley EH, Rumsfeld JS, Krumholz HM. Relation between door-to-balloon times and mortality after primary percutaneous coronary intervention over time: a retrospective study. Lancet. 2015;385(9973):1114–22.
8. Jollis JG, Al-Khalidi HR, Roettig ML, Berger PB, Corbett CC, Doerfler S, Fordyce CB, Henry TD, Hollowell L, Magdon-Ismail Z, Kochar A, McCarthy JJ, Monk L, O'Brien PK, Rea TD, Shavadia J, Tamis-Holland J, Wilson BH, Ziada KM, Granger CB. Impact of regionalization of ST elevation myocardial infarction care on treatment times and outcomes for emergency medical services transported patients presenting to hospitals with percutaneous coronary intervention: Mission: Lifeline Accelerator-2. Circulation. 2018;137(4):376–87. https://doi.org/10.1161/CIRCULATIONAHA.117.032446.
9. Fordyce CB, Al-Khalidi HR, Jollis JG, Roettig ML, Gu J, Bagai A, Berger PB, Corbett CC, Dauerman HL, Fox K, Garvey JL, Henry TD, Rokos IC, Sherwood MW, Wilson BH, Granger CB. Association of rapid care process implementation on reperfusion times across multiple ST-segment–elevation myocardial infarction network. Circ Cardiovasc Interv. 2017;10:e004061.
10. Glickman S, Lytle BL, Ou FS, Mears G, O'Brien S, Cairns CB, Garvey JL, Bohle DJ, Peterson ED, Jollis JG, Granger CB. Care processes associated with quicker door-in/door-out for patients with ST-elevation myocardial infarction requiring transfer: results from a statewide regionalization program. Circ Cardiovasc Quality Outcomes. 2011;4:382–8.

11. French WJ, Reddy VS, Barron HV. Transforming quality of care and improving outcomes after acute MI: lessons from the National Registry of myocardial infarction. JAMA. 2012;308:771–2.
12. Bagai A, Jollis JG, Dauerman HL, Peng SA, Rokos IC, Bates ER, French WJ, Granger CB, Roe MT. Emergency department bypass for ST-segment-elevation myocardial infarction patients identified with a prehospital electrocardiogram: a report from the American Heart Association mission: lifeline program. Circulation. 2013;128:352–9.
13. Kaul P, Federspiel JJ, Dai X, Stearns SC, Smith SC Jr, Yeung M, Beyhaghi H, Zhou L, Stouffer GA. Association of Inpatient vs outpatient onset of ST-elevation myocardial infarction with treatment and clinical outcomes. JAMA. 2014;312:1999–2007.

22 Strategies for Reducing Myocardial Infarct Size Following STEMI

Valeria Paradies, Mervyn Huan Hao Chan, and Derek J. Hausenloy

22.1 Introduction

In the context of ST-segment elevation myocardial infarction (STEMI), early and successful myocardial reperfusion by primary percutaneous coronary intervention (PPCI) is the most powerful intervention for reducing myocardial infarct (MI) size, preserving left ventricular (LV) systolic function and preventing the onset of heart failure. However, despite continual improvements in acute care, the mortality and morbidity rates following STEMI remain significant, with 7% death and 22% rehospitalisation for heart failure, at 1 year. Although timely reperfusion of the occluded vessel by PPCI is essential to minimise the acute ischaemic time (a major

V. Paradies
National Heart Research Institute Singapore, National Heart Centre, Singapore, Singapore

M. H. H. Chan
National Heart Research Institute Singapore, National Heart Centre, Singapore, Singapore

Cardiovascular and Metabolic Disorders Program, Duke-National University of Singapore Medical School, Singapore, Singapore

D. J. Hausenloy (✉)
National Heart Research Institute Singapore, National Heart Centre, Singapore, Singapore

Cardiovascular and Metabolic Disorders Program, Duke-National University of Singapore Medical School, Singapore, Singapore

Yong Loo Lin School of Medicine, National University Singapore, Singapore, Singapore

The Hatter Cardiovascular Institute, Institute of Cardiovascular Science, University College London, London, UK

The National Institute of Health Research, University College London Hospitals Biomedical Research Centre, London, UK

Barts Heart Centre, St Bartholomew's Hospital, London, UK
e-mail: derek.hausenloy@duke-nus.edu.sg

T. J. Watson et al. (eds.), *Primary Angioplasty*,
https://doi.org/10.1007/978-981-13-1114-7_22

determinant of MI size) and salvage viable myocardium, the process of reperfusion itself, paradoxically, induces additional myocardial injury and cardiomyocyte death, a phenomenon which has been termed 'myocardial reperfusion injury'. This has been shown to contribute to up to 50% of the final MI size, making it an important therapeutic target to reduce MI size in STEMI patients reperfused by PPCI. However, the translation of novel cardioprotective strategies for targeting myocardial reperfusion injury to reduce MI size following STEMI has been both challenging and disappointing. In this chapter, we provide an overview of myocardial reperfusion injury, discuss the challenges facing the investigation of treatment strategies for reducing MI size following STEMI and highlight future cardioprotective therapies for potentially improving clinical outcomes in STEMI patients.

22.2 Myocardial Reperfusion Injury: A Residual Target for Cardioprotection in STEMI

There is currently no effective therapy for reducing myocardial reperfusion injury, making it an important therapeutic target for reducing MI size following PPCI in STEMI patients. It is characterised by:

1. *Reperfusion arrhythmias*—these are often short-lived and easily treated.
2. *Myocardial stunning*—this is reversible impairment in myocardial contractile function and is due to oxidative stress and calcium dysregulation.
3. *Microvascular obstruction (MVO)*—this manifests as coronary no-reflow at the time of PPCI and refers to the inability to perfuse the myocardium at the level of the coronary microvasculature, despite a patent epicardial coronary artery. It has a multifactorial aetiology which includes coronary microembolisation, platelet activation and external compression of coronary microvasculature by swollen endothelial cells and cardiomyocytes. In severe cases of MVO, damage to the endothelium allows the extravasation of red blood cells into the myocardium (termed 'intramyocardial haemorrhage' or IMH). Both MVO and IMH have been shown to be independent predictors of adverse LV remodelling and clinical outcomes following STEMI.
4. *Cardiomyocyte death*—this lethal form of myocardial reperfusion injury contributes to the final MI size and is due to several factors including abrupt changes in intracellular pH, ATP depletion, oxidative stress, mitochondrial and cytosolic calcium overload, cardiomyocyte hypercontracture and mitochondrial dysfunction.

A number of other proponents also contribute to the pathophysiology of myocardial reperfusion injury, and these include endothelial dysfunction, platelet activation and inflammation. The strongest evidence for the existence and importance of myocardial reperfusion injury is the demonstration that acute MI size can be reduced by applying an intervention solely at the onset of reperfusion. However, given the complex pathophysiology underlying myocardial reperfusion injury, and the fact it manifests in the first few minutes of reperfusion, it is probably no surprise that it has been challenging to target reperfusion injury to reduce MI size following STEMI (see later section).

22.3 Strategies for Targeting Reperfusion Injury to Reduce MI Size Following STEMI

A large number of treatment strategies, shown to be effective in the experimental setting, have been tested in the clinical setting of STEMI over the years, and many have failed to show any benefit in terms of reducing MI size and/or improving clinical outcomes (Table 22.1), and the reasons for this are discussed in a later section. In this section, we review the most recent interventions which have been tested as cardioprotective strategies for reducing MI size in STEMI patients (Table 22.1). These can be divided into mechanical interventions and pharmacological therapies—the signalling pathways these cardioprotective therapies target in the cardiomyocyte are depicted in Fig. 22.1.

Table 22.1 Major recent clinical trials investigating strategies to reduce myocardial infarct size in STEMI patients

Treatment	Study	Patients (*n*)	Endpoints	Results
Ischaemic postconditioning	Staat et al.	30	Infarct size (72-h AUC total CK)	36% reduction in infarct size in IPC group
Ischaemic postconditioning	Hofsten et al. (DANAMI-3)	2000	Composite of death from any cause and hospitalisation for HF at 2 years	No difference in primary endpoint
Remote ischaemic conditioning	Soth et al.	333	Composite of all-cause mortality, MI, readmission for HF and ischaemic stroke/TIA	Significantly lower primary endpoint in remote ischaemic conditioning group
Remote ischaemic conditioning	CONDI-2/ ERIC-PPCI NCT01857414 NCT02342522	4300	Composite of cardiac death and hospitalisation for HF at 12 months	Ongoing
Hypothermia	Erlinge et al. CHILL-MI	120	Infarct size (4 days of CMR)	No differences in infarct size between the two groups Subgroup analysis showed smaller MI in early presenter (< 4 h) with anterior STEMI

(continued)

Table 22.1 (continued)

Treatment	Study	Patients (*n*)	Endpoints	Results
Statins	Lyu et al. Meta-analysis	1058	Myocardial perfusion measured by angiographic parameters (cTFC and MBG)	Significantly lower cTFC and trend towards lower MBG in statin arm
Adenosine	Ross et al.	2118	Infarct size Composite of CHF, rehospitalisation for CHF and death at 6 months	IS reduction in adenosine group No difference in clinical endpoint
Adenosine vs. nitroprusside vs. placebo	Nazir et al. REFLO-STEMI	247	Infarct size and MVO (1–4 days of CMR) Angiographic measures Composite of death, TLR, recurrent MI, severe HF and cerebrovascular events at 1 month	High-dose intracoronary adenosine and nitroprusside did not reduce infarct size or MVO measured by CMR Adenosine may adversely affect mid-term clinical outcome
Cangrelor	PITRI trial NCT03102723	210	Infarct size (3 days of CMR)	Ongoing
Cyclosporine	Piot et al.	58	Infarct size (6 months of CMR)	Reduction in infarct size in cyclosporine group
Cyclosporine	Latini et al. CYCLE	410	ST-segment resolution ≥70% 1 h after PPCI	No differences in primary endpoint between the two groups
Cyclosporine	Cung et al. CIRCUS	970	Composite endpoint of death, HF and adverse LV remodelling at 1 year	No differences in clinical outcomes between the two groups
MTP-131	Chakrabarti et al. EMBRACE-STEMI	118	Infarct size (72-h AUC total CK-MB)	No differences in primary endpoint between the two groups
TRO40303	Atar et al. MITOCARE	163	Infarct size (72-h AUC total CK-MB/ troponin-T)	No differences in primary endpoint between the two groups

Table 22.1 (continued)

Treatment	Study	Patients (n)	Endpoints	Results
Metoprolol	Roovlink et al. EARLY BAMI	408	Infarct size (30 days of CMR)	No differences in primary endpoint between the two groups. Metoprolol group had less malignant arrhythmias in the acute phase
IV sodium nitrite	Siddiqi et al. NIAMI	229	Infarct size (72-h AUC total CK-MB)	No differences in primary endpoint between the two groups
Inhaled nitric oxide	NOMI NCT01398384	248	Infarct size (2–3 days of CMR)	No differences in primary endpoint between the two groups
N-acetylcysteine + IV NTG vs. IV NTG	Pasupathy et al. NACIAM	112	Infarct size (3–7 days of CMR)	Infarct size reduced by 30% in N-acetylcysteine + IV NTG group

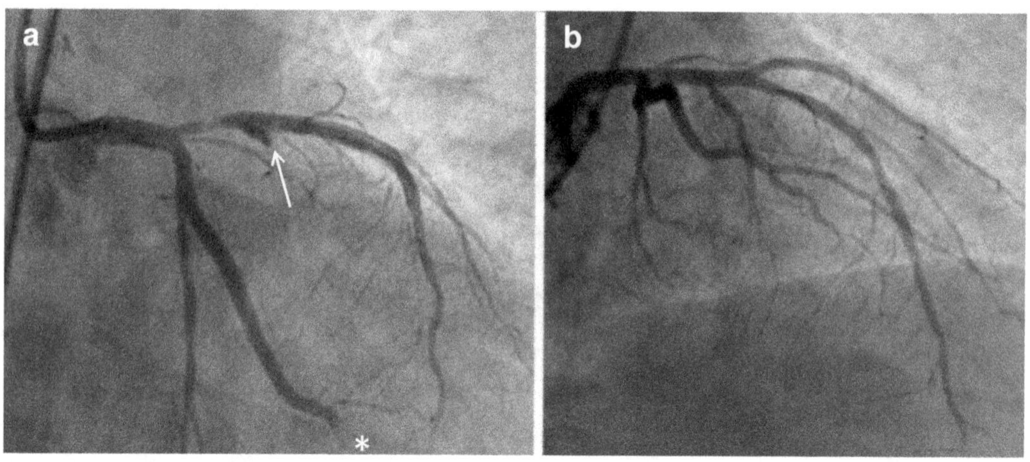

Fig. 22.1 Some of the major signalling pathways underlying ischaemic conditioning and the potential targets of cardioprotective therapies to reduce myocardial infarct size in ST-segment elevation myocardial infarction (STEMI) patients are depicted. The signalling cascade underlying cardioprotection begins at the cardiomyocyte plasma membrane with the activation of G-protein-coupled or cytokine receptors by autocoids such as adenosine, bradykinin or opioids (released in response to the ischaemic postconditioning [IPost] or remote ischaemic conditioning [RIC] stimulus). As a consequence, the reperfusion injury salvage kinase (phosphatidylinositol 3-kinase-Akt (PI3K-Akt) and mitogen-activated protein kinase 1/2-extracellular signal-regulated kinase 1/2 (MEK1/2-Erk1/2)), survivor activator factor enhancement (SAFE), Janus kinase and signal transducer and activator of transcription (JAK-STAT) and the PKG pathways are recruited. These pro-survival signalling pathways activate mediators such as endothelial nitric oxide synthase (eNOS), glycogen synthase kinase (GSK)-3, protein kinase C-ε (PKC-ε) and the mitochondrial ATP-dependent potassium channel (KATP), which then mediate an inhibitory effect on mitochondrial permeability transition pore (MPTP) opening

22.3.1 Ischaemic Postconditioning: Interrupting Reperfusion to Reduce MI Size Following STEMI

Experimental studies have demonstrated that following a sustained coronary artery occlusion, interrupting myocardial reperfusion with short-lived episodes of alternating coronary artery occlusion and reflow (four 30-s cycles) in the first few minutes of reflow reduced MI size in small and large animal models of acute myocardial infarction, a phenomenon which has been termed ischaemic postconditioning (IPost). The signalling pathways which mediate the cardioprotective effects of IPost in the cardiomyocyte are depicted in Fig. 22.1.

In the STEMI patient, IPost has been applied at the onset of reperfusion by PPCI using alternating low-pressure inflations and deflations of an angioplasty balloon (four 60-s cycles) positioned upstream of the directly deployed stent within the infarct-related artery, a manoeuvre which has been shown to reduce MI size by 30–40% and preserve LV systolic function. However, the results of the clinical studies have been mixed with positive, neutral and even negative studies in terms of MI size. Furthermore, two large clinical trials of IPost in STEMI patients were neutral. IPost (four 1-min inflations/deflations of coronary angioplasty balloon following PPCI) failed to improve ST-segment resolution when compared to control in a 700 STEMI patient study, and in the 460 STEMI patient LIPSIA trial, no difference was found between IPost (four 1-min inflations/deflations of coronary angioplasty balloon following PPCI) and control with respect to MRI-determined MI size and clinical outcomes at 6 months (death, re-infarction and new congestive heart failure).

The reasons for the discordant results of IPost in STEMI remain unclear, but they may be due to key factors: patient selection (STEMI patients most likely to benefit are those presenting with a fully occluded coronary artery and treated by direct stenting) and delivery of the IPost protocol (the most effective protocol should be four 60-s angioplasty inflations/deflations, delivered upstream of the deployed stent to avoid potential coronary thromboembolism). The largest clinical study of IPost to date, the multicentre DANAMI 3-iPOST trial, tested the effect of IPost on major clinical endpoints in 1234 STEMI patients treated by PPCI, and it found no difference between IPost (four 30-s inflations/deflations of coronary angioplasty balloon following PPCI) and control with respect to clinical outcomes (all-cause death, re-infarction and hospitalisation for heart failure), after an extended median follow-up of 3.8 years. However, this trial was likely underpowered (the primary event rate was lower than expected), may have used a suboptimal IPost stimulus (four 30-s angioplasty balloon inflations/deflations instead of standard four 60-s protocol) and included patients who were reperfused not using direct stenting.

In summary, IPost in the setting of STEMI is an invasive cardioprotective strategy which requires stringent patient selection and careful delivery of the IPost protocol to be effective. Whether IPost can improve clinical outcomes following STEMI remains unclear.

22.3.2 Remote Ischaemic Conditioning: Transient Arm Ischaemia to Reduce MI Size Following STEMI

IPost requires an invasive intervention to be administered directly to the heart thereby hampering its application in STEMI patients. Therefore, the phenomenon of remote ischaemic conditioning (RIC), which allows the cardioprotective intervention to be applied away from the heart, has greatly facilitated the translation of ischaemic conditioning into the clinical setting. Experimental studies have shown that RIC could be applied to the hindlimb of animals (using a tourniquet to induce cycles of brief ischaemia and reperfusion), and clinical studies have gone on to show that RIC could be non-invasively applied to human volunteers and patients by simply inflating a standard blood pressure cuff placed on the upper arm or thigh to induce cycles of brief ischaemia and reperfusion. The signalling pathways which mediate the cardioprotective effect of RIC in the cardiomyocyte are depicted in Fig. 22.1.

In patients presenting with a STEMI, the application of limb RIC to either the arm or leg prior to or even at the onset of PPCI has been shown in several proof-of-concept clinical studies to reduce MI size (assessed by serum cardiac biomarkers, myocardial nuclear imaging or cardiac MRI) and preserve LV ejection fraction. Only one recent study has been neutral, but this may have been due to the non-standardised and unorthodox limb RIC protocol used in this study, which comprised variable numbers of cycles of RIC (5 to 11 5-min cycles of lower limb cuff inflations/deflations), initiated prior to PPCI and continued to the end of the PCI procedure. Extended follow-up of a cohort of STEMI patients treated by limb RIC reported a 51% reduction in the combined clinical endpoint of all-cause mortality, non-fatal MI, transient ischaemic attack or stroke and hospitalisation for heart failure, when compared to control, although this study was not originally designed to test the effect of limb RIC on these clinical endpoints. In this regard, the 5200 STEMI CONDI2/ERIC-PPCI patient prospective study is currently investigating whether limb RIC (four 5-min inflations and deflations of a cuff placed on the upper arm administered prior to PPCI) can reduce cardiac death and hospitalisation for heart failure at 12 months—the results for this study are expected in the summer of 2019.

In summary, limb RIC provides a non-invasive, low-cost strategy for reducing MI size and has the therapeutic potential to improve clinical outcomes in STEMI patients.

22.3.3 Therapeutic Hypothermia: Cooling the Heart to Reduce MI Size Following STEMI

Therapeutic hypothermia has been shown to reduce MI size in preclinical studies by reducing myocardial metabolic demands, preventing platelet aggregation and limiting the inflammatory response. Large animal studies have shown that hypothermia to 32 °C is cardioprotective if initiated during ischaemia but not at reperfusion. Early clinical studies (ICE-IT, COOL-MI) failed to demonstrate a benefit of hypothermia, possibly due to slow cooling. The combination of cold saline and endovascular cooling induced a faster temperature decline and reduced MI size in a 20-patient pilot trial (RAPID MI-ICE). However, the larger CHILL-MI trial failed to demonstrate a significant reduction in MI size, although patients presenting within 4 h with an anterior STEMI had a reduction in MI size and there was also a significant reduction in heart failure. It was hypothesised, therefore, that faster cooling may be beneficial in anterior STEMI patients. However, the recently published COOL AMI EU Pilot Trial which recruited anterior STEMI patients only ($N = 50$), and used the ZOLL Proteus Intravascular Temperature Management System device to achieve rapid hypothermia (33.6 °C at the time of PPCI), failed to significantly reduce MI size, and the intervention resulted in a 17-min delay in reperfusion and increased the rates of paroxysmal atrial fibrillation.

As such, the role of therapeutic hypothermia to reduce MI size following STEMI remains unproven, and it is associated with logistical challenges to implement into the clinical pathway and has side effects.

22.3.4 Thrombus Aspiration to Improve Microvascular Reperfusion Following STEMI

Whether routine manual thrombus aspiration at the time of PPCI can reduce distal embolisation and improve microvascular perfusion in STEMI patients has been heavily debated in recent years following positive results in the TAPAS trial (Thrombus Aspiration During Percutaneous Coronary Intervention in Acute Myocardial Infarction Study) which showed that routine thrombus aspiration improved microvascular perfusion and reduced mortality at 1 year. However, two major randomised multicentre trials, TASTE (Thrombus Aspiration in ST-Elevation Myocardial Infarction in Scandinavia) and TOTAL (Trial of Routine Aspiration Thrombectomy with PCI vs. PCI Alone in Patients with STEMI), failed to confirm any beneficial effects of routine thrombus aspiration use during PPCI and found that it may increase the risk of stroke. As a result, the routine use of thrombus aspiration has been changed from a IIa to III recommendation in the latest 2017 ESC STEMI guidelines. Whether selective use of thrombus aspiration in STEMI patients with high thrombus burden is beneficial in terms of improving coronary microvascular perfusion and clinical outcomes remains to be elucidated. Further in-depth discussion of this chapter is available in Chap. 10.

22.3.5 GLP-1 Agonists to Reduce MI Size Following STEMI

The anti-diabetic agent, glucagon-like peptide-1 (GLP-1), has been demonstrated in experimental animal studies to reduce MI size when administered at the onset of reperfusion by mechanisms independent of increased insulin levels. As a therapeutic strategy, the GLP-1 analogue, exenatide, has also been shown to protect against myocardial reperfusion injury in small and large animal MI models. In the clinical setting, an intravenous infusion of exenatide initiated prior to PPCI has been shown to reduce MI size in patients presenting with an acute STEMI, especially in those patients presenting with short ischaemic times from symptom onset (<132 min). Another GLP-1 analogue, liraglutide, when administered prior to PPCI and continued for 7 days, has been shown in a study of 85 STEMI patients to improve LV systolic function. However, not all studies have been favourable with neutral effects on MI size in two recently published using exenatide in STEMI patients.

On the basis of these conflicting results, further clinical studies are required to determine whether this therapeutic approach is beneficial as adjunctive therapy to PPCI to reduce MI size in STEMI patients.

22.3.6 Adenosine to Reduce MI Size Following STEMI

Experimental studies have demonstrated that adenosine administered prior to index ischaemia can reduce MI size—however, whether it can also reduce MI size when administered at the time of reperfusion has been contentious. Unsurprisingly then, the results of clinical studies investigating adenosine as an adjunct to PPCI have been inconsistent, and this may in part relate to patient selection, the different doses used and the route of administration (intravenous versus intracoronary). Some studies have reported reductions in MI size with high-dose intravenous adenosine administered as a 3-h infusion initiated prior to reperfusion in STEMI patients presenting within 3 h of chest pain onset, with other studies using lower doses of IV adenosine or boluses of intracoronary adenosine being less successful at reducing MI size. The recently published REFLO-STEMI trial has recently shown that high-dose intracoronary adenosine during PPCI did not reduce MI size or MVO measured by cardiac magnetic resonance imaging (CMR) in 247 STEMI patients when compared to conventional treatment. Furthermore, the investigators reported that adenosine may adversely affect mid-term clinical outcomes.

On the basis of these conflicting results, the role of adenosine as adjunctive therapy to PPCI to reduce MI size in STEMI patients remains unclear.

22.4 Anti-platelet and Anti-thrombotic Strategies to Reduce MI Size Following STEMI

Anti-platelet and anti-thrombotic agents form the cornerstone of therapy for STEMI patients treated by PPCI. A number of studies have investigated new approaches to optimise anti-platelets and anti-thrombotic therapy to reduce MI size following STEMI.

It has been shown that current oral P2Y12 platelet inhibitors, such as prasugrel and ticagrelor, administered to STEMI patients prior to PPCI, can take 4–6 h to achieve maximal platelet inhibition, meaning that at the time of reperfusion, the platelets are not maximally inhibited—this may be expected to result in an increased risk of MVO and worsened clinical outcomes following STEMI. The intravenous (IV) P2Y12 platelet inhibitor, cangrelor, which has a rapid onset of action and induces maximal platelet inhibition within 1–2 min of administration, has been shown in the CHAMPION studies to reduce stent thrombosis and prevent MACE in ACS patients when administered at the time of PCI, when compared to oral clopidogrel. The administration of cangrelor prior to PPCI might be expected to offer complete platelet inhibition at the time of reperfusion, thereby reducing the risk of developing MVO following STEMI. Moreover, a number of experimental small and large animal studies have demonstrated that administrating cangrelor prior to reperfusion has the ability to reduce MI size through a direct cardioprotective effect on the cardiomyocyte involving the activation of established pro-survival signalling cascades. These findings suggest that administering cangrelor prior to reperfusion in STEMI patients has the therapeutic potential to target myocardial reperfusion injury through two distinct mechanisms—maximal platelet inhibition at time of PPCI, thereby preventing MVO, and a direct cardioprotective effect on the cardiomyocyte, thereby reducing MI size. The ongoing multicentre randomised controlled trial "Platelet Inhibition to Target Reperfusion Injury" (PITRI) (ClinicalTrials.gov NCT03102723) is currently investigating whether initiating a cangrelor infusion prior to PPCI can reduce MI size and prevent MVO in STEMI patients treated by PPCI.

The INFUSE-AMI trial demonstrated that an intracoronary bolus of the GPIIb/IIIa inhibitor, abciximab, reduced MI size on cardiac MRI at 30 days in anterior STEMI patients when compared to placebo, suggesting that potent platelet inhibition delivered locally to the infarct lesion site may be beneficial. Whether administering an intracoronary bolus of abciximab is more effective at reducing MI size and preventing MVO, when compared to using an intravenous bolus, had been unclear. However, the large randomised AIDA-STEMI trial failed to demonstrate significant differences in the primary composite outcome of all-cause mortality, re-infarction and new congestive heart failure between intracoronary and intravenous administration of abciximab. Current European guidelines recommend GPIIb/IIIa inhibitor administration only for bailout, evidence of no-reflow or thrombotic complications.

In order to target the thrombus within the infarct-related coronary artery following PPCI, the ongoing T-TIME trial (Trial of Low-dose Adjunctive alTeplase During prIMary PCI) is currently investigating the effect of low-dose intracoronary alteplase infusion initiated after reperfusion with aspiration thrombectomy ± angioplasty but before stenting, on the extent MVO on cardiac MRI in STEMI patients treated by PPCI.

22.5 Targeted Mitochondria to Reduce MI Size Following STEMI

The immunosuppressant, cyclosporin-A (CsA), has been shown to have a protective effect on mitochondrial function and reduce MI size when administered at the onset of reperfusion in a number of small and large animal experimental studies. Although an initial small proof-of-concept studies found that administering an IV bolus of CsA prior to PPCI reduced MI size in STEMI patients treated by PPCI, two subsequent large clinical trials (CYLCE and CIRCUS) failed to find any benefit with this therapeutic approach in terms of ST-segment resolution, enzymatic infarct size and clinical endpoints.

The mitochondria-targeting peptide, MTP-131, which optimises mitochondrial energetics and attenuates the production of ROS by selectively targeting cardiolipin in the inner mitochondrial membrane, has been reported in small and large animal experimental studies to reduce MI size when administered at the onset of reperfusion and prevent adverse LV remodelling following MI. However, in the 117-patient EMBRACE-STEMI clinical trial, intravenous MTP-131 administered prior to PPCI failed to reduce enzymatic MI size in a carefully selected population of anterior STEMI patients with ischaemic time < 4 h, no collaterals and fully occluded coronary artery.

Finally, the mitochondrial targeting drug, TRO40303, which binds to the translocator protein in the outer mitochondrial membrane, has been reported in small animal experimental studies to reduce MI size when administered at time of reperfusion. However, in a clinically relevant large animal MI model, it failed to reduce MI size in the porcine heart. In the 163 STEMI patient MITOCARE study, this agent failed to reduce MI size despite careful patient selection (completely occluded infarct-related artery, large area-at-risk). Prior experimental studies had revealed ambiguous cardioprotective capacity, and the formulation and dosage of TRO40303 used in the clinical study differed from experimental studies, which may in part explain the neutral findings of the MITOCARE study. Finally, more adverse events were reported in patients receiving TRO40303 when compared to the placebo arm, thereby limiting the clinical application of this therapeutic approach.

As such, the current evidence does not support a role for these three mitoprotective agents as an adjunct to PPCI to reduce MI size following STEMI.

22.6 Metoprolol: Beta-Blocker Therapy to Reduce MI Size Following STEMI

Intravenous metoprolol administered prior to reperfusion has been shown to reduce MI size and preserve LV systolic function in the porcine heart. The mechanisms underlying this cardioprotective effect are currently being investigated and appear to extend beyond their effects on haemodynamics and myocardial oxygen consumption. In the 270 anterior STEMI patient METOCARD-CNIC trial, intravenous metoprolol administered in the ambulance prior to PPCI reduced MI size, prevented LV adverse remodelling, preserved LV systolic function and lowered hospital readmissions for heart failure. However, the larger EARLY BAMI trial failed to show any benefit with IV metoprolol on MI size by cardiac MRI or clinical outcomes in a non-selected cohort of 683 STEMI patients.

As such, the current evidence does not support a role for IV metoprolol as an adjunct to PPCI to reduce MI size following STEMI.

22.7 Nitric Oxide Donors to Reduce MI Size Following STEMI

Although there have been experimental studies demonstrating reduced MI size with intravenous nitrite administered at the onset of reperfusion to release nitric oxide, the National Heart, Lung, and Blood Institute (NHLBI) Consortium for preclinicAl assESsment of cARdioprotective therapies (CESAR) Network failed to demonstrate MI size reduction with nitrite using a multicentre approach in small and large animal MI models. Two recent clinical studies have failed to demonstrate a significant reduction in MI size with nitrite administered by either the intravenous or intracoronary routes in STEMI patients treated by PPCI. However, there was a borderline increase in myocardial salvage index and reduced MI size in a subgroup of patients presenting with a fully occluded coronary artery. The 250-patient NOMI study investigated the role of inhaled nitric oxide (vasoKINOX 450) as an adjunct to PPCI to target myocardial reperfusion injury in STEMI patients also failed to reduce MI size (day 3 cardiac MRI), although a post-hoc subgroup analysis revealed that there was a significant reduction in MI size in those patients who had not received nitrates in the ambulance. Recently, the NACIAM trial demonstrated that the co-administration of two old drugs, the nitric oxide donor, nitroglycerin, and the anti-oxidant, N-acetylcysteine (NAC), reduced MI size on cardiac MRI, but had no beneficial effects on LV remodelling in 112 all-comers STEMI patients.

As such, the current evidence is mixed over whether there is a role for nitric oxide donors as an adjunct to PPCI to reduce MI size following STEMI.

22.8 Optimising the Translation of Cardioprotection into the Clinical Setting

Given the numerous examples of failed translation of cardioprotective therapies to reduce MI size and improve clinical outcomes following STEMI, new approaches are required to optimise the preclinical and clinical testing of future cardioprotective therapies—these include the following.

22.8.1 More Rigorous Preclinical Evaluation of the Cardioprotective Strategy Before Clinical Testing

A number of clinical trials may have failed to demonstrate benefit with some cardioprotective therapies due to inconsistent and/or insufficient experimental data. In general, most treatment strategies have only been studied in healthy, young animals, and preclinical studies in adult or older animals, with comorbidities and concomitant medication usually received by patients with STEMI, have been lacking.

Thus, clinical testing of novel cardioprotective strategies should only be performed after consistent demonstration of efficacy and absence of safety concerns obtained in adequate small and large animal models in different laboratories using standardised methods.

22.8.2 Optimising Clinical Study Design

(a) *Patient selection:* It is important to select those STEMI patients who are more likely to benefit from a strategy applied at the onset of reperfusion to reduce MI—this includes those STEMI patients presenting with:
  - Short ischaemic time (<2–3 h)
  - Large area-at-risk (>30–40% of LV) such as proximal LAD STEMI
  - Fully occluded coronary artery prior to PPCI (TIMI flow <1)
  - No significant coronary collaterals

(b) *Dosing the intervention:* A failure to ascertain the most efficacious dose of the cardioprotective strategy, whether it be a mechanical or pharmacological one, may have contributed to the failure to translate cardioprotection in some of the clinical STEMI studies.

(c) *Timing the intervention*: There is consistent preclinical evidence that the intervention to target myocardial reperfusion injury might reduce final MI size when administered prior or at the onset of reperfusion, and it has achieved sufficient concentrations in the blood in the first few minutes of reperfusion.

22.9 Future Perspectives

Translating cardioprotective therapies for targeting myocardial reperfusion injury to reduce MI size following STEMI has been extremely challenging. The failure to find an effective agent for preventing myocardial reperfusion injury thus far, however, does not question the existence of myocardial reperfusion injury as a valid target for cardioprotection—rather it underscores the need to better understand the mechanisms underlying myocardial reperfusion injury and investigate novel strategies for cardioprotection. These should include combination therapy to (1) target different cardioprotective signalling pathways within the cardiomyocyte in order to provide additive cardioprotection and (2) target the different players involved in myocardial reperfusion injury (cardiomyocyte, microvasculature, inflammatory cells, and platelets). These experimental and clinical studies are currently under way and should allow more effective targeting of myocardial reperfusion injury, thereby reducing MI size in reperfused STEMI and preventing the onset of heart failure.

22.10 Case Report: Strategies for Reducing Myocardial Infarct Size Following STEMI

Valeria Paradies, Mervyn Huan Hao Chan, and Derek J. Hausenloy

22.10.1 Case Report

This 41-year-old male with diabetes was referred to our hospital for primary percutaneous coronary intervention (PPCI) for acute onset of chest pain and anterolateral ST-segment elevation myocardial infarction (STEMI) on ECG. He was recruited into the PITRI trial which is currently investigating the effect of an intravenous infusion of the P2Y12 inhibitor, cangrelor, initiated prior to PPCI, on myocardial infarct size and microvascular obstruction (MVO), in STEMI patients treated by PPCI. Right coronary angiography demonstrated the absence of both atherosclerotic lesions and collaterals towards the left coronary artery. Left coronary angiography revealed a critical lesion in the proximal left descending artery (LAD) with evidence of acute thrombus. Distal coronary embolisation and abrupt occlusion of a big septal branch, apical LAD and first marginal branch were detected (Fig. 22.2a). Thrombus aspiration of the septal branch was initially performed with restoration of the flow. The procedure continued with PPCI of the culprit lesion and drug-eluting stent implantation in the proximal LAD. The procedure was completed with thrombectomy of the marginal branch and this achieved good final angiographic result (Fig. 22.2b). Cardiac MRI performed at day 4 after PPCI revealed normal left ventricular (LV) size with severely impaired LV systolic function with akinesia of the LAD territory and mid lateral segment with a dyskinetic apical cap. Late gadolinium enhancement (LGE) images showed transmural infarction in the LAD territory in the basal to mid septum, mid

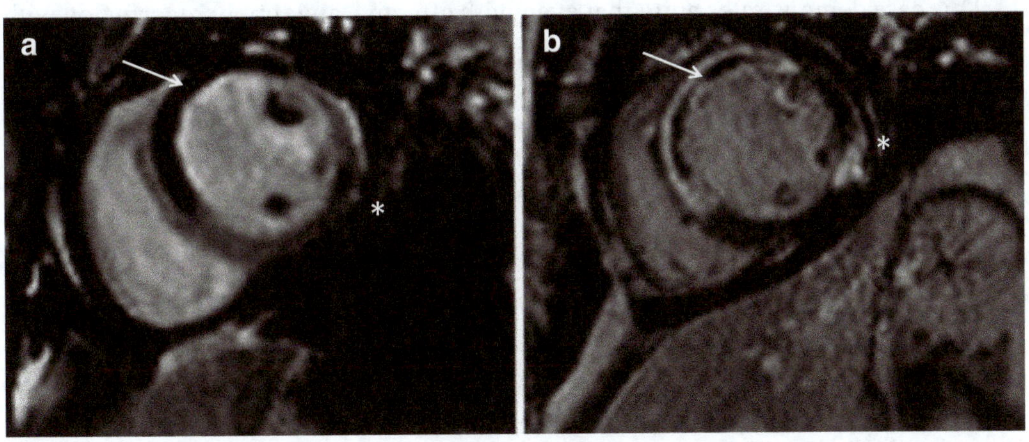

Fig 22.2 Coronary angiogram in acute LAD STEMI patient. (**a**) Left coronary angiography showing culprit lesion in proximal LAD and distal embolisation in septal branch (arrow), distal LAD and marginal branch (asterisk). (**b**) Angiographic result after PPCI with proximal LAD, thrombectomy of septal and marginal branches

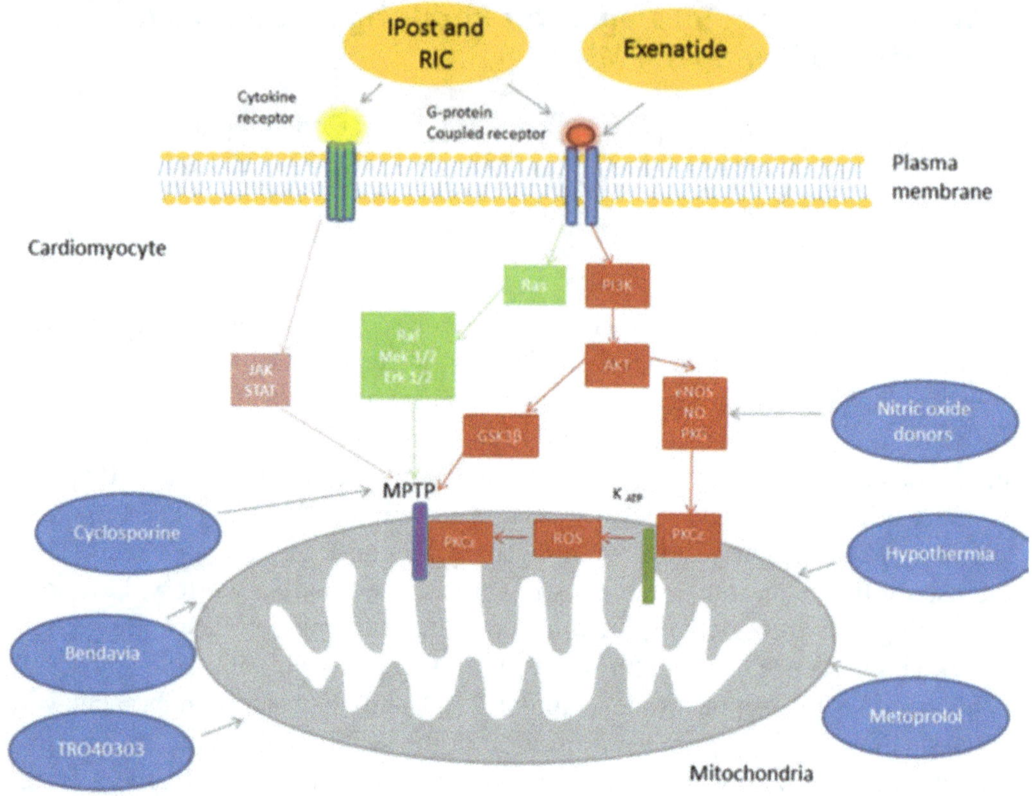

Fig. 22.3 Cardiac MRI scan in acute LAD STEMI patient. (**a**) Mid LV short-axis slice showing MVO on early gadolinium enhancement (EGE) contrast MRI images in mid septal, anterior (arrow) and lateral LV segments (asterisk). (**b**) Mid LV short-axis slice showing myocardial infarction on late gadolinium enhancement (LGE) contrast MRI images in mid septal, anterior (arrow) and lateral LV segments (asterisk), with hypointense core representing MVO

anterior, mid lateral and apical segments. MVO was detected at the mid septum and mid lateral LV segments (Fig. 22.3a, b).

This case demonstrates aptly that even with effective and timely reperfusion with PPCI for STEMI, the insult to the myocardium is often substantial, and effective interventions to protect the myocardium from myocardial reperfusion injury (which can contribute up to 50% of final infarct size) are urgently needed.

Conflicts of Interest None.

Further Readings

Fröhlich GM, Meier P, White SK, Yellon DM, Hausenloy DJ. Myocardial reperfusion injury: looking beyond primary PCI. Eur Heart J. 2013;34(23):1714–22.

Hausenloy DJ, Botker HE, Engstrom T, Erlinge D, Heusch G, Ibanez B, Kloner RA, Ovize M, Yellon DM, Garcia-Dorado D. Targeting reperfusion injury in patients with ST-segment elevation myocardial infarction: trials and tribulations. Eur Heart J. 2016;38(13):935–41.

Hausenloy DJ, Garcia-Dorado D, Bøtker HE, Davidson SM, Downey J, Engel FB, Jennings R, Lecour S, Leor J, Madonna R, Ovize M, Perrino C, Prunier F, Schulz R, Sluijter JPG,

Van Laake LW, Vinten-Johansen J, Yellon DM, Ytrehus K, Heusch G, Ferdinandy P. Novel targets and future strategies for acute cardioprotection: position paper of the European Society of Cardiology Working Group on cellular biology of the heart. Cardiovasc Res. 2017;113(6):564–85.
Hausenloy DJ, Yellon DM. Ischaemic conditioning and reperfusion injury. Nat Rev. Cardiol. 2016;13(4):193–209.
Yellon DM, Hausenloy DJ. Myocardial reperfusion injury. N Engl J Med. 2007;357(11):1121–35.

Primary PCI: Outcomes and Quality Assessment

23

John S. Douglas

23.1 Introduction

ST-segment elevation myocardial infarction (STEMI) and patients with equivalent findings (true posterior MI, hyper-acute T-wave changes, anterior ST depression with ST elevation in lead aVR, and new left bundle branch block with Sgarbossa concordance criteria or hemodynamic instability) account for 30–50% of myocardial infarctions (MI) and are associated with substantial short- and long-term morbidity and mortality [1, 2]. Reperfusion of ischemic myocardium is the primary therapeutic goal and can be accomplished by primary angioplasty with stent implantation or intravenous fibrinolytic therapy. Timely PCI (≤90 min from first medical contact) is the preferred approach in PCI-capable hospitals (ACC/AHA class I recommendation, level of evidence A) resulting in more complete reperfusion and lower rates of early death, reinfarction, and bleeding, including intracranial hemorrhage, compared to fibrinolysis.

When hospital transfer for primary PCI involves a delay of more than 120 min, fibrinolytic therapy, if not contraindicated, is an ACC/AHA class I recommendation, level of evidence A. Following fibrinolytic therapy, subsequent transfer to a PCI-capable hospital is recommended. This reperfusion strategy (Fig. 23.1) has resulted in reductions in in-hospital mortality from over 20% to less than 5% in patients treated without significant delays due to need for non-cardiac diagnostic testing or other nonsystem delays. Evaluation of the care received by the STEMI patient requires an assessment of events extending from initial symptom onset to reperfusion to hospital discharge and return home [3]. Outcome data must be

J. S. Douglas
Department of Medicine, Emory University Hospital, Atlanta, GA, USA

Interventional Cardiology Fellowship Program, Emory University School of Medicine, Emory University Hospital, Atlanta, GA, USA
e-mail: jdoug01@emory.edu

T. J. Watson et al. (eds.), *Primary Angioplasty*,
https://doi.org/10.1007/978-981-13-1114-7_23

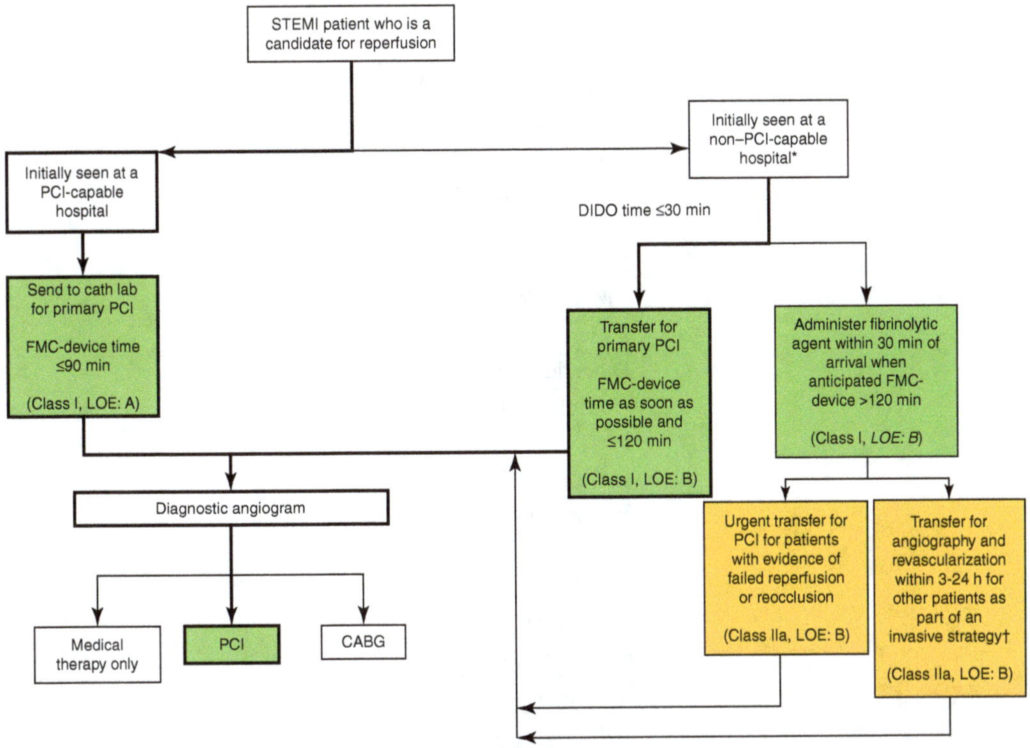

Fig. 23.1 Reperfusion therapy for patients with STEMI. The bold arrows and boxes are the preferred strategies. Performance of PCI is dictated by an anatomically appropriate culprit stenosis. *Patients with cardiogenic shock or severe heart failure initially seen in a non-PCI-capable hospital should be transported for cardiac catheterization and revascularization as soon as possible, DIDO, door-in-door-out. Source: O'Gara PT, Kushner FG, Ascheim DD, et al. 2013 ACCF/AHA guideline for the management of ST-elevation myocardial infarction: a report of the American College of Cardiology Foundation/American Heart Association Task Force on Practice Guidelines. J Am Coll Cardiol 2013; 61(4):e78-e140

risk-stratified as complications of death, acute kidney injury, and bleeding are highly influenced by baseline patient characteristics as well as subsequent clinical events. ACC/AHA STEMI guidelines give a class I recommendation for an active quality assessment and improvement program which is judged to be essential to optimize application of evidence-based reperfusion strategies and improve outcomes in all STEMI patients irrespective of gender, age, race, education, insurance status, and income.

23.2 Quality Assessment

Three components of quality assessment (QA) in healthcare have been conceptualized: (1) structure, (2) processes of care, and (3) outcomes (Table 23.1). In the STEMI patient, *structural components* include prehospital emergency medical services (EMS), emergency rooms, cardiac catheterization laboratories, inpatient

Table 23.1 Quality domains in primary angioplasty

Structural components
STEMI/cath lab QA committee: chairman and staff, regular meeting
Analysis of times to treatment including EMS, emergency department, and cath lab
Monthly-quarterly-annual reporting
Credentialing
Standardized forms and order sets
Process domain
Patient care issues
Procedural indications
Complication management
Medications
Infection control
Radiation safety
Outcomes
Mortality, risk adjusted
Procedural success
Complications
Radiation exposure
Length of stay
Hospital- and physician-specific data
NCDR and AHA registries, comparative results

hospital facilities, and medical personnel. Cath lab QA committees perform surveillance of times to treatment and initiate improvement activities needed to provide optimal STEMI care. *Process measures* include those actions performed by providers in the delivery of care to STEMI patients ideally using proven diagnostic and therapeutic strategies advocated by clinical guideline statements and appropriate use criteria. Writing committees of the ACC/AHA have established specific measures that assess essential aspects of care in STEMI patients [4, 5]. The AHA/ACC Task Force on Performance Measures was charged with updating performance and quality measures in patients hospitalized with STEMI in order to benchmark and improve the care of these patients. In 2017, this committee published a comprehensive measure set that included 22 total measures related to STEMI patients (Table 23.2). Seventeen were performance measures (those with the strongest supporting evidence such as administration of aspirin) and five quality measures (strong but less robust supporting evidence such as inappropriate in-hospital use of nonsteroidal anti-inflammatory drugs). The chair of the writing committee stated, "Implementation of this measure set by health care providers, physician practices and hospital systems will enhance the quality of care and likely improve *outcomes* of patients hospitalized with a heart attack." Important in-hospital outcomes of patients with STEMI are substantially less favorable than with non-STEMI (Fig. 23.2) and include procedural success and complications, death, reinfarction, heart failure, shock, and stroke (Table 23.3).

Table 23.2 2017 AHA/ACC STEMI clinical performance and quality measures

Measure title	Measure region
Performance measures	
Aspirin at arrival	Effective clinical care
Aspirin prescribed at discharge	Effective clinical care
Beta blocker prescribed at discharge	Effective clinical care
High-intensity statin prescribed at discharge	Effective clinical care
Evaluation of LVEF	Effective clinical care
ACEI or ARB prescribed for LVSD	Effective clinical care
Time to fibrinolytic therapy	Communication and care coordination
Time to primary PCI	Communication and care coordination
Reperfusion therapy	Effective clinical care
Time from ED arrival at STEMI referral facility to ED discharge from STEMI referral facility in patients transferred for primary PCI	Communication and care coordination
Time from FMC (at or before ED arrival at STEMI referral facility) to primary PCI at STEMI receiving facility among transferred patients	Communication and care coordination
Cardiac rehabilitation patient referral from an inpatient setting	Communication and care coordination
P2Y12 receptor inhibitor prescribed at discharge	Effective clinical care
Immediate angiography for resuscitated out-of-hospital cardiac arrest in STEMI patients	Effective clinical care
Noninvasive stress testing before discharge in conservatively treated patients	Efficiency and cost reduction
Early cardiac troponin measurement (within 6 h of arrival)	Efficiency and cost reduction
Participation in ≥1 regional or national registries that include Patients with Acute Myocardial Infarction Registry	Community, population, and public health
Quality measures	
Therapeutic hypothermia for comatose STEMI patients with out-of-hospital cardiac arrest	Effective clinical care
Aldosterone antagonist prescribed at discharge	Effective clinical care
Inappropriate in-hospital use of NSAIDs	Patient safety
Inappropriate prescription of prasugrel at discharge in patients with history of prior stroke or TIA	Patient safety
Inappropriate prescription of high-dose aspirin with ticagrelor at discharge	Patient safety

Abbreviations: *ACC* American College of Cardiology, *ACEI* angiotensin-converting enzyme inhibitor, *AHA* American Heart Association, *ARB* angiotensin receptor blocker, *ED* emergency department, *FMC* first medical contact, *LVEF* left ventricular ejection fraction, *NSAIDs* nonsteroidal anti-inflammatory drugs, *PCI* percutaneous coronary intervention, *PM* performance measures, *QM* quality measures, *LVSD* left ventricular systolic dysfunction, *STEMI* ST-elevation myocardial infarction, *TIA* transient ischemic attack

Source: adapted from Jneid et al. [4]

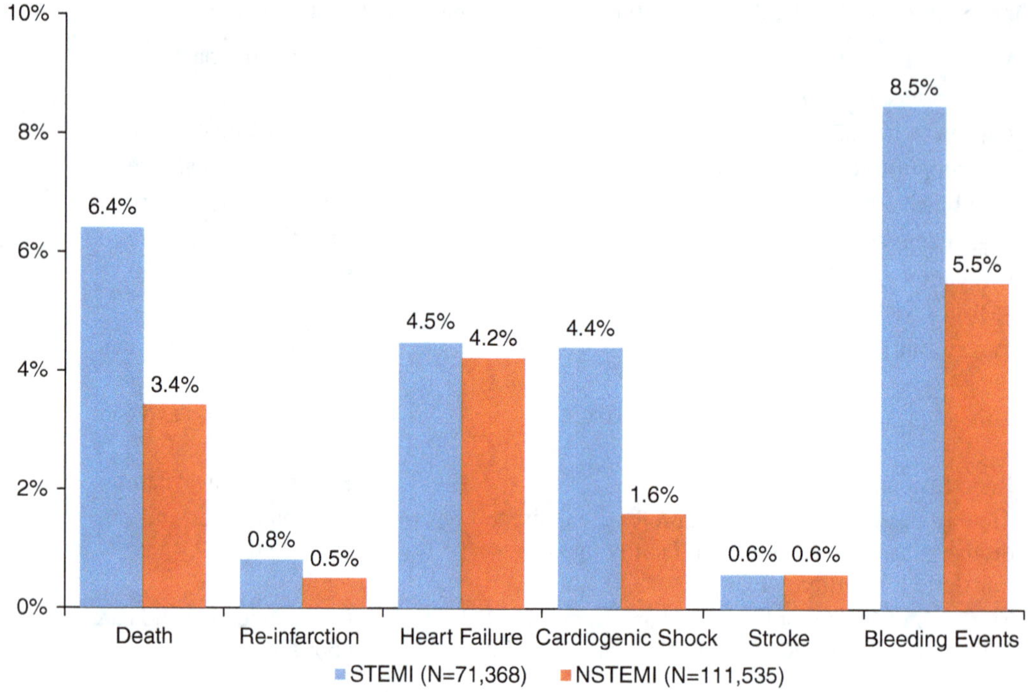

Fig. 23.2 In-hospital outcomes of the ACTION-GWTG Program 2014. Rates of death, reinfarction, heart failure, cardiogenic shock, stroke, or bleeding during hospitalization for patients with STEMI and NSTEMI. Source: Masoudi MD, Ponirakis A, de Lemos JA et al. Trends of US Cardiovascular Care. J Am Coll Cardiol 2017; 69:1427–50

Table 23.3 Characteristics and in-hospital outcomes of 10,730 patients with STEMI transported by EMS to 132 PCI-capable hospitals in 2015–2017

Median age	62 years
Male	70%
Prior MI	20%
Prior PCI	17%
Prior CABG	5%
Diabetes	27%
Symptoms to FMC	50 min
ED dwell time	30 min
Shock presentation	10%
Cardiac arrest	11%
Heart failure	9%
Primary PCI	90%
FMC to device ≤90 min	54%
In-hospital death	8.3%
Stroke	1%
Major bleeding	5.1%
Reinfarction	1%

Source: Data from Jollis et al. [3]

23.3 Risk Assessment and Adjustment

The risk associated with STEMI is highly dependent on demographic features such as age, acuity of presentation, baseline comorbidities (diabetes, peripheral vascular and chronic lung disease), left ventricular function, and findings at coronary angiography. High-risk angiographic findings include large culprit vessel size and distribution (left main, LAD). A number of risk scores have been developed to estimate the threat to life that STEMI poses to the individual patient. Although the majority of high-risk patients survive primary PCI without a complication, risk assessment models such as the NCDR CathPCI Registry Bedside Risk Scoring System (Table 23.4) allow the physician to estimate the risk of primary PCI, counsel the patient and family, and correlate clinical features and in-hospital mortality. In addition to the risk of ischemic complications, bleeding risk can be estimated. Bleeding risk has a different temporal pattern than ischemic risk (Fig. 23.3). Among patients presenting with STEMI to US hospitals and captured in the NCDR ACTION Registry between 2007 and 2009, the CRUSADE bleeding risk score predicted a fivefold difference in the risk of bleeding based on eight criteria (hematocrit, creatinine, heart rate, sex, heart failure, systolic blood pressure, prior vascular disease, and diabetes) (Fig. 23.4). Although the bleeding risk associated with the use of bivalirudin is lower than unfractionated heparin, fewer stent thromboses and lower costs favored the frequent use of unfractionated heparin which is documented in this figure and supported by the VALIDATE-SWEDEHEART randomized comparison of these two agents in 25 Swedish PCI centers and reported in 2017. The most important bleeding avoidance strategy, the use of radial artery access, is described below.

Among the highest risk patients are those experiencing out-of-hospital cardiac arrest. Only a small minority survive to reach the hospital. Those reaching the hospital have a significant risk of failure to recover neurologically. In a study of out-of-hospital cardiac arrest in North Carolina during 2012–2014, among 1507 patients with prehospital return of circulation, survival to discharge was approximately threefold higher in those transported to a PCI center even if the transport time exceeded 30 min [6]. However, survival to discharge in both groups was quite low (33% and 14.6%, respectively).

Cardiogenic shock is the most common cause of in-hospital death in patients with STEMI, and, disappointingly, mortality rates still approach 50% and are not decreasing in spite of early invasive strategies, better technology, and the availability of improved mechanical circulatory support devices [7, 8]. Risk scores have been proposed which allow early risk stratification (Fig. 23.5). In an adequately powered randomized trial, the use of intra-aortic balloon pump (IABP) compared to control showed no benefit with respect to mortality or hemodynamic parameters [9]. These findings led to downgrading of recommendations for the use of IABP in guideline statements (class III in the European STEMI guidelines) [10]. In three small randomized trials, the Impella 2.5 hemodynamic

Table 23.4 NCDR CathPCI Registry Bedside Risk Scoring System

Scoring response categories							Total points	Risk of inpatient mortality (%)
STEMI	No	Yes					0	0
	0	6					5	0
							10	0.1
Age	<60	60–70	70–80	≥80			15	0.1
	0	4	9	15			20	0.2
							25	0.3
BMI	<20	20–30	30–40	≥40			30	0.6
	5	1	0	3			35	0.9
							40	1.4
CVD	No	Yes					45	2.3
	0	2					50	3.7
							55	5.9
PAD	No	Yes					60	9.2
	0	3					65	14.2
							70	21.2
Chronic lung disease	No	Yes					75	30.4
	0	3					80	41.5
							85	53.6
Prior PCI	No	Yes					90	65.2
	3	0					95	75.3
							100	83.2

(continued)

Table 23.4 (continued)

Scoring response categories							Total points	Risk of inpatient mortality (%)
Diabetes mellitus	No	Noninsulin	Insulin				105	88.9
	0	2	3				110	92.9
							115	95.5
GFR	Renal failure	30–45	45–60	60–90	≥90		120	97.2
	16	11	7	3	0		125	98.2
							130	98.9
EF	<30	30–40	40–50	≥50			135	99.3
	9	4	2	0			139	99.5
Cardiogenic shock/PCI status	Sustained shock and salvage	Sustained shock alone or salvage alone	Transient shock but not salvage	Emergency PCI without shock/salvage	Urgent PCI without shock/salvage	Elective PCI without shock/salvage		
	54	43	37	22	11	0		
NYHA class within 2 weeks	NYHA class IV	NYHA class <IV	No HF					
	7	3	0					
Cardiac arrest within 24 h	No	Yes						
	0	13						

Source: From Brennan JM, Curtis JP, Dai D et al. Enhanced mortality risk prediction with a focus on high-risk percutaneous coronary intervention. J Am Coll Cardiol Interv 2013; 6: 790–9

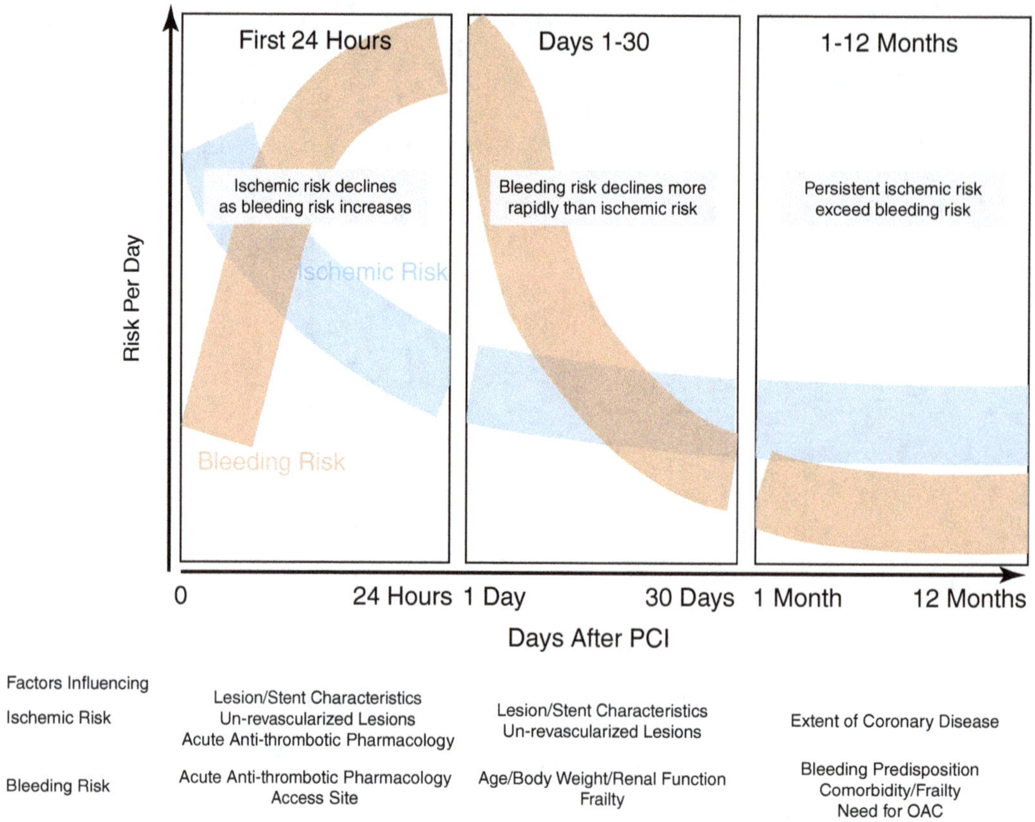

Fig. 23.3 Conceptualizing the temporal risk of ischemic and bleeding risk of PCI in STEMI. Ischemic risk is influenced by culprit and non-culprit lesion characteristics, antithrombotic therapy, and extent of coronary disease. Bleeding risk is affected by bleeding risk of the patient, access site, antithrombotic pharmacology, duration of antithrombotic therapy, and need for anticoagulation with warfarin. Source: Chew DP and Bhatt DL. J Am Coll Cardiol 2017; 70:1858–60

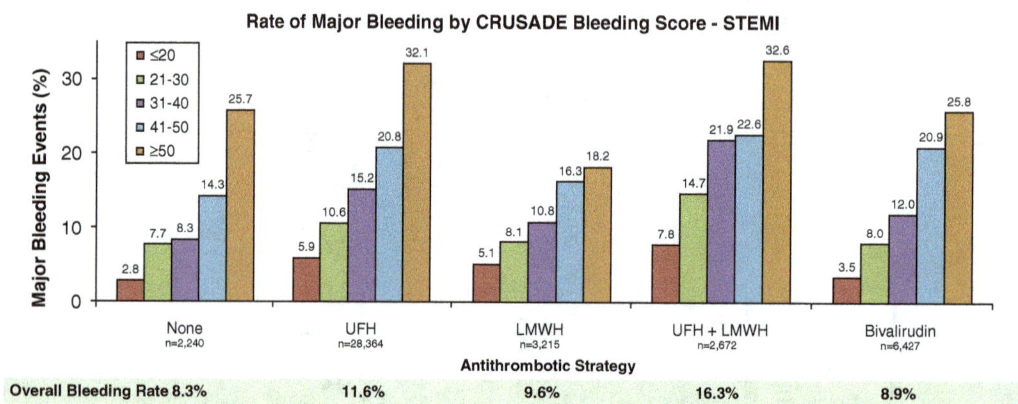

Fig. 23.4 Rates of major bleeding according to anticoagulation regimen and the CRUSADE BLEEDING RISK SCORE in patients with STEMI. Source: Kadakia MB, Desai NR, Alexander KP et al. Use of anticoagulant agents and risk of bleeding among patients admitted with myocardial infarction J Am Coll Cardiol 2010; 3:1166–77

Score	
Variable	Points
Age >73 years	1
History of stroke	2
Glucose >10.6 mmol/l (191 mg/dl)*	1
Creatine >132.6 μmol/l (1.5 mg/dl)*	1
Arterial Lactate >5 mmol/l*	2
TIMI flow grade <3 after PCI	2
Maximum	9

Risk categories	
Category	Points
Low	0-2
Intermediate	3/4
High	5-9

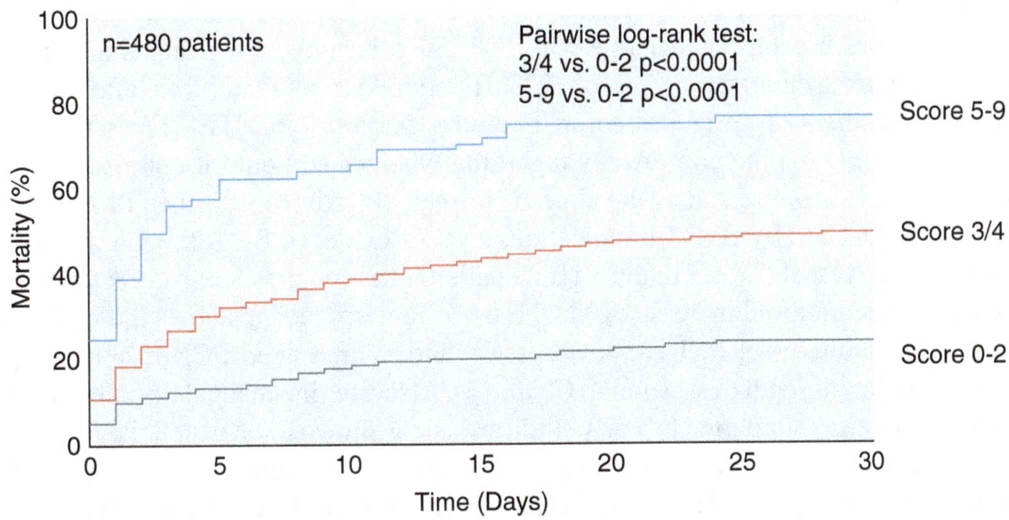

Fig. 23.5 Cardiogenic shock complicating acute myocardial infarction: IABP-SHOCK II RISK SCORE. The scoring system attributed one or two points per variable. Source: Pöss J, Köster J, Fuervan G, et al. J Am Coll Cardiol 2017; 69:1913–20

support device compared to IABP improved hemodynamics but was associated with more complications, and there was no difference in mortality. In a recently published randomized comparison of the Impella CP left ventricular support device (maximum output of about 3.7 L/min) and IABP in 48 STEMI patients with cardiogenic shock, there was no difference in mortality at 30 days or in serum lactate [11]. This study was underpowered but there was no signal, suggesting benefit with Impella CP use. It has been estimated that a trial of approximately 2500 cardiogenic shock patients would be required to confirm a significant mortality benefit of 4% with a strategy such as left ventricular support. In a randomized trial of patients with cardiogenic shock due to acute myocardial infarction and multivessel disease [7], the guideline-supported strategy of progressing to PCI of non-culprit arteries in patients with persisting shock resulted in worse outcomes than culprit-only PCI, suggesting that a change in the guideline statement may be needed. A recent AHA scientific statement reviewed efforts to study this thorny and resistant clinical problem [8].

23.4 Procedural Outcomes

In patients undergoing primary PCI for treatment of STEMI, complete reperfusion with development of TIMI 3 flow is achieved in over 90% of patients compared to 50–60% of patients treated with fibrinolytic therapy. Patients who achieve less than TIMI 3 flow with PCI are frequently late presenters, have large thrombus burden, and have poorer outcomes. No reflow due to microcirculation injury and/or distal embolization is a particularly unfavorable prognostic finding. With the advent of intracoronary stents, the need for emergency coronary bypass surgery has plummeted to 6% of STEMI patients according to the NCDR CathPCI Registry, but surgery may be required in advanced triple vessel or left main coronary artery disease that does not appear treatable with PCI. Surgery may be needed as the initial emergency revascularization (3% of STEMI patients) or at a later time after percutaneous treatment of the culprit coronary artery lesion (2% of STEMI patients).

There is an ongoing controversy regarding whether non-culprit coronary artery stenoses should be treated at the time of primary PCI in the absence of ongoing ischemia (ACC/AHA class IIb indication, level of evidence B). Although the presence of multivessel disease in the STEMI patient is an independent risk factor associated with a threefold increase in MACE on follow-up, recent studies indicate that immediate multivessel PCI is not necessary and favor staged PCI of non-culprit lesions (more in-depth discussion in Chap. 13). Also, routine manual thrombus aspiration which was supported by early studies was not shown to be beneficial in recent reports and was associated with a small increase in the risk of stroke (more in-depth discussion in Chap. 10). However, thrombus aspiration may be indicated in patients with large thrombus burden or thrombotic complications. Bleeding complications, most commonly access site bleeding, occur in 5–10% of patients and are a major source of morbidity and occasionally mortality. Increased use of radial artery access has occurred, especially in Europe (Fig. 23.6), and the use of fibrinolytic therapy has diminished dramatically both in Europe and the United States. Randomized trials have demonstrated that compared to femoral access, the use of radial artery access in STEMI patients leads to lower rates of bleeding, major adverse cardiac events, and in-hospital mortality (more in-depth discussion in Chap. 7). Recent studies indicate that, in experienced hands, radial artery access does not result in the use of more contrast media or increased radiation exposure of patients or operators. In spite of these advantages, the use of radial artery access in the United States remained less than 50% in early 2017 as reported by the NCDR CathPCI Registry. The failure to use radial artery access in higher-risk patients (e.g., elderly female patients) has been described as a "risk-treatment paradox." Although the 2013 ACCF/AHA guideline statement supports implantation of either drug-eluting or bare-metal stents in patients with STEMI, the 2017 European guideline statement endorses the use of drug-eluting stents (more in-depth discussion in Chap. 11). The use of second-generation drug-eluting stents has become the standard practice in most US centers. The critical role of antithrombotic therapy in treatment of STEMI

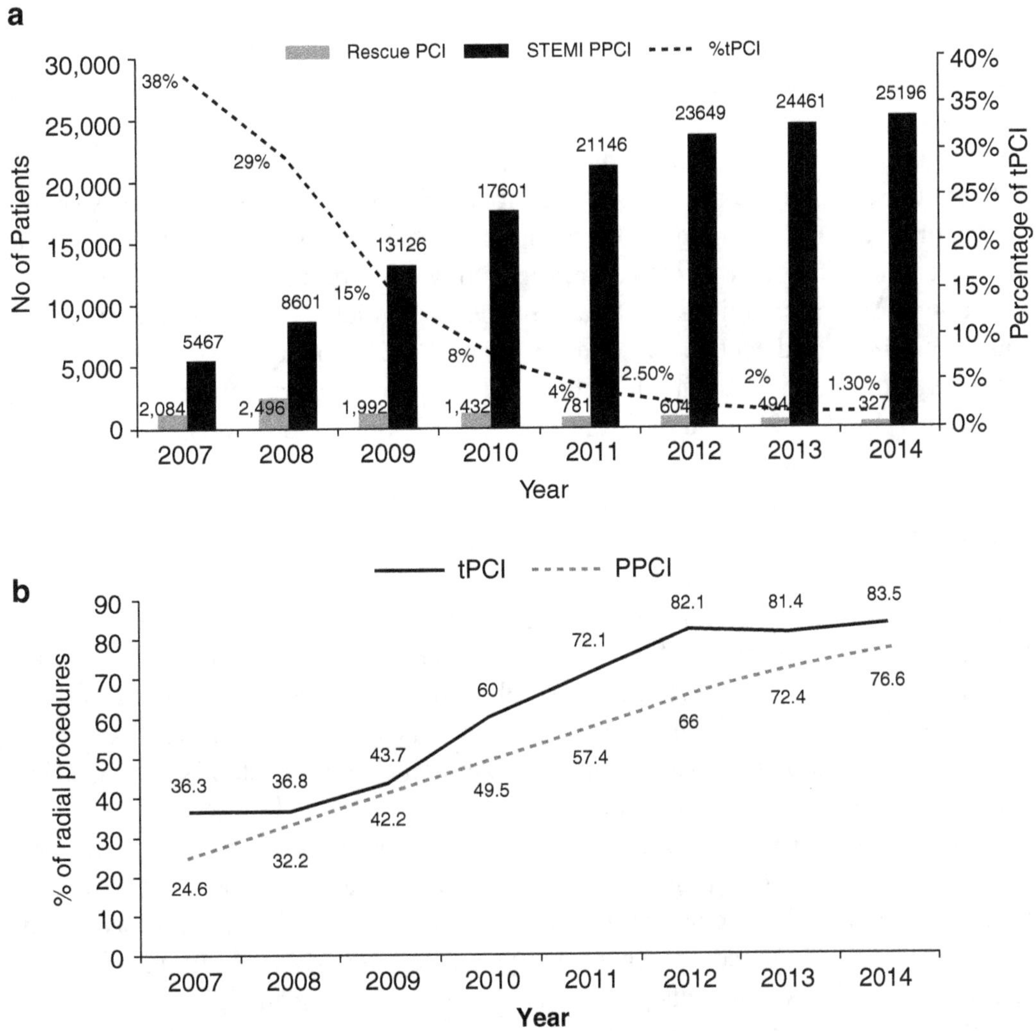

Fig. 23.6 Temporal trends in the thrombolytic and PCI activity and the use of radial access in STEMI in the United Kingdom. (**a**) Decrease in the use of fibrinolytic therapy and increase in radial artery access. (**b**) The use of radial access from 2007 to 2014. Source: Rashid et al. J Am Coll Cardiol Interv 2017; 22;2258–65

has been recognized. In addition to aspirin, an oral $P2Y_{12}$ inhibitor (clopidogrel, prasugrel, or ticagrelor) is recommended pre-procedure and to be taken for 1 year (more in-depth discussion in Chap. 8). Ticagrelor and prasugrel are more effective antiplatelet agents than clopidogrel but are associated with more bleeding necessitating a risk-benefit analysis and are more expensive, which becomes a factor in the uninsured patient. Glycoprotein IIb/IIIa platelet receptor inhibitors currently have a limited role in primary PCI being primarily reserved for treatment of thrombotic complications. Following primary PCI, STEMI patients have an increased risk of thrombotic events such as deep vein thrombosis and/or pulmonary embolism. Although anticoagulation with unfractionated heparin has been frequently used for several days post-PCI, data from HORIZONS-AMI and EUROMAX trials indicate that this practice is associated with more bleeding with no reduction in ischemic or thrombotic events (more in-depth discussion in Chap. 9). Consequently, routine post-PCI anticoagulation should be avoided unless there is a clear indication for its use. With early reperfusion and better techniques, the results of primary PCI have improved substantially. In stented patients with early reperfusion and preserved left ventricular function, hospitalizations as short as 3 days are possible. In less fortunate patients, more prolonged hospitalizations are required to allow recovery of left ventricular function and monitor for complications and for titration of medical therapy. Treatment of heart failure symptoms may be required in large myocardial infarctions. Warfarin anticoagulation is needed when left ventricular aneurysms or mural thrombus is detected. Importantly, in all STEMI patients, education is provided regarding risk factor modification, activity, smoking cessation, medications, and follow-up planning, and referral to cardiac rehabilitation is accomplished.

23.5 Audit

There is a wide variation in treatment of patients with STEMI around the world. To improve quality of care, the US and European STEMI guideline statements indicate that measurable quality indicators be established (see Table 23.2), that routine data collection be carried out, and that routine audits be performed. The American College of Cardiology and American Heart Association have established registries, the NCDR CathPCI and ACTION Registries by the ACC, and the Mission: Lifeline program by the AHA. These registries provide parallel opportunities for collection of the important data relating to the STEMI patient and quarterly update on the performance of healthcare providers and systems aimed at reducing time to reperfusion and improving outcomes. In an analysis of quarterly AHA Mission: Lifeline reports in over 10,000 patients [3], it was shown that enhanced regional efforts can significantly reduce time to reperfusion and lead to a significant reduction in in-hospital mortality. Inpatient death was reduced from 4.4 to 2.3% ($p = 0.001$), a remarkable and encouraging outcome.

23.6 Conclusion

Primary PCI is the preferred reperfusion strategy in STEMI. Timely delivery of this strategy requires well-honed local and regional networks of dedicated professionals and institutions aimed at achieving the earliest possible reperfusion which has been shown to save lives in a significant number of patients presenting with STEMI.

23.7 Case Presentation

A 62-year-old female with a history of hypertension developed crushing chest pain and called emergency medical services. About 15 min before the ambulance reached the emergency room (ER), ventricular fibrillation occurred that was effectively

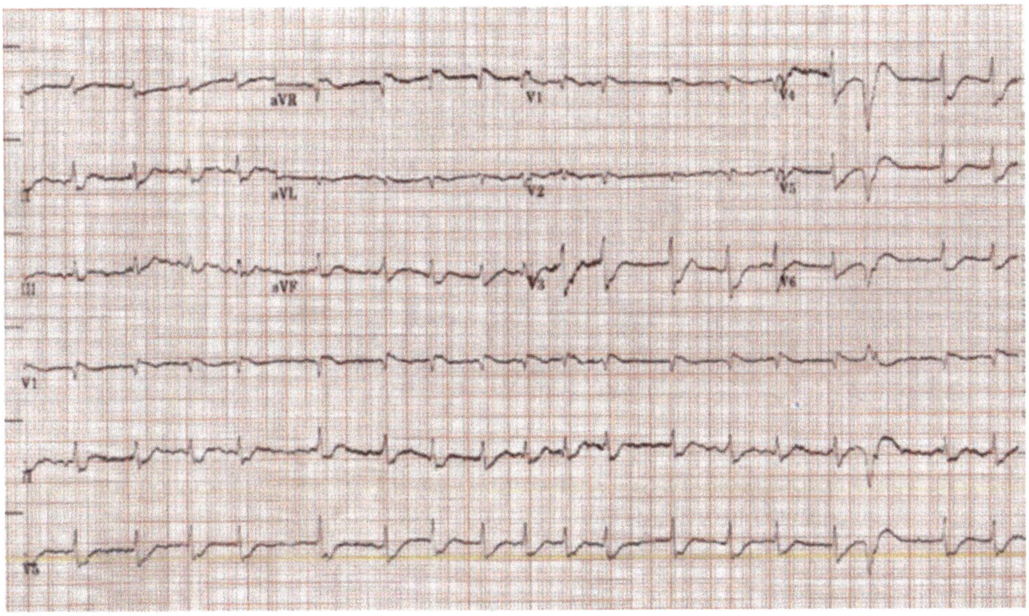

Fig. 23.7 Electrocardiogram following multiple cardioversions suggests diffuse subendocardial ischemia with ST-segment elevation in lead aVR and ST-segment depression in anterior leads

terminated with a shock. As the ambulance was nearing the hospital, ventricular fibrillation recurred which did not immediately respond to cardioversion, and the patient entered the ER with ongoing cardiopulmonary resuscitation (CPR). Tracheal intubation was performed and CPR continued. Amiodarone bolus plus infusion was initiated, but ventricular fibrillation recurred repetitively requiring over 20 shocks. Abnormal lab results included arterial blood pH 6.91 and serum lactate 18.9 mmol/L. Blood pressure was 70–80/30–40 mm Hg in spite of norepinephrine infusion. The ECG is shown (Fig. 23.7).

After 90 min of CPR, the rhythm stabilized long enough to rush the patient to the cardiac catheterization laboratory where ventricular fibrillation recurred twice. An intra-aortic balloon pump was inserted. Coronary angiography revealed moderate diffuse left coronary artery disease (Fig. 23.8a) and total occlusion of the proximal right coronary artery (Fig. 23.8b). Following placement of two drug-eluting stents in the right coronary artery, flow was restored (Fig. 23.8c). Cardiac rhythm stabilized and blood pressure increased to 100/60 mm Hg. The patient was treated with hypothermia and mechanical ventilation for 48 h and made a complete recovery.

Although the presence of refractory ventricular fibrillation, shock, and markedly elevated serum lactate are poor prognostic signs, observed cardiac arrest and even prolonged resuscitation can result in complete recovery. While the use of the intra-aortic balloon pump has not been shown to improve outcomes, its use is not contraindicated in ACCF/AHA guidelines, is thought by some experienced operators to provide assistance, and can be performed in a few minutes. Mechanical left ventricular assist devices provide more hemodynamic support but require longer times to insert and also have not been shown to save lives in randomized studies of shock in patients with STEMI [11].

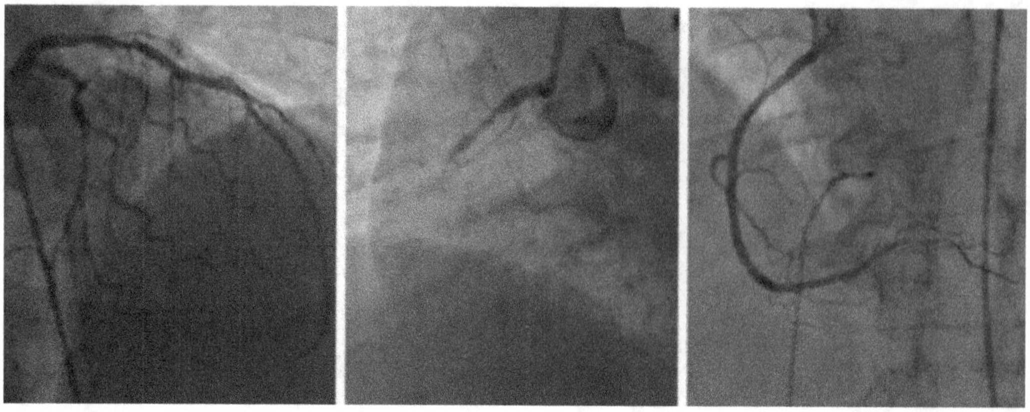

Fig. 23.8 Left coronary angiogram in the right anterior oblique view (**a**). Right coronary artery angiogram showing total occlusion (**b**). Right coronary angiogram after implantation of two drug-eluting stents and restoration of TIMI 3 flow (**c**)

References

1. Levine GN, O'Gara PT, Bates ER, Blankenship JC, Kushner FG, Ascheim DD, et al. 2015 ACC/AHA/SCAI focused update on primary percutaneous coronary intervention for patients with ST-elevation myocardial infarction: an update of the 2011 ACCF/AHA/SCAI guideline for percutaneous coronary intervention and the 2013 ACCF/AHA guideline for the management of ST-elevation myocardial Infarction: a report of the American College of Cardiology/American Heart Association task force on clinical practice guideline and the Society for Cardiovascular Angiography and Interventions. J Am Coll Cardiol. 2016;67:1235–50.
2. Pera VK, Larson DM, Sharkey SW, Garberick RF, Solie CJ, et al. New or presumed new left bundle branch block in patients with suspected STEMI. Eur Heart J Acute Cardiovasc Care. 2017;1:1–10.
3. Jollis JG, Al-Khalidi HR, Roettig ML, Berger PB, Corbett CC, Doerfler S. Impact of regionalization of ST elevation myocardial infarction care on treatment time and outcomes for emergency medical services transported patients presenting to hospitals with percutaneous coronary intervention: Mission: Lifeline Accelerator-2. Circulation. 2018;137(4):376–87.
4. Jneid H, Addison D, Bhatt DL, Fonarow GC, Gokak S, Grady KL. 2017 AHA/ACC Clinical performance and quality measures for adults with ST-elevation and non-ST-elevation myocardial infarction: a report of the American College of Cardiology/American Heart Association Task Force on performance measures. J Am Coll Cardiol. 2017;70:2048–90.
5. Patel MR, Calhoun JH, Dehmer GJ, Grantham JA, Maddox TM, Maron DJ, Smith PK. ACC/AATS/AHA/ASE/ASNC/SCAI/SCCT/STS 2017 appropriate use criteria for coronary revascularization in patients with acute coronary syndromes: a report of the American College of Cardiology appropriate use criteria task force, American Association for Thoracic Surgery, American Heart Association, American Society of Echocardiography, American Society of Nuclear Cardiology, Society for Cardiovascular Angiography and Interventions, Society of Cardiovascular Computed Tomography, and Society of Thoracic Surgeons. J Am Coll Cardiol. 2017;69:570–91.
6. Jollis JG, Granger CB. Improving care of out-of-hospital cardiac arrest. Circulation. 2016;134:2040–2.
7. Thiele H, Akin I, Sandri M, Fuernau G, de Waha S, Meyer-Saraei R, et al. PCI strategies in patients with acute myocardial infarction and cardiogenic shock. N Engl J Med. 2017;376:1–13.

8. Van Diepen S, Katz JN, Albert NM, Henry TD, Jacobs AK, Kapur NK et al.; on behalf of the American Heart Association Council on Clinical Cardiology; Council on Cardiovascular and Stroke Nursing; Council on Quality of Care and Outcomes Research; and Mission: Lifeline. Contemporary management of cardiogenic shock: a scientific statement from the American Heart Association. Circulation. 2017;136:e232–68.
9. Thiele H, Zeymer U, Neumann FJ, et al. Intra-aortic balloon counterpulsation in acute myocardial infarction complicated by cardiogenic shock (IABP-SHOCK II). Final 12 month results of a randomized open-label trial. Lancet. 2013;382:1638–45.
10. Ibanez B, James S, Agewall S, Antunes MJ, Buccianrelli-Ducci C, Bueno H, et al. 2017 ESC Guidelines for the management of acute myocardial infarction in patients presenting with ST-segment elevation. Eur Heart J. 2018;39(2):119–77.
11. Ouweneel DM, Eriksen E, Sjauw KD, et al. Percutaneous mechanical circulatory support versus intra-aortic balloon pump in cardiogenic shock after acute myocardial infarction. J Am Coll Cardiol. 2017;69:278–87.

www.ingramcontent.com/pod-product-compliance
Lightning Source LLC
LaVergne TN
LVHW060056220926
848484LV00008BA/1959
* 9 7 8 1 0 1 3 2 7 4 3 7 4 *